Color Atlas of Emergency Trauma

This full-color atlas presents nearly 700 images from the largest and busiest trauma center in North America. The images bring the reader to the bedside of patients with the full spectrum of common and uncommon traumatic injuries including motor vehicle accidents, falls, lacerations, burns, impalements, stabbings, and gunshot wounds. The clinical, operative, and autopsy photographs; x-ray, ultrasound, magnetic resonance imaging, and angiography radiographs; and original illustrations depicting injury patterns will help guide clinicians in recognizing, prioritizing, and managing trauma patients. Organized by major body regions into separate chapters on the head, face, neck, chest, abdomen, musculoskeletal system, spine, and soft tissue, this thorough text discusses management guidelines, emergency workup protocols, and common pitfalls. The *Color Atlas of Emergency Trauma* is an essential resource for those involved in trauma care.

Diku P. Mandavia, MD, is Attending Staff Physician in the Department of Emergency Medicine at Los Angeles County-USC Medical Center and at Cedars-Sinai Medical Center in Los Angeles. As Clinical Associate Professor of Emergency Medicine at the University of Southern California's Keck School of Medicine, Dr. Mandavia specializes in emergency ultrasound and trauma care.

Edward J. Newton, MD, is the former Vice Chairman and current Interim Chairman of the Los Angeles County-USC Medical Center's Department of Emergency Medicine. Dr. Newton is also Associate Professor of Clinical Emergency Medicine at the University of Southern California's Keck School of Medicine.

Demetrios Demetriades MD, PhD, is Professor of Surgery at the University of Southern California's Keck School of Medicine. Dr. Demetriades is also Director of the Trauma Program and Surgical Intensive Care Unit at the Los Angeles County-USC Medical Center, the largest trauma center in the United States.

COLOR ATLAS OF
EMERGENCY TRAUMA

Diku P. Mandavia, MD, FACEP, FRCPC

Clinical Associate Professor of Emergency Medicine
Keck School of Medicine
University of Southern California

Attending Staff Physician
Department of Emergency Medicine
Los Angeles County-USC Medical Center
Department of Emergency Medicine
Cedars-Sinai Medical Center
Los Angeles, California

Edward J. Newton, MD, FACEP, FRCPC

Associate Professor of Clinical Emergency Medicine
Keck School of Medicine
University of Southern California

Interim Chairman
Department of Emergency Medicine
Los Angeles County-USC Medical Center
Los Angeles, California

Demetrios Demetriades, MD, PhD, FACS

Professor of Surgery
Keck School of Medicine
University of Southern California

Director
Division of Trauma and Critical Care
Los Angeles County-USC Medical Center
Los Angeles, California

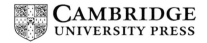
CAMBRIDGE
UNIVERSITY PRESS

PUBLISHED BY THE PRESS SYNDICATE OF THE UNIVERSITY OF CAMBRIDGE
The Pitt Building, Trumpington Street, Cambridge, United Kingdom

CAMBRIDGE UNIVERSITY PRESS
The Edinburgh Building, Cambridge CB2 2RU, UK
40 West 20th Street, New York, NY 10011-4211, USA
477 Williamstown Road, Port Melbourne, VIC 3207, Australia
Ruiz de Alarcón 13, 28014 Madrid, Spain
Dock House, The Waterfront, Cape Town 8001, South Africa

http://www.cambridge.org

First published 2003

Printed in Singapore

Typefaces Goudy 11/13 pt. and Stone Sans   *System* QuarkXPress™   [HT]

A catalog record for this book is available from the British Library.

Library of Congress Cataloging in Publication Data

Mandavia, Diku P., 1965–
    Color atlas of emergency trauma / Diku P. Mandavia, Edward J. Newton,
        Demetrios Demetriades.
        p.   cm.
    Includes bibliographical references and index.
    ISBN 0-521-78148-5 (hardback)
    1. Medical emergencies—Atlases. 2. Emergency medical services—Atlases. 3.
Wounds and injuries—Atlases. I. Newton, Edward, 1950–II. Demetriades,
Demetrios, 1951–III. Title.
    [DNLM: 1. Wounds and Injuries—Atlases. 2. Emergencies—Atlases. WO 517
M271c 2003]
    RC86.7 M3478 2003
    616.02′5′0222—dc21   2002191221

ISBN 0 521 78148 5   hardback

To my parents, my brother Sujal, my precious daughter Neela, and especially to my loving wife Katina who has supported me throughout my career.

DM

Dedicated with thanks to my family and colleagues.
To my students of trauma and emergency care, may the collected experience contained in this text assist your pursuit of excellence.

EN

To my parents, my wife Elizabeth, my daughters Alexis and Stefanie, and my son Nicky.

DD

Contents

Photographic Acknowledgments

Major Contributor

Marie Russell, MD
Los Angeles County–USC Medical Center

The authors thank Dr. Marie Russell for her generous photographic contributions to the text.

Photographic Contributors

Joel Aronowitz, MD
Cedars-Sinai Medical Center

Paul Carter, MD
Los Angeles County-USC Medical Center

Jeff Cohen, MD
Los Angeles County-USC Medical Center

John L. Go, MD
Los Angeles County-USC Medical Center

Jason Greenspan, MD
Los Angeles County-USC Medical Center

Anthony Joseph, MD
Royal Northshore Hospital, Sydney, Australia

Cindy Kallman, MD
Cedars-Sinai Medical Center

Larry Khoo, MD
Los Angeles County-USC Medical Center

William Mallon, MD
Los Angeles County–USC Medical Center

Sujal Mandavia, MD
Cedars-Sinai Medical Center

John Michael, MD
Boston, Massachusetts

Peter Mishky, MD
Naval Medical Center, San Diego, California

Jack Pulec, MD
Pulec Ear Clinic, Los Angeles

Paul Prendiville, MD
Laguna Beach, California

Bronwyn Pritchard, MD
Laguna Beach, California

Jeff Sipsey, MD
Los Angeles County-USC Medical Center

Mark Tiara, MD
Los Angeles County-USC Medical Center

James Tourge, MD
Cedars-Sinai Medical Center

Forewords

Though many texts are written in medicine, few have the impact of an atlas that can capture the presence of being at the bedside. The authors share the visual aspects of trauma care and allow the reader to more readily understand textual descriptions. They have produced a comprehensive atlas of trauma that is an excellent reference for physicians involved in trauma care.

The experienced trauma clinicians writing this text present their collective experience in a visual manner that represents many years of dedicated image collection and collaborative efforts from the Department of Emergency Medicine and the Division of Trauma at Los Angeles County-University of Southern California Medical Center. This Center is one of the busiest and most active trauma centers in the world.

Gail V. Anderson Sr., MD
Professor and Chairman
Department of Emergency Medicine
University of Southern California

There is no end to the writing of books, and their shelf life is limited by the march of understanding. Surgical atlases are less common and their effect lasts longer. Perhaps this is due to their dependency on the experience of the authors. Time is required between simply performing a procedure and becoming intimately familiar with the procedure. It is the latter that provides technical insights and make the atlas of value.

Most atlases consist of an artist's conception of the procedures involved. They are a step removed from the real world and there are concerns of authenticity. A danger exists that the illustrations will encourage action without a thorough understanding of the pathophysiological principles involved. The latter differentiates knowledge *about* from knowledge *of* the procedure being described and the problems it is designed to correct. The best atlases combine a short written description of the principles involved with the actual operative photographs. They bring the reader a step closer to the actual encounter.

Such is the atlas produced by the Division of Trauma and the Department of Emergency Medicine at the University of Southern California Keck School of Medicine. The authors have produced an atlas on trauma consisting of color photographs and accompanied by text that focuses on the principles involved. Being familiar with the impediments to stopping during an operative procedure or a resuscitative effort to record the pathology on camera gives one an appreciation for the efforts employed in accomplishing such a task. The authors of this atlas get my highest commendation. I encourage those interested in the subject to enjoy this work while also being educated by it.

Tom R. DeMeester, MD
Professor and Chairman
Department of Surgery
University of Southern California

Preface

Good trauma care requires a substantial knowledge base and clinical skill. The comprehension and intuition required to treat trauma injury is gained over many years of clinical experience at the bedside of critically injured patients. The aim of this atlas is to share the experience of the authors from the largest trauma center in the United States and provide a solid companion to the many well-written textbooks on trauma management.

This project represents many decades of collective clinical experience. We have assembled one of the largest collections of trauma images to help bring the reader "to the bedside" of the patients. The majority of the photographs originate from the Los Angeles County–University of Southern California Trauma Center though some special photographs were donated from outside centers. The acquisition and final assembly of this collection of images was a difficult process and they were acquired with the gracious cooperation of our patients. We regularly use these images in our clinical teaching and hope this atlas will supplement other instructional resources in trauma management.

Diku P. Mandavia, MD
Edward J. Newton, MD
Demetrios Demetriades, MD, PhD

Acknowledgments

Illustrations and Digital Imaging by:

Robert S. Amaral, MA
Medical Illustrator
Instructional Imaging Center
Keck School of Medicine
University of Southern California

Our appreciation to the following:

Burn Unit, Los Angeles County-USC Medical Center
Department of Radiology, Los Angeles County-USC Medical Center
Department of Imaging, Cedars-Sinai Medical Center

And to the staff and residents of:

Department of Emergency Medicine & Division of Trauma
Los Angeles County-USC Medical Center
Department of Emergency Medicine & Division of Trauma
Cedars-Sinai Medical Center

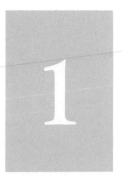

Head Injury

Introduction

Head injury accounts for the majority of deaths and severe disabilities due to trauma, and complicates the management of injury to other systems. Blunt head injury is most commonly the result of motor vehicle crashes, auto versus pedestrian collisions, or falls from significant heights. Gunshot wounds cause the vast majority of penetrating head injuries, although stab wounds and impalement injuries may also be seen.

Clinical Examination

Head injury is classified into mild, moderate, and severe categories, depending on the patient's Glasgow Coma Scale (GCS) (see Table 1.1) at the time of presentation. Mild head injury patients have a GCS of 14–15. Typically these injuries include concussion or transient loss of neurologic function, usually a transient loss of consciousness. Concussion does not result in any gross pathologic abnormalities of the brain, but subtle changes have been described using electron microscopy. Although the neurologic examination is usually normal in terms of quantifiable deficits, post-concussive neuropsychiatric symptoms are very common. These include amnesia for the event, headache, loss of concentration, dizziness, sleep disturbance, and a host of related symptoms. These symptoms resolve within two weeks for the vast majority of patients but may persist for many months in a small percentage. "Hard" neurologic findings such as diplopia, motor weakness, pupillary abnormalities, and other cranial nerve deficits are never due to post-concussive syndrome and demand further investigation.

Moderate head injury (GCS 8–14) and severe head injury (GCS <8) comprise a spectrum of injuries including cerebral contusion, diffuse cerebral edema, axonal shear injury, subarachnoid hemorrhage (SAH), and extra-axial lesions (subdural hematoma and epidural hematoma). The GCS is determined by the severity of the lesion and its time course.

A rapid but thorough neurologic examination is done prior to administering paralytic agents. The head is inspected for signs of trauma including lacerations, areas of skull depression, raccoon eyes, Battle's sign, hemotympanum, rhinorrhea, and otorrhea. The pupils are examined for symmetry and reaction to light; the extraocular movements and other cranial nerve functions are assessed; motor and sensory function is assessed for symmetry. The GCS is useful in categorizing patients as to severity of head injury but is not sufficient to determine the presence or absence of neurologic injury, as it does not assess pupils, subtle changes in mentation, cranial nerve injury, or skull fractures.

Patients with increased intracranial pressure (ICP) inevitably have some diminution in their typical level of alertness. As ICP increases further, herniation of the uncus across the tentorium can occur, resulting in compression of the ipsilateral cerebral peduncle and ipsilateral oculomotor nerve. Consequently, ipsilateral ptosis, restricted extraocular movement, and pupillary dilation occur, along with contralateral motor posturing (decorticate, followed by decerebrate, and finally flaccid paralysis). Once this process begins, there is a very brief interval for effecting a reversal by lowering ICP.

Skull fractures are common sequelae of both blunt and penetrating head trauma. Although it may be an isolated finding, skull fracture is frequently associated with intracranial injury. Closed simple linear fractures of the cranial vault are relatively benign in themselves but signify that substantial force has been applied to the cranium, putting its more delicate cerebral contents at risk. Skull fractures are particularly dangerous in certain anatomic locations, such as across the middle meningeal arterial groove, across dural sinuses, or in the occipital area because the intracranial bleeding associated with these fractures may be life threatening.

Table 1.1. Glasgow Coma Scale

EYES (E)		
Open	Spontaneously	4
	To verbal command	3
	To pain	2
No Response		1
BEST VERBAL RESPONSE (V)		
	Oriented & converses	5
	Disoriented & converses	4
	Inappropriate words	3
	Incomprehensible sounds	2
	No response	1
BEST MOTOR RESPONSE (M)		
To verbal stimuli	Obeys	6
To painful stimulus	Localizes pain	5
	Flexion-withdrawal	4
	Abnormal flexion (decorticate rigidity)	3
	Extension (decerebrate rigidity)	2
	No response (flaccid)	1
	Total:	3–15

As with fractures of other bones, skull fractures are classified as open or closed, simple or comminuted, and displaced or undisplaced. Open fractures of the skull may result in direct introduction of contaminants such as hair, skin, or foreign debris into the cranial vault. Subsequent infection can produce meningitis, osteomyelitis, or, more commonly, brain abscess. Consequently, open wounds of the cranium must be carefully debrided, irrigated, and closed to prevent such complications. Fractures of the paranasal sinuses that communicate with the dura are at high risk for ascending infection of the meninges and brain and are sometimes difficult to detect.

Isolated skull fractures may result in headache and local tenderness. Clinical findings with basilar skull fracture depend on which fossa of the cranium is involved. Frontobasilar fractures may present with raccoon eyes, rhinorrhea, and anosmia; middle fossa fractures present with hemotympanum, otorrhea, vertigo, or Battle's sign; posterior fossa fractures may present with ataxia and nystagmus.

Investigations

All patients with GCS <14 require evaluation by head computerized tomography (CT) without contrast. Selected patients may require further investigation by CT with contrast, magnetic resonance imaging (MRI),

or, rarely, cerebral angiography. Multiple trauma patients may have injuries to the chest or abdomen that require immediate operative intervention and take precedence over head injury. In these cases CT of the head may be deferred, although some patients may be stable enough to undergo a modified CT scan of the head with only a few cuts to identify an extra-axial hematoma. If one is identified, simultaneous evacuation of the brain hematoma can be done while a laparotomy or thoracotomy is in progress. In patients who are too unstable to undergo even a modified CT scan of the head and who show signs of neurologic deterioration, intraoperative burr holes can be placed to evacuate a hematoma.

Skull x-rays are seldom indicated because CT scan is equally sensitive in identifying skull fractures and provides much more information regarding any underlying brain injury. Skull x-rays can be useful in locating foreign bodies (e.g., bullet fragments) or intracranial air, and as part of a skeletal survey in suspected child abuse.

Cervical spine injury is frequently associated with blunt head trauma, and the evaluation of the spine is difficult in a patient whose mental status is diminished because of head injury. Consequently, it is essential to immobilize the spine and evaluate the integrity of the spinal column by plain radiographs and by CT scan if questions remain about possible spinal column injury. The cervical spine should remain immobilized in unresponsive patients until they are conscious enough to report persistent neck pain or paresthesias.

General Management

The goal of cerebral resuscitation in the emergency department (ED) is to prevent secondary injuries to the brain such as hypoxia, hypotension, seizures, hyperthermia, and hypercarbia. Subsequently, interventions to decrease elevated ICP are indicated.

Cerebral resuscitation and treatment are performed in the context of overall resuscitation and are guided by advanced trauma life support (ATLS) principles. Patients with severe head injury tend to hypoventilate and are at risk for aspiration of oral secretions. Consequently, securing an airway and ensuring adequate ventilation are the highest priorities. A brief neurologic examination should be performed prior to using paralytic drugs for rapid sequence intubation (RSI) to secure the airway. Patients with a GCS <8 require intubation, although patients with a higher GCS may also need intubation.

Maintaining adequate cerebral perfusion pressure is important in the face of increased ICP to prevent secondary ischemic injury. Consequently, measures to maintain adequate systemic blood pressure are essential and include crystalloid infusion, blood transfusion, thoracotomy, laparotomy, and pressors as indicated.

For patients with evidence of increased ICP or clinical signs of actual or impending transtentorial herniation, immediate measures to decrease ICP are indicated. Hyperventilation to reduce pCO_2 to a level of 30–35 mm Hg decreases cerebral blood flow and thus decreases intracranial blood volume, allowing a temporary decrease in ICP. Osmotic diuresis with mannitol and use of loop diuretics such as furosemide dehydrate all tissues including brain, again allowing more space for an expanding hematoma and lowering ICP. These medications must be used with extreme caution if at all in multiply injured patients, as severe systemic hypotension may result. Positioning the head at 30 degrees elevation can decrease ICP once the spine has been cleared radiographically. Placement of a ventriculostomy to drain cerebrospinal fluid (CSF) has been shown to be effective not only in treating elevated ICP but also in following the progress of the patient's condition. Use of hypertonic saline, cerebral or systemic mild hypothermia, and administration of magnesium sulfate have been shown experimentally to improve outcome from severe head injury.

Definitive treatment for head injury depends on the nature of the lesion. Closed skull fractures require no specific treatment, but open fractures should be irrigated, debrided, and closed. Depressed skull fractures require elevation of the fragment if it is depressed greater than one bone width, and debridement if the wound is grossly contaminated. Basilar skull fractures usually heal uneventfully, but patients with rhinorrhea or otorrhea require careful follow-up to ensure that the fistula closes. Most CSF leaks stop within two weeks, but persistent leaks may require a formal dural closure. Most epidural hematomas (EDHs) require surgical evacuation, although those that are <1 cm can be treated by observation and repeat CT scan if the patient is asymptomatic. Larger EDHs require craniotomy for evacuation. Subdural hematoma (SDH) is rarely asymptomatic, and surgical treatment is almost invariably needed to evacuate the hematoma. Subarachnoid hemorrhage is treated with nimodipine to decrease surrounding vasospasm, and measures to decrease rebleeding are undertaken. Intraventricular hemorrhage may require ventriculostomy to remove blood and CSF, but the prognosis usually remains poor. Patients requiring surgery and those with depressed skull fracture and cerebral contusion should be started on a course of anticonvulsant medication.

Common Mistakes and Pitfalls

1. Certain patients are at higher risk for intracranial injury from even relatively minor mechanisms of injury. These include the elderly, chronic alcoholics, infants, patients with cerebral atrophy, and those with coagulopathy. A low threshold for obtaining a head CT scan should be maintained in these patients.

2. Altered mental status, seizures, and focal neurologic deficits should not be ascribed to intoxication, dementia, or other chronic conditions if there is a history or evidence of head trauma present.

3. Excessive hyperventilation (to a pCO_2 <30 mm Hg) should be avoided because it lowers cerebral blood flow to a point that cerebral ischemia can occur.

4. Delayed presentation of SDH and EDH can occur, often with subtle neurologic signs. Obtaining a repeat CT scan or initial CT scan even weeks after the injury is appropriate in selected cases.

5. Subacute SDH may appear isodense with surrounding brain five to ten days after the injury. Altering the density values of the CT or use of contrast will demonstrate the lesion.

6. Coagulopathy is common with serious head injury and may result in more severe bleeding, hemorrhage from other noncerebral sites, and disseminated intravascular coagulopathy (DIC). A baseline coagulation profile should be obtained in patients with serious head injury and repeated periodically during admission.

7. Child abuse must be suspected in cases of intracerebral injury or skull fracture in infants and children.

1.1 Scalp Injuries

Commentary

The scalp is a tough, mobile, multilayered covering of the skull. It is composed of epidermis, dermis and a strong fibrous layer of subdermal tissue, a muscle layer, and the galea or periosteal covering of the skull. The scalp is highly vascular, and vessels are fixed within the scalp and unable to retract and constrict when lacerated. Conse-quently, scalp wounds frequently bleed profusely and can result in hemorrhagic shock. In scalping type injuries careful attention must be paid to ensuring that there are not also skull fractures associated with the soft tissue injury. A completely avulsed scalp can be replaced and usually heals well because of its extensive vascularity.

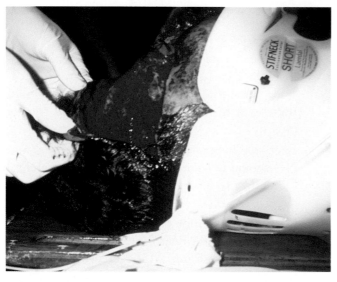

1.1A. Photograph of a patient with severe facial and scalp avulsion.

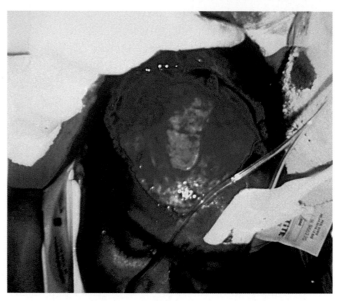

1.1B. Photograph of a patient with avulsion of the apical scalp.

1.2 Linear Skull Fracture

Commentary

Linear skull fracture results from a direct blow to the head. Motor vehicle crashes cause the majority of these injuries, although the incidence of serious head injury from this source has decreased as a result of the use of motorcycle helmets, seatbelts, and airbags. Other causes of linear skull fractures include falls and assaults. Linear skull fractures account for approxi-mately 80% of all skull fractures, and the vast majority (85%) occur in males.

Skull fractures are relatively common in children in spite of the greater pliability of their skulls. Skull frac-tures in infants are commonly due to child abuse, and the circumstances surrounding the injury need to be carefully investigated. Skull fractures in neonates can also occur in association with a cephalohematoma as a result of a difficult delivery and use of forceps. Management of these injuries is generally conservative unless the skull fragments are depressed. A "growing" skull fracture occasionally occurs in children as a result of the interposition of a leptomeningeal cyst between the fracture edges, and it may require surgery. Healing of a skull fracture takes place over many months, so children should be rechecked approximately six months following a fracture to ensure that proper healing has occurred.

A skull fracture may occasionally become apparent on physical examination while a scalp laceration is explored. It is felt as a step-off of the normally smooth skull surface. These fractures should be treated as any other open fracture with debridement, irrigation, and closure of each layer of the scalp, including the galea. Antibiotic prophylaxis is indicated, and CT scan should be obtained to delineate the extent of the fracture and to determine if intracranial injury has occurred.

On plain radiographs a linear skull fracture appears as a straight or minimally branched lucency if the fragments are distracted or as a hyperdensity if the fragments overlap. A fracture must be distinguished from suture lines and vascular grooves. Suture lines have a characteristic zigzag appearance and are located in predictable locations. They are of near uniform width throughout their course. Vascular grooves have sequential bifurcations. Fracture lines can cross either of these structures and typically are wider in their center, tapering in width toward either end. Plain radiography of the skull is rarely obtained in the current era as CT scan has largely replaced it. Plain radiography may still be useful in the assessment of depressed skull fractures or location of foreign bodies within the cranium, such as bullet fragments or impaled objects. Detection of a fracture on plain films or on physical examination is an indication for obtaining a CT scan of the head. The incidence of brain injury in the presence of a skull fracture is as high as 12%. Fractures across the middle meningeal vascular groove are associated with epidural hematoma in a small percent of cases, but 80% of epidural hematomas are associated with a skull fracture.

CT scan will reveal a linear fracture as a gap in the skull and has the advantage of demonstrating any underlying injury to the brain. The sensitivity for detection of skull fracture with CT scan is very high and comparable to the accuracy of plain radiographs. Patients with linear skull fracture can be discharged if they have no other intracerebral injury, a normal neurologic examination, and reliable follow-up, although children are generally admitted for observation.

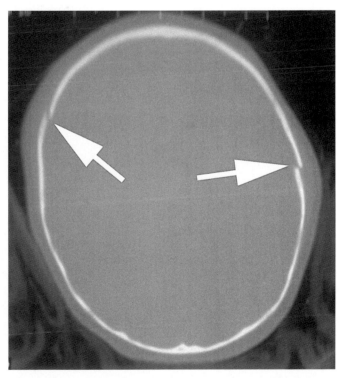

1.2A. AP skull radiograph showing linear skull fracture (arrow B) caused by a gunshot wound (GSW) to the right temporal area (arrow A).

1.2B. CT scan with bone windows showing right frontal and left parietal skull fractures (arrows).

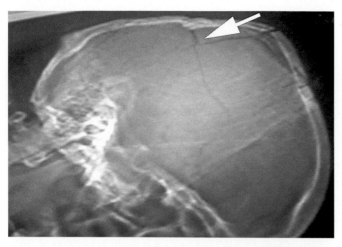

1.2C. Lateral skull radiograph showing a comminuted fracture of the apex of the skull (arrow).

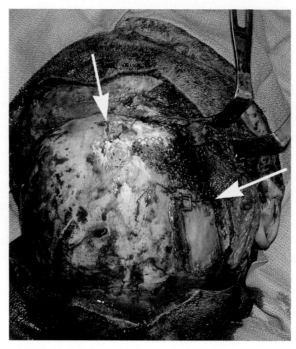

1.2E. Photograph of a semicircular linear skull fracture at craniotomy (arrows).

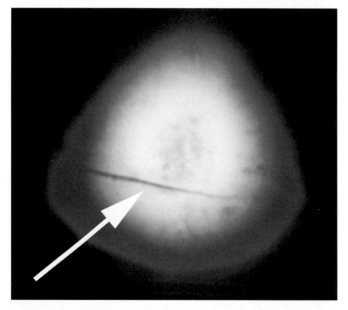

1.2D. Linear skull fracture on CT in a patient with a machete injury.

1.3 Depressed Skull Fracture

Commentary

The typical depressed skull fracture occurs when a large amount of force is applied to a small area of the skull (e.g., a blow with a hammer) that results in a stellate fracture with a depressed center. Physical examination of the skull may reveal a depression in the skull, but more commonly the fracture is not palpable because of overlying soft tissue swelling. Unless the view is exactly tangential, plain radiographs may not reveal the extent of bone depression. CT scan is highly sensitive and accurate in detecting depressed skull fracture as well as underlying brain injury.

Patients with depressed skull fractures have an increased incidence of post-traumatic seizures because the impact of the fragments on the cortex of the brain results in areas of scarring that ultimately become seizure foci. Consequently, anticonvulsant prophylaxis is begun in the ED and continued for one week. Management of a closed depressed skull fracture is contro-versial. Some advocate conservative treatment for all of these fractures; others recommend surgical eleva-tion of the fragments if the depression is greater than one bone width (from inner to outer table). Open, contaminated depressed fractures clearly require surgi-cal debridement.

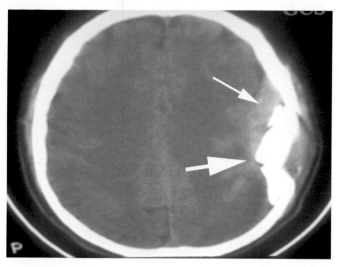

1.3A. CT scan showing deformity and depressed skull fracture of the left parietal area (large arrow) with underlying SDH (small arrow).

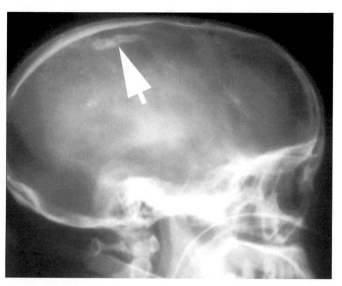

1.3C. Lateral radiograph of the skull showing hyperdensity due to overlapping bone fragments (arrow) at the apical-parietal skull.

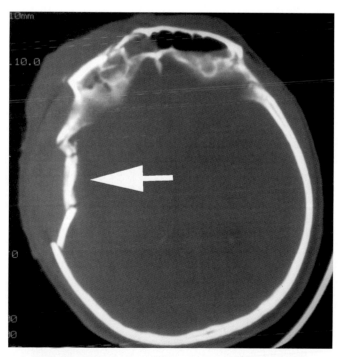

1.3B. CT scan bone windows showing right temporoparietal comminuted depressed fracture (arrow) and associated soft tissue swelling. There is also a fracture of the right frontal sinus. This patient suffered a concomitant epidural hematoma.

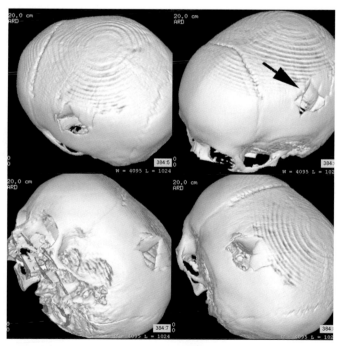

1.3D. CT scan showing 3-D reconstruction of left parietal depressed skull fracture (arrow).

1.4 Open Skull Fracture

Commentary

Open skull fracture can result from penetration of both the scalp and the skull from blunt or penetrating trauma or from fracture of air-filled sinuses that communicate with the intracranial space. Although pneumocephalus can rarely result in a mass effect and displacement of intracranial contents, more commonly its significance is the creation of a communication between the CSF and the environment that often leads to the development of meningitis or brain abscess. Open skull fracture should be treated as any open fracture, with surgical debridement, irrigation, and appropriate parenteral antibiotics.

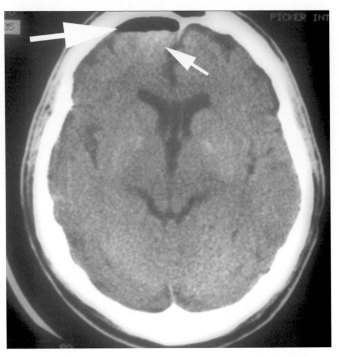

1.4B. CT scan showing right frontal intracranial air (large arrow) with a small SAH in the frontal lobe (small arrow).

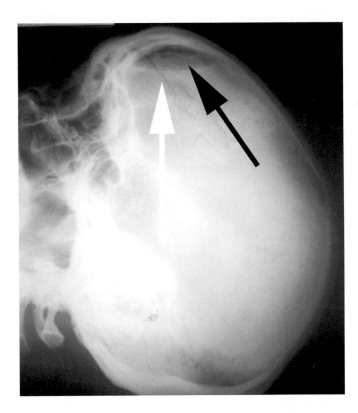

1.4A. Lateral radiograph of the skull showing a frontal linear skull fracture (white arrow) and accumulation of frontal intracranial air (pneumocephalus) (black arrow).

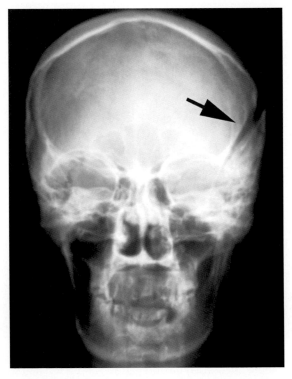

1.4C. AP skull radiograph showing a large oblique skull defect on the left (arrow) secondary to a blow from an axe.

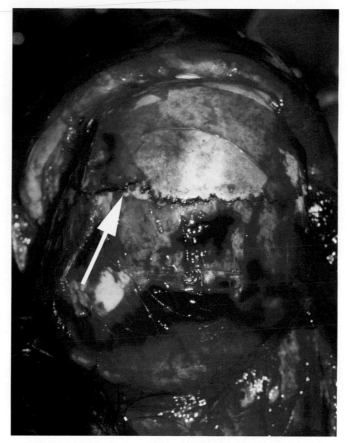

1.4D. Photograph of an open linear skull fracture.

1.5 Basilar Skull Fracture

Commentary

The skull base is divided into three compartments, and the clinical presentation differs depending on the location of the fracture. Basilar skull fracture is a clinical diagnosis based on physical findings of raccoon eyes, Battle's sign, CSF rhinorrhea or otorrhea, or hemotympanum. Injury to cranial nerves that exit the base of the skull is common, and a careful neurologic examination is required to seek out these injuries. Occasionally, plain radiographs or CT scan will make the diagnosis in the absence of these clinical findings, although neither imaging technique is highly sensitive. The fracture line may be visualized directly or by indirect evidence such as blood in the sphenoid sinus, the mastoid air cells, or the auditory canal or fracture of the posterior wall of the maxillary sinus. On plain radiographs, an air-fluid level may be seen in the sphenoid sinus lying anterior to the pituitary fossa, or the fracture line may be visualized directly.

Because fracture fragments often tear the underlying dura, leakage of CSF through the nose (rhinorrhea) or ear canal (otorrhea) is common. If the tympanic membrane remains intact, a hemotympanum may be seen. Battle's sign occurs because of tracking of blood through the mastoid air cells to the skin behind the ear, which appears ecchymotic. This sign is often delayed many hours and may not be apparent on initial examination. Similarly, raccoon eyes appear sooner but become increasingly evident with time and may not be apparent on initial examination.

Treatment of a basilar skull fracture is conservative unless cranial nerve injury mandates surgical decompression. Although meningitis can ensue from a persistent CSF leak, prophylactic antibiotics are not indicated, as 90% of the dural tears heal within one week. Persistent leakage beyond two weeks may require operative repair with a dural patch.

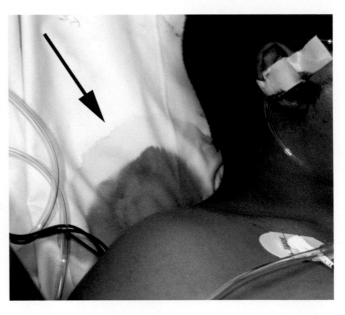

1.5D. Photograph of the CSF double ring sign on bed sheet.

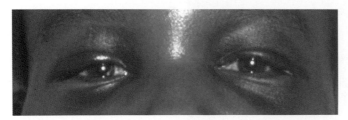

1.5A. Photograph of a patient with raccoon eyes due to a frontobasilar skull fracture.

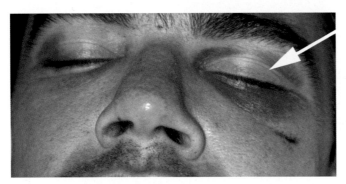

1.5B. Close-up photograph of raccoon eyes showing tarsal plate sparing (arrow).

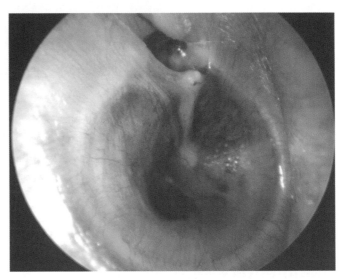

1.5E. Photograph of a hemotympanum. (with permission from Pulec, JL and Deguine: *Atlas of Otoscopy.* Singular/Thompson Learning. 2001. p. 151).

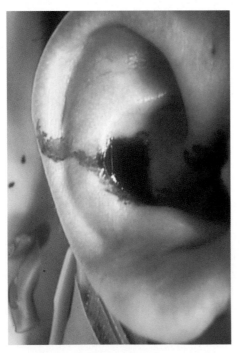

1.5C. Photograph of otorrhea following basilar skull fracture with rupture of the tympanic membrane.

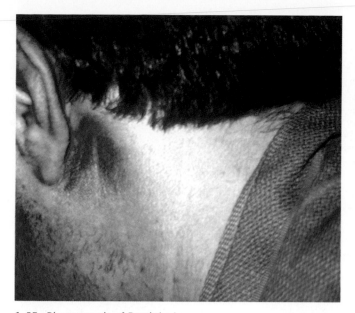

1.5F. Photograph of Battle's sign.

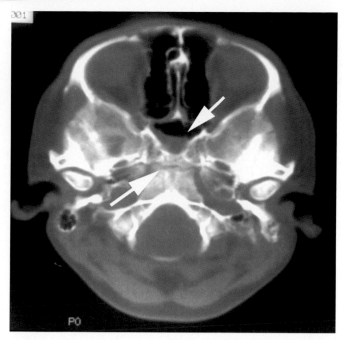

1.5G. CT scan of the base of the skull showing a basilar skull fracture (bottom arrow) and an isolated air-fluid level in the sphenoid sinus (top arrow), which is characteristic of basilar skull fracture.

1.6 Epidural Hematoma

Commentary

EDH accounts for approximately 10–15% of severe head injuries, with the peak incidence in young adult males between the ages of 15 and 24. Common etiologies include motor vehicle accidents, auto versus pedestrian accidents, and sports injuries. The typical EDH is unilateral and occurs as a result of a temporoparietal skull fracture that transects the course of the middle meningeal artery. Blood accumulates outside the dura mater, dissecting the dura from the inner table of the skull and compressing underlying brain as it expands under arterial pressure.

The classical pattern is that of an initial head trauma with loss of consciousness due to concussion, followed by a lucid interval as the patient recovers from the concussion, with a subsequent decreased level of consciousness due to mass effect from the accumulating EDH. However, only 30% of patients with EDH demonstrate this classical pattern. The duration of the lucid interval is highly variable, and most patients are not completely asymptomatic during this interval. Because the bleeding is under arterial pressure, it generally accumulates quickly, causing a mass effect with shift of the ipsilateral hemisphere and, eventually, transtentorial herniation. Some small EDHs never progress to this stage and can be managed conservatively.

The diagnosis of EDH is based on CT scan that reliably demonstrates the typical hyperdense accumulation of blood in a lenticular shape at the periphery of the cerebrum, indenting the cerebral cortex and brain parenchyma. Outside of the posterior fossa, the hematoma will not cross suture lines, as the dura is tightly adherent at suture lines. CT scan is indicated in patients who have a history of a potentially severe mechanism of head injury with loss of consciousness, evidence of a skull fracture, or a less than normal GCS on initial examination.

The diagnosis may not be apparent on the initial CT scan if the patient suffers from severe anemia (lowering the density of the hematoma on CT scan) or has severe hypotension (which reduces the rate of arterial blood loss), or if the CT scan is obtained too soon after the trauma (before a significant amount of blood has accumulated). Approximately 8% of EDHs are detected after a significant delay. Occasionally EDH may result from tears of venous sinuses or veins, and the accumulation of blood occurs more slowly.

Treatment of EDH is surgical evacuation of the clot and repair of the vessels or dural sinus involved. Patients who are not in coma at the time of presentation usually recover very well, as often there is little underlying brain damage. Mortality ranges from none to 20% in various series.

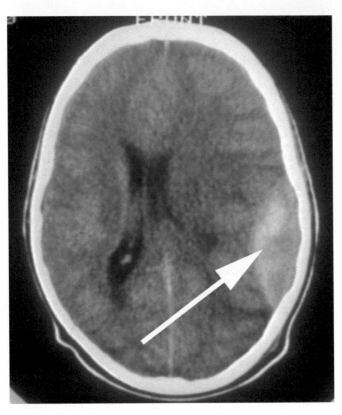

1.6A. CT scan showing typical epidural hematoma in the left posterior parietal area (arrow) with significant shift of cerebral contents across the midline.

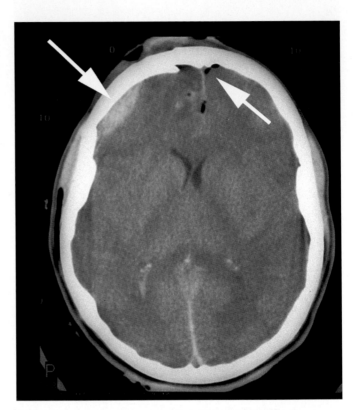

1.6B. CT scan showing a small right frontal epidural hematoma (left arrow), intracranial air in the frontal area (right arrow), an overlying fracture of the frontotemporal skull, and evidence of increased intracranial pressure (obliteration of the ventricles and cisterns and loss of definition of the sulci).

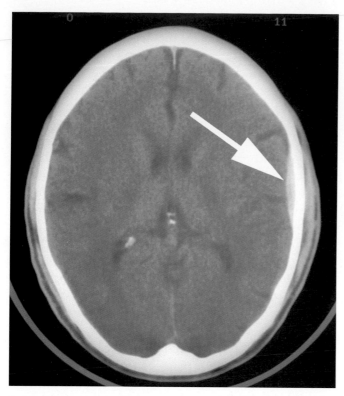

1.6C. CT scan of a subtle left parietal epidural hematoma (arrow) without mass effect.

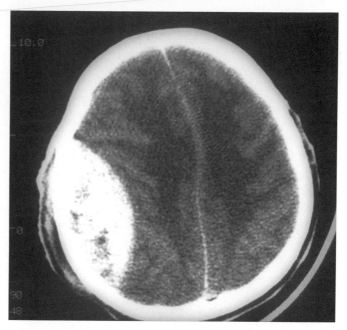

1.6D. CT scan of a massive, acute right parietal epidural hematoma showing the typical swirling appearance of the acute hematoma with a mass effect and increased intracranial pressure.

1.7 Subdural Hematoma

Commentary

SDH is divided into three categories based on the time elapsed since the injury. These categories are acute SDH (0–24 hours), subacute SDH (1–7 days), and chronic SDH (>7 days). The importance of this distinction is that the appearance of the hemorrhage on CT scan varies with time as it moves from a solid hyperdense clot (acute SDH) to an intermediate or isodense phase in which the hematoma is often indistinguishable from adjacent normal brain tissue (subacute SDH). After approximately 5–10 days a chronic phase begins in which the cellular elements of the hematoma break down and are reabsorbed, leaving a fluid-filled encapsulated hypodense mass (chronic SDH). Radiographic interpretation has to take these sequential changes into account.

SDH accounts for approximately 40% of cases of severe head injury. It is found in all age groups, but certain populations are at higher risk for SDH, including the elderly, chronic alcoholics, patients who are anticoagulated, and infants (shaken baby syndrome).

Symptoms of SDH depend on multiple variables, including the size and location of the SDH, the rate of accumulation of blood, the degree of underlying brain injury, the extent of cerebral atrophy, and the premorbid level of functioning. Acute SDH results from either a direct blow to the head or acceleration/deceleration forces applied to the brain. The movement of the brain within the skull stretches bridging veins from the dura to the surface of the brain, resulting in accumulation of blood beneath the dura. This collection of blood is seen on CT scan as a hyperdense semilunate (crescent-shaped) hematoma that conforms to the convexity of the cerebral hemisphere. Depending on the size of the hematoma and the degree of underlying cerebral edema, a mass effect will occur with obliteration of the ventricles and cisterns and shift of cerebral structures across the midline that may culminate in transtentorial herniation. Because of underlying cortical damage, patients will often demonstrate contralateral focal neurologic deficits consistent with the location of the SDH. Additional symptoms include altered mental state, headache, nausea and vomiting, and other symptoms related to increased intracranial pressure.

As the SDH persists beyond 5–7 days, resorption of cellular elements results in loss of density of the hematoma. At some point (usually from 5–10 days), the density of the hematoma will be very similar to that of the adjacent brain parenchyma, making it difficult to distinguish with standard CT scan exposures. In some cases, only subtle evidence of mass effect such as compression of the ipsilateral ventricle will suggest the presence of an SDH. Slight differences in density can be magnified by altering the Hounsfield units of the CT scan exposure, and these "subdural windows" may be diagnostic. Alternatively, a contrast-enhanced CT scan can be done in which the isodense hematoma will appear less dense than the contrast-enhanced adjacent brain. Symptoms at this stage include headache, diminished concentration and alertness, and variable focal neurologic deficits.

As the process of resorption continues beyond two weeks, the SDH enters a chronic phase. The SDH releases osmotically active cellular elements as it breaks down that cause the hematoma to expand. Symptoms may be very subtle or may be suggestive of increased intracranial pressure. Chronic SDH occurs more commonly in patients with significant preexisting cerebral atrophy, so that changes in mental state such as increasing confusion, disorientation, lethargy, and depression may be difficult to detect. In fact, the original head trauma may have been relatively minor and completely forgotten by the time the patient presents for care. There is a high risk of rebleeding into a chronic SDH so that a sudden decompensation may be the presenting complaint when this occurs. CT scan reveals a hypodense semilunate collection of fluid with a surrounding hyperdense capsule and variable amounts of cellular debris in the dependent portion of the SDH. Rebleeding is seen as a hyperdense collection of blood superimposed on an encapsulated chronic hematoma.

Treatment for a large SDH in the acute or subacute stages is evacuation via craniotomy. Small hematomas can be managed conservatively with close neurologic observation. The decision regarding management of a chronic SDH depends on the premorbid function of the individual, size of the SDH, and current symptoms. Seizure prophylaxis should be provided in all cases for the first week to decrease the incidence of early post-traumatic seizures.

Acute Subdural Hematoma

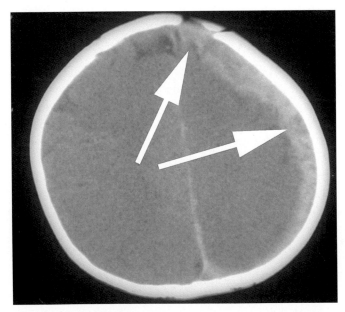

1.7A. CT scan showing acute large left SDH (lower arrow) and a left frontal skull fracture (upper arrow) in a case of shaken baby syndrome.

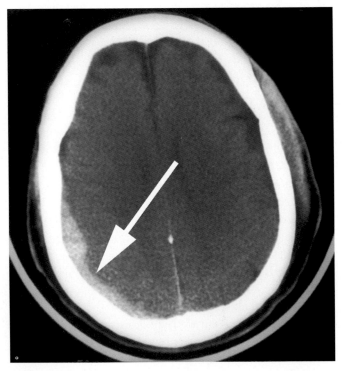

1.7B. Smaller right parieto-occipital acute SDH without mass effect (arrow).

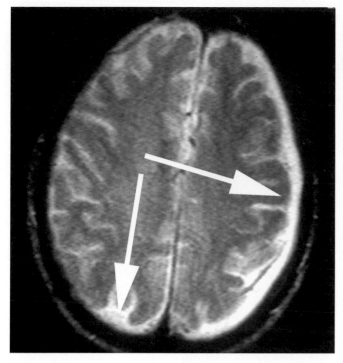

1.7C. T2 weighted MRI showing large left SDH (upper arrow) with right occipital contrecoup subarachnoid hemorrhage injury (lower arrow)

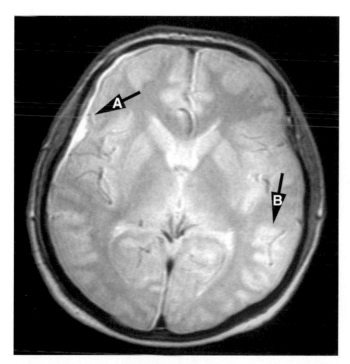

1.7D. T2 weighted MRI showing small right frontotemporal "rim subdural" (arrow A) with left parieto-occipital contrecoup contusion (arrow B).

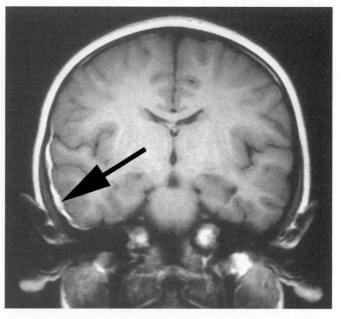

1.7E. T1 weighted MRI showing a temporal rim SDH in the coronal plane (arrow).

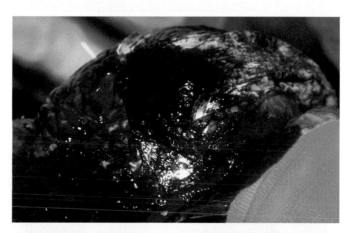

1.7F. Autopsy photograph of a subdural hematoma.

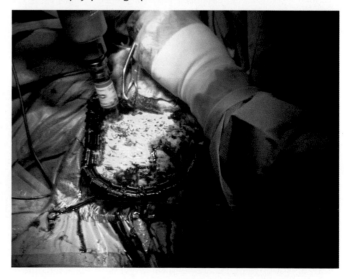

1.7G. Photograph of burr hole creation in progress.

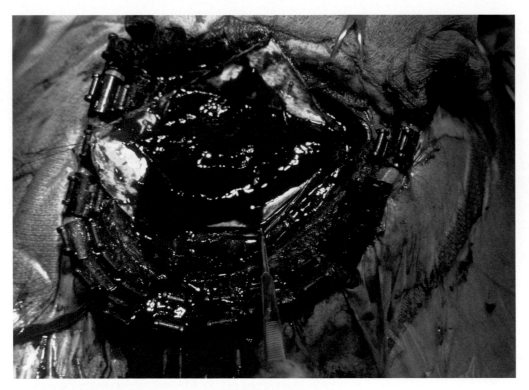

1.7H. Photograph of removal of acute SDH at craniotomy.

Subacute Subdural Hematoma

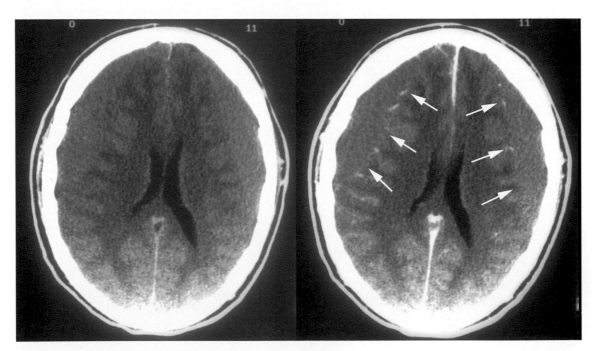

1.7I. CT scan that appears almost normal (left) and CT scan of the same patient using intravenous contrast (right). Bilateral isodense SDHs are seen (arrows) with early capsule formation medially and minimal mass effect (compression of the right lateral ventricle).

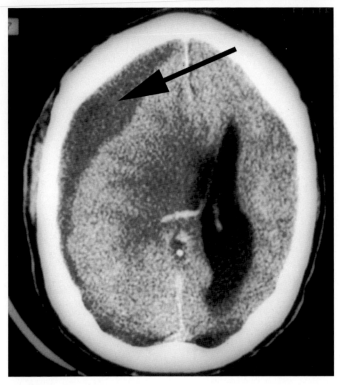

1.7J. CT scan of a right subacute SDH (arrow) at a later stage of development (less density of the hematoma) with severe mass effect.

Chronic Subdural Hematoma

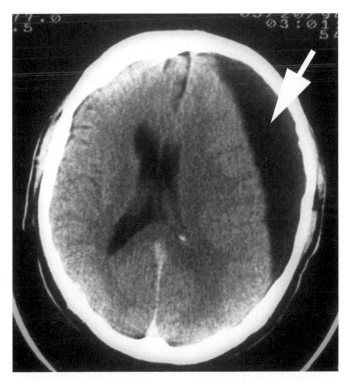

1.7K. CT scan with large chronic left SDH (arrow) with mass effect.

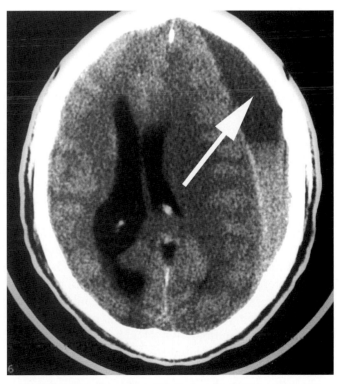

1.7L. CT scan with unilateral left chronic SDH (arrow) with acute rebleeding seen in the dependent (lower) aspect of the SDH, and significant shift of intracerebral contents across the midline.

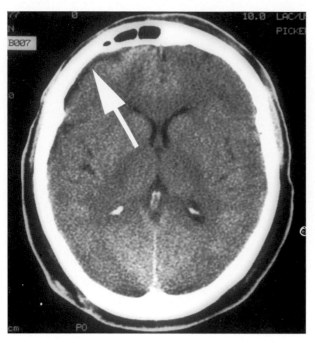

1.7M. CT scan with subtle right frontal chronic SDH (arrow) without mass effect.

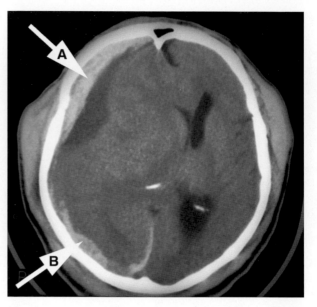

1.7N. CT scan with chronic right frontal SDH, rebleeding in the right frontal (arrow A) and occipital areas (arrow B), and midline shift.

1.8 Traumatic Subarachnoid Hemorrhage

Commentary

Most SAHs occur spontaneously as a result of a rupture of an arteriovenous malformation (AVM) or berry aneurysm. However, head trauma can also result in SAH and tends to have a worse outcome than nontraumatic SAH. The SAH appears as a hyperdense collection of blood that tracks along the outer edge of the brain parenchyma beneath the arachnoid membrane. On CT scan it is seen tracking into sulci, usually in the frontal lobes. The CT scan appearance may be very subtle, and the SAH is easily missed. Often SAH is associated with intraventricular, subdural, and intraparenchymal bleeding, as well as with mass lesions such as SDH. The exact patient presentation depends on the location of the hemorrhage but often includes headache, altered level of consciousness, nausea and vomiting, nuchal rigidity, coma, and, rarely, retinal subhyaloid hemorrhage.

Treatment of an isolated traumatic SAH is conservative. There is less risk of rebleeding than with SAH caused by aneurysm rupture, but trauma patients should be observed for this complication as well. During the acute phase, intense vasospasm caused by subarachnoid blood may worsen symptoms and outcome

by causing ischemia in adjacent normal brain. Use of calcium channel blockers has shown some utility in reducing this vasospasm. Long-term sequelae include obstructive hydrocephalus that may require creation of a ventriculoperitoneal shunt for decompression.

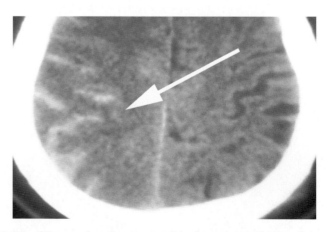

1.8A. CT scan showing traumatic subarachnoid hemorrhage (SAH). Arrow shows collection of blood in the sulci of the posterior parietal lobe.

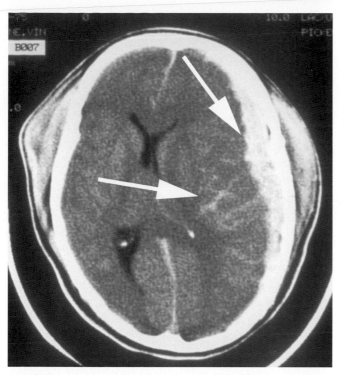

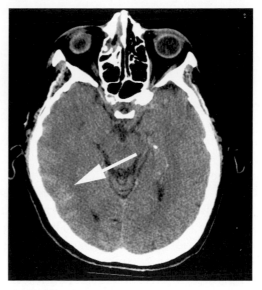

1.8C. Subtle traumatic SAH in an elderly patient with a ground level fall.

1.8B. CT scan showing acute left SDH (upper arrow) with a left parietal SAH (lower arrow), effacement of the posterior horn of the left lateral ventricle, and midline shift.

1.8D. Photograph of diffuse and focal SAH (arrow) at craniotomy.

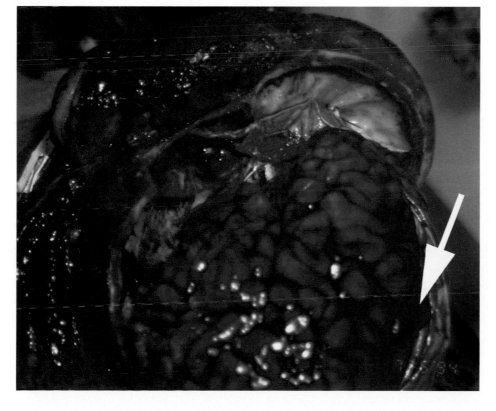

1.9 Cerebral Contusion

Commentary

Cerebral contusion occurs as the brain parenchyma strikes fixed portions of the skull during sudden deceleration or acceleration. It is often associated with a coup-contrecoup injury and may be found relatively distant from the site of head impact. Certain locations are particularly prone to contusion: The frontal lobe striking the anterior skull and the temporal lobe striking the projections of the sphenoid bone are the two most common locations for cerebral contusion.

The clinical presentation depends on the size and location of the contusion. Frontal lobe contusions are characterized by agitation, confusion, perseveration or repetitive questioning, impaired short-term memory, and aggressiveness that often requires physical or chemical restraint. Cerebral contusions, especially frontal or temporal, are also characterized by a high incidence of post-traumatic seizures. Because of this, neurosurgeons often recommend routine prophylactic treatment with anticonvulsants (e.g., phenytoin) for approximately seven days following injury.

Initially the contusion is primarily hemorrhagic. Over a period of hours to days, localized cerebral edema develops, causing a mass effect that potentially can result in transtentorial herniation. Management with diuresis and intracranial pressure monitoring is helpful with contusions that develop a mass effect. Glucocorticoids are not helpful because the edema is vasogenic in nature. Eventually the edema regresses and the hematoma reabsorbs completely or liquefies, leaving a cystic fluid-filled structure.

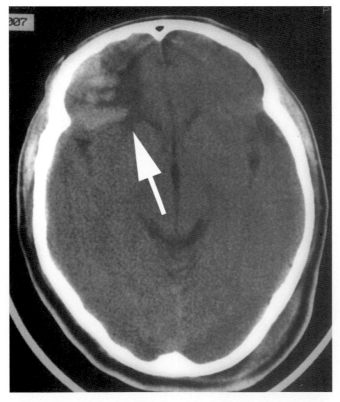

1.9A. CT scan showing right frontal lobe contusion (arrow) with surrounding edema.

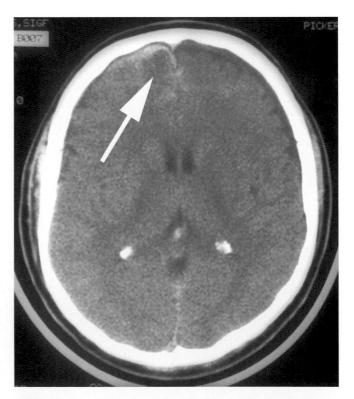

1.9B. CT scan showing subtle right frontal lobe contusion (arrow) with small associated SAH and no surrounding edema.

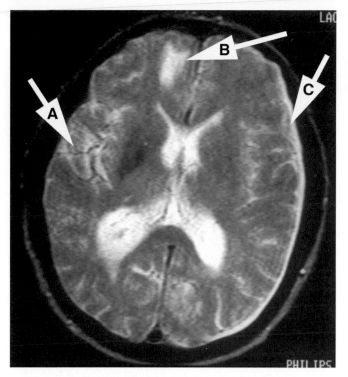

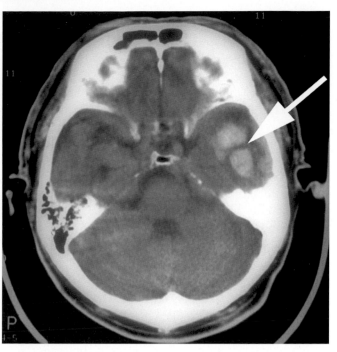

1.9E. CT scan showing a left temporal lobe contusion (arrow) with surrounding edema.

1.9C. T2 weighted MRI showing right frontal lobe contusion (arrow B), with a large rim SDH on the left (arrow C) and contrecoup contusion of the left temporal lobe (arrow A).

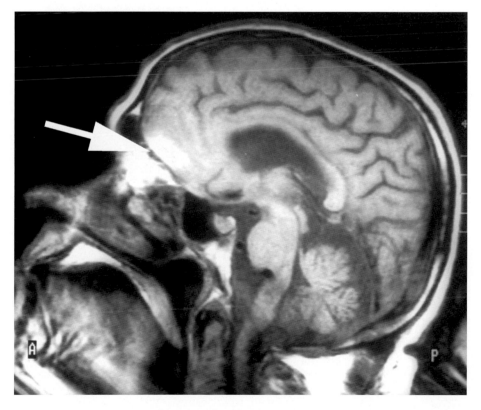

1.9D. T1 weighted sagittal-view MRI showing a frontobasilar contusion (arrow).

1.10 Penetrating Head Injury

Commentary

The vast majority of penetrating head wounds involve GSWs. These are devastating injuries that frequently result in death or profound disability in survivors. As a bullet enters the skull, it produces multiple high-velocity fragments (both from shattered skull bony fragments and from bullet fragmentation) that cause multiple injuries. Although the skull absorbs some kinetic energy, the bullet retains sufficient energy to cause a pressure wave once it enters brain parenchyma. This produces a rapidly expanding cavity and subsequent recoil of brain tissue. The abrupt deformation of brain tissue results in laceration and contusion of brain parenchyma, accumulation of blood in the epidural or subdural spaces, intraparenchymal bleeding, and direct laceration of brain tissue by bullet and bone fragments. Because of the high kinetic energy imparted to the brain, subsequent cerebral edema is common.

Other types of penetrating injuries involve less kinetic energy and have a better prognosis. Stab wounds, impalement injuries, and low-velocity shrapnel wounds can produce all of the same injuries but most commonly result in open skull fracture and direct laceration of brain parenchyma. Impaled objects result from both accidental trauma and intentional injury. Many different objects may be involved, but knives and metal rods are the most common. A careful physical examination is indicated with stab wounds of the scalp to ensure that the knife blade has not broken off inside the cranium. Wounds associated with these injuries may appear very innocuous and may be missed altogether as they are often covered with matted hair. Surprisingly, many of these patients are relatively asymptomatic and often have a normal neurologic examination in spite of a dramatic presentation. Plain AP and lateral radiographs of the skull will accurately delineate the location and depth of penetration of radiopaque impaled objects. If the patient can fit into the CT scan gantry without disturbing the impaled object, the CT scan will demonstrate underlying brain injury, although metal artifact may be problematic. Impaled foreign bodies should be removed only in the operating room, where prompt vascular control can be obtained once the object is removed.

Management depends on the overall condition of the patient. Frequently, GSW victims have multiple wounds of the chest, neck, or abdomen that may take priority in terms of restoring hemodynamic stability to the patient. As with open skull fractures, bleeding from a GSW of the head may be profuse, but hemorrhagic shock is uncommon with isolated head injuries, and other associated injuries should be sought to explain the shock. Because there is open communication with the environment, an epidural hematoma associated with a penetrating injury may decompress spontaneously. Surgical debridement and control of cerebral hemorrhage may be life saving. The incidence of post-traumatic seizures is more than 50%, and use of anticonvulsant medication is routine in these cases.

Patients with exposed brain matter, GSW that crosses the midline of the brain, severe coagulopathy, or early transtentorial herniation invariably die of their wounds and should be considered as potential organ donors.

Gunshot Wound

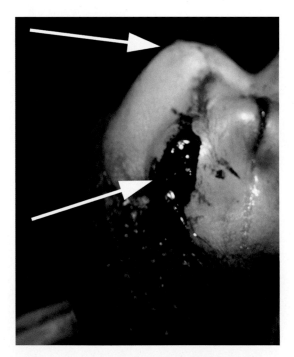

1.10A. Photograph of a patient with a GSW entry wound on the right temporal area (lower arrow) with bulging deformity of the forehead due to comminuted frontal bone fractures (upper arrow).

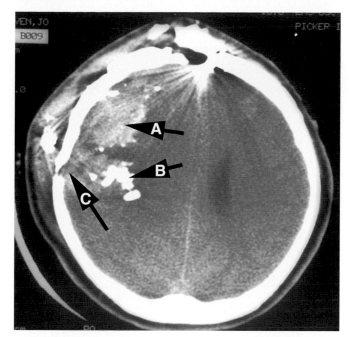

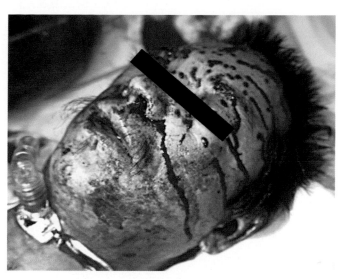

1.10B. CT scan showing a GSW of the right frontotemporal skull and brain. Findings include a subdural hematoma, intraparenchymal hemorrhage (arrow A) and intraparenchymal bullet fragments in the right parietal area (arrow B), and an open frontotemporal skull fracture (arrow C).

1.10C. Photograph of a patient with fatal close-range buckshot shotgun wound (SGW) of the face.

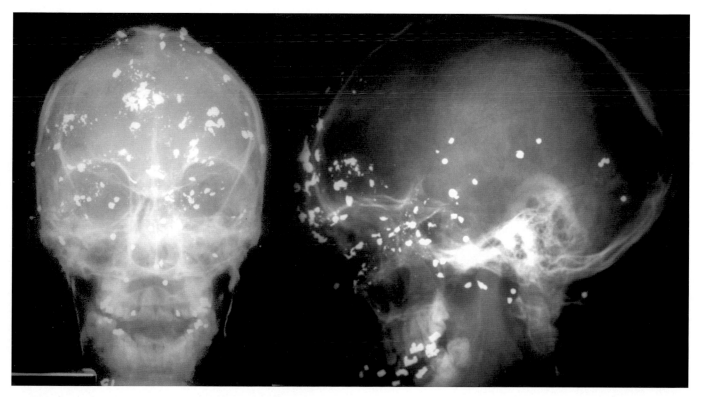

1.10D. AP and lateral radiograph of the skull in the same patient showing multiple buckshot shotgun pellets of the face and skull.

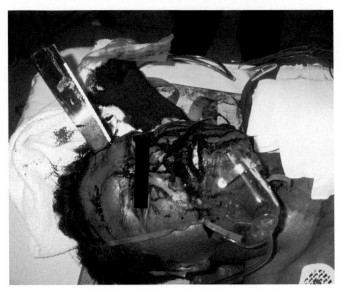

1.10E. Photograph of an awake patient with an embedded knife in the frontal area.

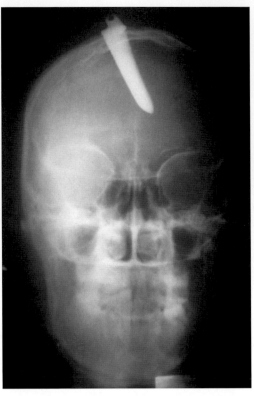

1.10F. AP skull radiograph showing a knife embedded in the cranium.

1.11 Transtentorial Herniation

Commentary

Herniation is the result of progressive expansion of one segment of the brain under the pressure of hemorrhage or edema formation, with the resultant compression and dysfunction of adjacent brain structures. If compression of the brainstem occurs, loss of vital functions such as respiration and vasomotor control result in rapid demise. There are four main types of herniation described:

1. Uncal herniation: The most common form of herniation results from edema or mass lesions (hemorrhage, tumor, abscess, etc.) in one cerebral hemisphere that causes a shift of that hemisphere across the midline, under the falx, and downward across the tentorium. The patient becomes somnolent or comatose. Compression of the ipsilateral cranial nerve III produces ipsilateral ptosis, loss of pupillary light reflex, and loss of extraocular movements. Compression of the ipsilateral cerebral peduncle results in weakness or abnormal posturing (decorticate, then decerebrate) of the contralateral limbs. In up to 30% of the cases the opposite cerebral peduncle is compressed, resulting in a false localizing sign (Kernohan's notch phenomenon). Respiratory abnormalities progress from central neurogenic hyperventilation to Cheyne-Stokes breathing, to ataxic breathing, and finally to apneustic respiration.

2. Central herniation: Compression of the brainstem by a frontal or apical mass lesion that expands downward produces pinpoint pupils, downward gaze preference, and other brainstem dysfunction described previously. Bilateral motor findings (posturing, paralysis) may occur.

3. Cingulate gyrus herniation: Pressure in one cerebral hemisphere may result in herniation of the ipsilateral medial cingulate gyrus under the falx.

4. Cerebellar tonsillar herniation: Mass lesions or edema of the cerebellum can result in expansion of the cerebellar tonsils into the foramen magnum, compressing the posterior brainstem. This presents as sudden loss of consciousness and loss of brainstem function with consequent apnea and hypotension. This condition has extremely high mortality, so cerebellar lesions must be recognized before the onset of herniation to salvage the patient.

Patients who achieve hemodynamic stability should be treated with a cerebral resuscitation protocol including rapid sequence intubation (RSI), moderate hyperventilation to a pCO_2 of 35 mm Hg, osmotic and loop diuresis, sedation with cerebrally protective agents (e.g., propofol, etomidate, pentobarbital), and mild elevation of the head once the cervical spine is "cleared." Early placement of a ventriculostomy is indicated for monitoring and control of intracranial pressure by removal of CSF. Emergency placement of burr holes on the side of pupillary dysfunction may be successful in draining an EDH. Cerebral perfusion pressure is maintained by infusion of fluids and pressors if needed. Complications include DIC that is often fatal, so a baseline coagulation profile is obtained in the ED. Once DIC occurs, transfu-

sion of fresh frozen plasma may be helpful, although the prognosis is dismal at this stage.

Cerebral blood flow (CBF) is governed by the relationship of mean arterial pressure (MAP) and intracranial pressure (ICP) as follows: CBF=MAP–ICP. Consequently, as ICP increases, every effort must be made to maintain or elevate MAP. Once ICP exceeds MAP no blood flow to the brain can occur and this is one definition of "brain death".

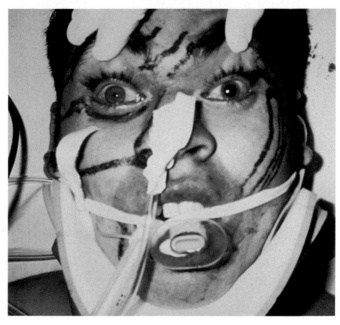

1.11B. Photograph of a patient with transtentorial herniation from blunt head trauma. The right pupil is constricted normally; the left pupil is fixed and dilated.

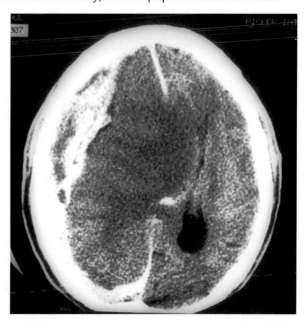

1.11C. CT scan of an acute right SDH with massive shift of cerebral contents across the midline, effacement of the right ventricles and cisterns, and compression of the left lateral ventricle.

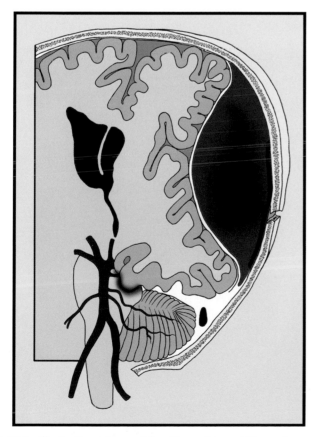

1.11A. Illustration of an epidural hematoma with acute mass effect and compression of the ipsilateral cerebral peduncle resulting in uncal herniation.

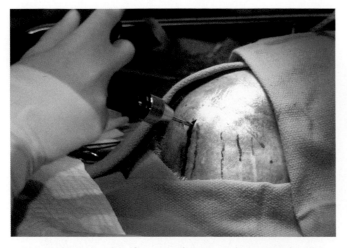

1.11D. Photographs of ventriculostomy placement for ICP monitoring and withdrawal of CSF to reduce ICP.

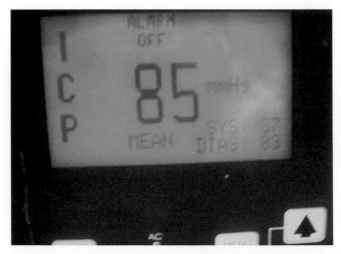

1.11E. Photograph of ICP monitor showing severe elevation of ICP.

1.12 Diffuse Cerebral Edema

Commentary

Occasionally blunt head trauma results in diffuse hyperemia or edema formation rather than mass lesions (epidural or subdural hematoma, cerebral contusion). In most cases the edema is primarily vasogenic in nature, resulting from the loss of autoregulation and subsequent exposure of cerebral arterioles to the full force of arterial pressure. Transudation of plasma fluid into the extracellular compartment results in an increase in cerebral water content and swelling of the affected part of the brain. Elevated venous pressure contributes to the process of edema formation by decreasing the resorption of brain water. Progression of edema can result in herniation with brainstem compression and death.

Diffuse cerebral edema may be associated with mass lesions or may occur in isolation. It is more common in children and infants than in adults. Cerebral contusions are prone to develop severe focal edema in the surrounding tissues. Treatment is directed at decreasing brain water content with osmotic and loop diuretics, while preserving cerebral blood flow and perfusion pressure. Removal of CSF through a ventriculostomy may be life saving.

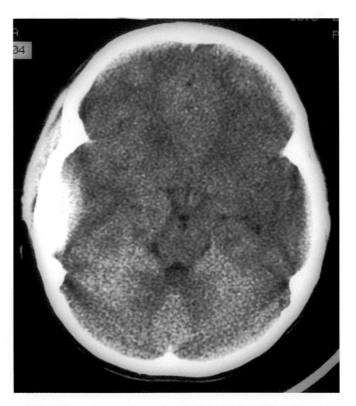

1.12A. CT scan showing diffuse edema with effacement of the lateral ventricles and sulci. The cisterns remain open. A right temporal epidural hematoma is also seen.

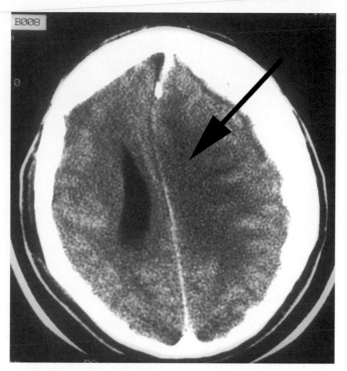

1.12B. CT scan showing severe edema of the left hemisphere (arrow) with shift across the midline from an acute left subdural hematoma. The left lateral ventricle is obliterated; the right lateral ventricle is open.

1.13 Pediatric Head Injury

Commentary

Children commonly sustain injury to the head for several reasons. First, young children in the course of exploring their environment are often oblivious to the dangers of certain situations (e.g., fall from a window or down a flight of stairs, wandering into traffic). Second, they are often less agile in escaping a dangerous situation than older children or adults. Third, the size and mass of a child's head relative to the body is much greater than in adults. Consequently, children are commonly thrust forward or fall headfirst, and the major impact is often onto the head. Finally, children are at the mercy of their caregivers and may be physically abused. Abuse in infants often takes the form of violent shaking of the baby and can result in characteristic patterns of injury known as the shaken baby syndrome or shaken impact syndrome.

Physiologically, the child's skull is more compliant than that of adults because it is less densely calcified and has unfused sutures that allow movement of one section of the skull on another. In spite of this, skull fractures are still relatively common in children. Because of the greater compliance of the skull, more kinetic energy can be transmitted directly to the brain during trauma. Cerebral contusion and subdural hematomas are common injuries. EDHs are relatively rare in very young children because of the tight adherence of the dura to the inner table of the skull.

Children are less susceptible to mass lesions than adults and more frequently develop diffuse cerebral hyperemia or diffuse edema as their principal injury pattern. Because of this propensity for diffuse hyperemia, mannitol is used with caution in young children with evidence of elevated ICP following head trauma. Mannitol causes a transient increase in cerebral perfusion and expands the vascular compartment temporarily before exerting its diuretic effect. Many authors recommend using loop diuretics and mild hyperventilation rather than mannitol when managing elevated ICP in a young child.

Another injury that occurs almost exclusively in children with head trauma is transient cortical blindness. The actual incidence of this complication is unknown but is thought to be secondary to vasospasm induced by trauma. Children also manifest cerebral concussion differently from adults. The "infant concussion syndrome" consists of the transient appearance of pallor, diaphoresis, vomiting, tachycardia, somnolence, and weakness, often occurring in an infant after relatively minor head trauma (e.g., falling off a changing table). CT scan is invariably normal, and the child often will make an equally dramatic recovery while still in the emergency department. Small infants may bleed sufficiently into the head to develop hemorrhagic shock, although this is rare. Separation of cranial sutures, a bulging fontanelle, or increasing head circumference may rarely be the initial clues to head injury in infants, but the diagnosis of serious head injury is generally made by CT scan.

The principal concern in evaluating children with head trauma is to consider the possibility of nonaccidental trauma. A history incompatible with the severity of injury or that involves activities that the child would be developmentally incapable of performing can be an initial clue that the injuries may be due to abuse.

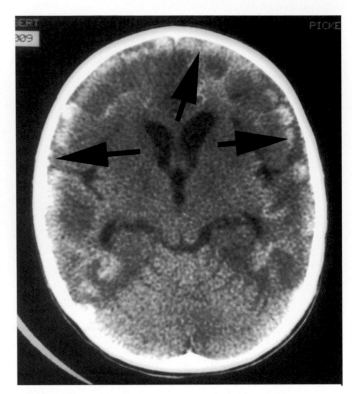

1.13B. CT scan of a child with shaken baby syndrome showing dilated ventricles and multiple cortical calcifications (arrows) suggestive of multiple previous SDHs.

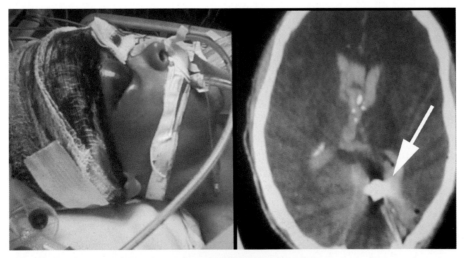

1.13A. Photograph and corresponding CT scan of a child with a GSW to the frontal area with massive hemorrhage. CT scan shows bullet fragment in left occipital area (arrow) with intraventricular and intraparenchymal hemorrhage.

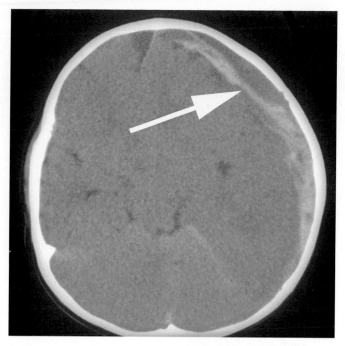

1.13C. CT scan of the head of a child with shaken baby syndrome showing a chronic SDH with acute rebleeding on the left, as well as diffuse cerebral edema and compressed ventricles.

1.14 Axonal Shear Injury

Commentary

Diffuse axonal injury results from disruption of neurons at the interface of gray matter and white matter in the brain due to sudden deceleration or acceleration injuries of the head. Gray matter has greater mass than white matter because of higher water content and, as a result of greater momentum during sudden deceleration, continues farther than white matter, producing shear forces at the gray-white interface. The resultant tearing of neurons produces profound neurologic dysfunction. Patients with extensive axonal shear injury present in profound coma that often continues as a persistent vegetative state. Initial diagnosis is difficult as many other causes of coma must also be considered, including intoxication, encephalopathy, hypoglycemia,

a postictal state, hypovolemic shock, and brainstem injury. Patients with less extensive areas of axonal shear injury may regain consciousness fairly rapidly (within 24 hours). More severe injuries may also heal over long periods of time, and occasionally a patient with this type of injury will awake after months of coma.

The CT scan in patients with diffuse axonal shear injury is often misleadingly normal or near normal. Findings include petechial hemorrhages seen mainly in the central part of the brain (corpus callosum, basal ganglia, and other medial structures). There may be additional, more evident injuries as well, such as EDH or SDH. MRI is more sensitive in delineating the extent of axonal disruption.

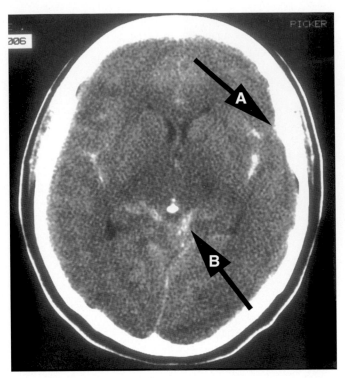

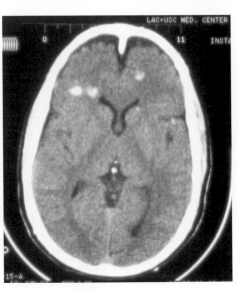

1.14B. CT scan showing focal petechial hemorrhages in the frontal lobe at the gray-white matter junction in a patient with axonal shear injury.

1.14A. CT scan showing a small left parietal SDH (arrow A), bilateral small SAH, and a cluster of petechial hemorrhages in the right pericisternal area (arrow B).

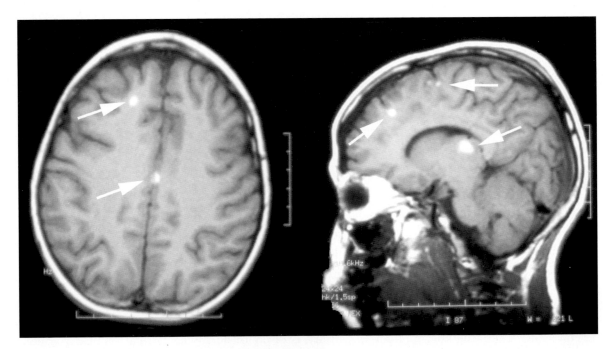

1.14C. T1 weighted MRI showing multiple high-intensity focal hemorrhages including those at the gray-white matter interface.

1.15 Intraventricular Hemorrhage

Commentary

Hemorrhage into the ventricular system is more common following hypertensive bleeds than after trauma. Occasionally blood from a traumatic lesion (e.g., SAH) will track into the ventricular system, or lacerations of the brain parenchyma may communicate directly with the ventricles. The prognosis of intraventricular hemorrhage is not as grim as in cases of spontaneous bleeding, and patients may recover well. Complications include obstructive hydrocephalus that may require placement of a ventriculoperitoneal shunt.

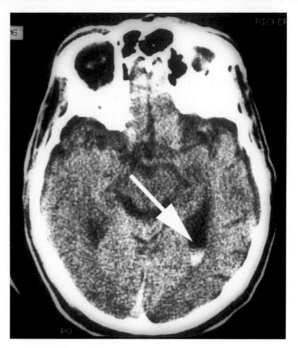

1.15A. CT scan showing a small collection of blood in the left posterior horn of the lateral ventricle (arrow).

1.16 Intraparenchymal Hemorrhage

Commentary

Direct laceration of the brain parenchyma by penetrating wounds or bone fragments may result in hemorrhage that is relatively confined to the brain parenchyma. Bleeding in these cases is usually tamponaded by surrounding tissue but may become extensive enough to produce a midline shift. Exposure of injured brain thromboplastin to the circulation results in activation of the coagulation cascade and frequently produces DIC, which is a poor prognostic sign.

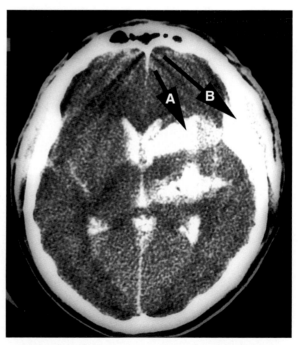

1.16A. CT scan showing accumulation of blood in all ventricles as well as intraparenchymal blood on the left (arrow A) and a left EDH (arrow B).

2 Facial Injury

Introduction

Soft tissue injuries of the face are common in modern society. The majority of serious injuries occur in the context of vehicular trauma or assaults. Use of seatbelts and airbags has decreased the frequency but not eliminated facial trauma produced by motor vehicle accidents. In addition to direct impact of the face against the windshield, steering wheel, or dashboard, broken glass fragments frequently produce lacerations and eye injuries.

The lower face and neck contain structures that define and maintain the patency of the airway. Consequently, facial injuries at times assume the highest priority in trauma management until airway patency and adequate ventilation can be established. Because facial tissues are highly vascularized, massive bleeding into the oral cavity can occlude the airway, especially when patients are obtunded from head injury or intoxication. In the presence of massive bleeding, airway compromise may be produced by placing the patient supine for spinal immobilization. Blood, secretions, fragments of teeth, and foreign bodies must be removed to avoid aspiration and airway occlusion. Although severe facial injuries are dramatic and often distract the inexperienced clinician from more critical tasks, treatment of most facial injuries can be safely deferred until life-threatening problems have been addressed.

The face and scalp also contain many structures that are essential for the function of special senses of sight, smell, taste, and hearing. Human communication is dependent not only on facial structures required for speech and hearing but also those involved in facial expression. In addition, many facial landmarks define human appearance, and their preservation as intact symmetrical structures is important cosmetically and psychologically. Injury to these structures can result in devastating disability that often can be avoided with early detection and repair.

Special attention is indicated in repairing facial injuries. Debridement of wound margins should be minimized, cartilaginous structures should be preserved,

and fine sutures with minimal inflammatory properties should be used in closing the wounds. Complex lacerations involving delicate and essential facial structures such as the eyelid should be referred to a specialist.

Clinical Examination

1. Examination of the face.

After completion of the primary survey, the face is examined for areas of swelling and tenderness that can indicate underlying fractures. Palpation of the facial bones for crepitus or abnormal motion can locate a fracture. Grasping the teeth and pulling forward can demonstrate Le Fort fractures with abnormal motion of the alveolar ridge, midface, or whole face. Lacerations are noted, and massive bleeding is tamponaded by direct pressure. Blind clamping of bleeding sites is dangerous in that it can injure nerves and other structures that run in proximity to vessels. Lacerations crossing the path of the parotid duct mandate examination of Stensen's duct in the mouth (discussed later). Facial asymmetry can be due to direct trauma but also to facial nerve injury, and an assessment of the muscles of facial expression and facial sensation is made. In comatose patients corneal reflexes should be tested to determine these functions.

2. Examination of the eye.

Anatomically, the orbit sits relatively protected by the orbital ridge, malar prominence, and nose. The ciliary and corneal reflexes rapidly close the eyelid, adding further protection to direct contact with the globe. Injuries to the eye range from minor (e.g., corneal abrasion) to critical (e.g., ruptured globe).

Examination of the eye and its adnexa is an important part of the secondary survey. Victims of motor vehicle crashes often have fragments of glass that can become embedded in the eye causing lacerations or corneal abrasions. Occasionally a patient's refractory agitation can be cured by treatment of a corneal abrasion or removal of glass fragments in the eye that were initially unsuspected. Often patients have massive soft tissue swelling around the eye that makes examination difficult. In these cases devices to hold the eyelids open must be used and can be improvised by bending paper clips into blunt retractors and gently retracting the lids. Formal measurement of visual acuity may not be possible in the early phases of resuscitation, but an initial estimate of vision can be made by having the patient count fingers or report light perception. Complete loss of vision in a previously normal eye requires immediate consultation with an ophthalmologist. The pupils are examined for symmetry and equality as well as reaction to light. The conjunctivae are assessed for foreign bodies and chemosis that can indicate rupture of the globe. A peaked pupil is highly suspicious for rupture of the globe, and the "peak" often points to the site of rupture. Visible scleral or corneal lacerations may indicate penetration of the globe by a foreign object and require radiographs or CT of the orbits to detect intraocular foreign bodies. The position of the globe in the orbit is noted for enophthalmos (blow-out fracture) or exophthalmos (retro-orbital hematoma). Inability to perform all extraocular movements may indicate a brain lesion, peripheral nerve injury, or entrapment of extraocular muscles. Lacerations involving the lacrimal duct and lid margins should be noted and referred to an ophthalmologist for repair. A brief fundoscopic examination is performed to assess the position of the lens and presence of blood in the anterior chamber (hyphema) or retina.

3. Examination of the ear.

The external ear is inspected for the presence of lacerations or hematoma. Cartilaginous lacerations or avulsions require particular attention. The ear canal is examined with an otoscope for bleeding or CSF otorrhea indicating a ruptured tympanic membrane and basilar skull fracture. The tympanic membrane is examined for perforations or accumulation of blood in the middle ear that is seen as hemotympanum. Although it may take many hours to appear, inspection of the mastoid area for Battle's sign is important in detecting basilar skull fracture.

4. Examination of the nose.

The nose is inspected for lacerations of overlying skin and of the cartilage. The presence of nasal fracture is often obvious clinically with deformity, crepitus, epistaxis, and tenderness to palpation. The nares are inspected for the presence of epistaxis or hematoma and for CSF drainage.

5. Examination of the mouth.

The mouth is inspected for lacerations, avulsion or fracture of teeth, swelling of the tongue and oral mucosa, and misalignment of teeth (indicating a mandible or maxilla fracture). Blood, loose teeth, and foreign bodies are removed manually or by suction. Simultaneously, an evaluation of the airway is made examining for stridor, dysphonia, gagging or drooling, and inability to handle oral secretions. The presence or absence of a gag reflex in obtunded patients often influences the decision to intubate the patient to protect against aspiration.

Investigations

After physical examination has indicated areas of likely injury, specific radiographs or CT scans may be indicated to delineate injuries. Plain radiographs are useful in detecting most facial fractures and in locating radiopaque foreign bodies, but CT scan can more accurately identify these if the patient is sufficiently stable to undergo this examination. Certain radiographic views are indicated to clarify specific clinical findings such as a submentovertex view to detect zygomatic arch fracture or Panorex views for suspected mandible fractures. Leakage of CSF from the nose or ear can be assessed by examining the drainage for the presence of glucose (indicating CSF) or for a double ring sign when the drainage is applied to filter paper. Suspicion of injury to the lacrimal duct is best confirmed by an ophthalmologist using fine probes. Instillation of fluorescein into the conjunctival sac and examination with a UV light source can demonstrate corneal abrasion, and Seidel's test can demonstrate leakage of aqueous humor from a ruptured globe. A detailed evaluation of the anterior chamber can be performed on stable patients using a slit-lamp examination. Patients with suspected post-traumatic glaucoma or retro-orbital hematoma should undergo tonometry to measure intraocular pressure, but this test should never be done if there is a posibility of a ruptured globe. Parotid duct laceration can be demonstrated by probing the duct or by performing a sialogram.

General Management

Airway management is of prime importance when facial injuries threaten the ability to ventilate the patient. Suction of secretions and manual removal of foreign bodies and blood clots may establish airway patency, but often endotracheal intubation is indicated. Nasotracheal intubation should not be attempted with nasal, basilar skull, or Le Fort fractures or in apneic patients. Patients with massive facial injuries present a special problem, and the management of the airway in these cases is controversial. Use of paralytic agents to facilitate intubation may cause loss of airway patency, as the patient's voluntary effort to maintain an airway is lost. Consequently, some advocate use of awake orotracheal intubation in these cases. This is an extremely difficult and often unsuccessful task in an agitated, possibly hypoxic patient with massive bleeding in the oropharynx. Others have demonstrated the safety and efficacy of using rapid-sequence intubation with paralytic drugs in this setting. Massive facial injuries that distort anatomic landmarks and produce severe bleeding may make orotracheal intubation impossible. Prolonged attempts at intubation are detrimental to the patient, and early use of cricothyrotomy is essential and often life saving. All physicians managing trauma should be familiar with this technique.

Facial injuries that do not threaten the airway can safely be deferred to the secondary survey and definitive care phases of trauma management. Active bleeding can usually be controlled by direct pressure or packing of wounds. However, prolonged bleeding from facial or scalp wounds can result in hemorrhagic shock and should not be ignored. Treatment of facial fractures can be deferred until the patient is hemodynamically stable.

Minor eye injuries (e.g., corneal abrasion, rust ring, eyelid laceration) can be deferred, but sight-threatening injuries should be dealt with immediately and consultation with an ophthalmologist is essential. Once the possibility of a ruptured globe has been established, the eye should be protected by use of a Fox shield or similar device to prevent further pressure on the globe. Retro-orbital accumulation of blood or air with deteriorating vision or massive elevation of intraocular pressure requires decompression by lateral canthotomy or creation of a communication from the retro-orbital space nto the maxillary sinus. Entrapment of extraocular muscles by fractures should be relieved urgently.

Penetrating trauma of the ear is relatively uncommon and is managed by minimal debridement, irrigation, and primary closure. Blunt trauma is more common and often results in perichondrial hematoma formation. Because ear cartilage is dependent on its skin covering for blood supply, an interposed hematoma can result in ischemic necrosis of the cartilage. Consequently, the ear must be examined for this condition, and a hematoma should be aspirated. A pressure dressing is applied to prevent reaccumulation of the hematoma or abscess formation.

Avulsed cartilage from the ear or nose should be preserved in saline, as it is difficult to re-create the shape of these organs with other tissues.

Most facial fractures can be repaired electively with operative fixation and bone grafting if necessary. Intraoral lacerations are repaired with absorbable sutures. Antibiotics are unnecessary for most facial lacerations, although open fractures require prophylactic coverage.

Common Mistakes and Pitfalls

1. Focusing on dramatic but not life-threatening facial injuries before assessing the primary survey and overall hemodynamic stability of the patient is a common error.

2. Injury to the cranial nerves is difficult to detect in severely injured patients, especially if they are comatose, intoxicated, or otherwise unable to cooperate with physical examination.

3. Leakage of CSF from the ear or nose may be difficult to detect when mixed with blood, and continued leakage after bleeding has stopped should suggest a basilar skull fracture.

4. Evidence of avulsed teeth that are not accounted for should prompt a search for possible aspiration of a tooth, which can produce a severe lung abscess.

5. Eye injury associated with use of power tools or "metal-on-metal" hammering should raise suspicion of a penetrating globe injury. Orbital CT scan is indicated to locate the foreign body. Seidel's test can indicate perforation of the globe.

6. Patients with orbital blow-out fracture should have extraocular muscles tested to detect entrapment of the inferior rectus muscle.

7. Trauma to the mouth and mandible can produce delayed airway occlusion from swelling or bleeding, and these patients must be observed carefully.

2.1 Corneal Abrasion

Commentary

In spite of brisk protective reflexes, corneal abrasion is common. The usual cause is the patient's own finger as the eye is rubbed to relieve itching or to remove a foreign body. Other causes are scraping by branches or twigs, broken glass, industrial injuries involving power grinders and saws, or welding without adequate eye protection. Clinically, the patient presents with a history of sudden onset of pain in the affected eye and the sensation of having a foreign body in the eye, with increased tearing and resultant blurred vision. Physical examination is often normal unless the eye is examined using a UV light source with magnification after fluorescein dye is instilled into the conjunctival sac. If the patient is capable of sitting, ideally the examination should be with a slit lamp. Otherwise, the examination can be made using a portable source of UV light such as a Wood's lamp. Areas of abrasion on the corneal surface show increased dye uptake and appear intensely fluorescent under UV light. The patient will experience complete relief of the pain after instillation of topical anesthetic drops onto the affected cornea. Treatment is supportive as most corneal abrasions heal within 48 hours. Antibiotic drops are prescribed, oral analgesia with nonsteroidal anti-inflammatory drugs (NSAIDs) is appropriate, and tetanus vaccination should be updated if necessary. The use of eye patches is controversial but generally considered unnecessary for small abrasions.

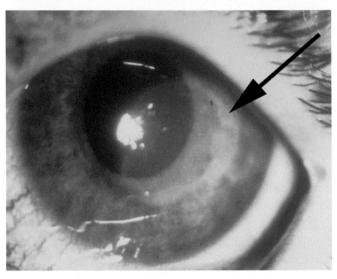

2.1A. Photograph of the eye after instillation of fluorescein dye showing bright yellow-green uptake of dye lateral to the pupil (arrow).

2.2 Ocular Foreign Bodies

Commentary

There are certain situations that merit special caution in dealing with apparent corneal abrasions. Patients who present with symptoms of corneal abrasion after high-speed grinding or hammering on metal should be suspected of having a perforated globe. Small fragments of metal can enter the eye at high speed, leaving only minimal evidence of their entry into the globe. CT scan of the orbit is indicated to locate these foreign bodies, as plain films are less sensitive. A metal foreign body that impacts the cornea at lower speed may become embedded in the cornea and produce a rust ring that can impair vision if it occurs in the visual axis. These should be removed electively after one to two days, when they are less adherent to the cornea. A retained wood foreign body is also important to detect, as fungal enophthalmitis can result.

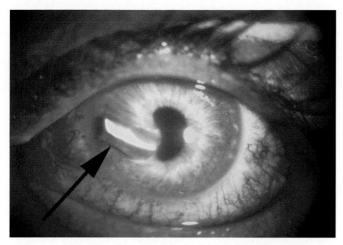

2.2A. Photograph of the eye showing a metallic foreign body on the cornea that is deforming the iris and pupil (arrow).

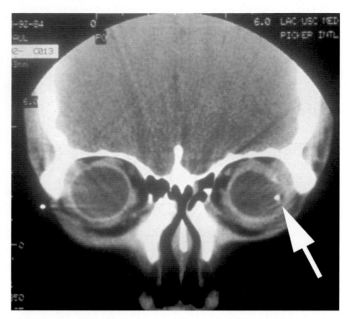

2.2C. CT scan of the orbit showing one small intraocular foreign body of the left eye (arrow) and another lateral to the right orbit.

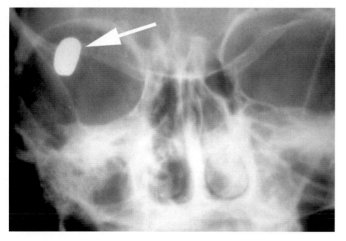

2.2B. Plain radiograph showing an intraocular bullet (arrow).

2.2D. Photograph of the eye showing a central rust ring in the cornea (arrow). This rust ring is in the visual axis and will seriously impair vision if not removed.

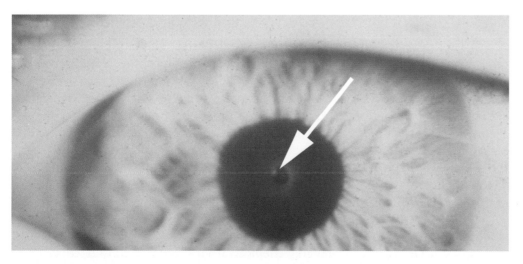

2.3 Hyphema

Commentary

Hyphema is the accumulation of blood in the anterior chamber of the eye. With the patient laying supine, the blood is less visible than in an upright position, when it forms a clearly visible layer of blood in the dependent portion of the anterior chamber. The initial bleeding usually resorbs without complication, but in up to a third of cases rebleeding will occur two to five days after the initial injury. Complications from hyphema include hemosiderin staining of the inner surface of the cornea with resulting loss of vision, as well as post-traumatic glaucoma due to fibrotic occlusion of the canals of Schlemm. Treatment is conservative and consists of bed rest with the head elevated, sedation, and monitoring of intraocular pressure. Surgery is required occasionally for evacuation of blood or to decompress the anterior chamber.

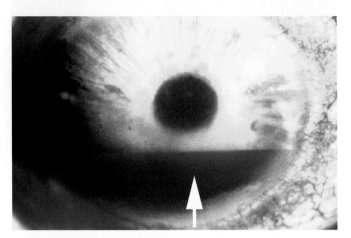

2.3A. Photograph of the eye showing a collection of blood pooled (hyphema) in the inferior aspect of the anterior chamber (arrow).

2.4 Ruptured Globe

Commentary

Rupture of the globe usually occurs after penetrating injury but can be caused by blunt trauma as well. Penetration of the sclera results in herniation of orbital contents through the wound and exposure of the choroid membrane, visible as a dark layer of tissue in the wound. Penetration of the cornea allows leakage of vitreous humor through the wound. In either case, distortion of the globe results in loss of functional vision at the time of injury, although light perception may be preserved. Patients report pain and often resist eye examination.

Signs of globe penetration include enophthalmos, loss of eyeball turgor, a peaked pupil that points toward the site of injury, loss of pupillary reactivity, and a positive Seidel's test. The latter is performed by instilling fluorescein dye into the conjunctiva and observing the dye clearing from the cornea or sclera in the area of rupture because of the flow of aqueous humor from the anterior chamber. Although intraocular pressure is reduced in the presence of a ruptured globe, tonometry and any other maneuver that increases pressure on the globe are contraindicated. The conjunctiva is very distensible and often becomes edematous after trauma, resulting in bulging chemosis that frequently limits complete examination. Because of its common association with rupture of the globe, bulging chemosis itself should be considered a sign of possible ruptured globe.

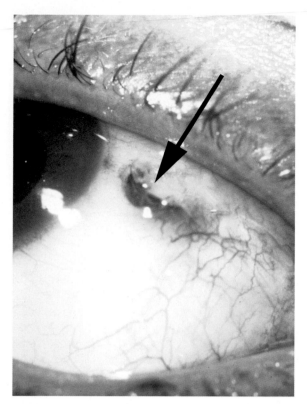

2.4A. Photograph of the eye showing a scleral laceration with exposure of the choroid (arrow). This is highly suggestive of rupture of the globe.

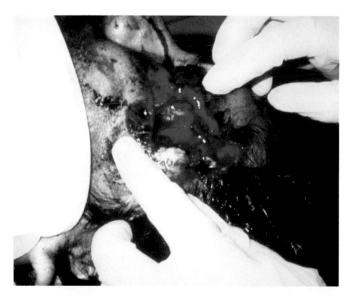

2.4B. Photograph of a patient with enucleation and destruction of the eye.

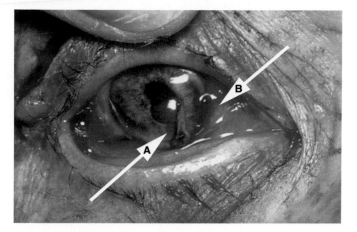

2.4C. Photograph of an irregular, peaked pupil (arrow A), bulging chemosis (arrow B), and laceration of the iris due to a ruptured globe.

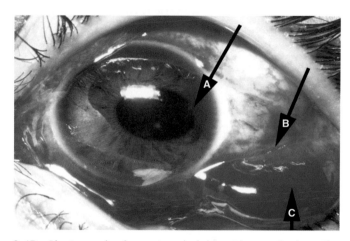

2.4D. Photograph of a ruptured globe with a peaked pupil (arrow A), laceration of the inferior/lateral sclera (arrow B), and bulging chemosis (arrow C). The peak in the pupil points toward the laceration.

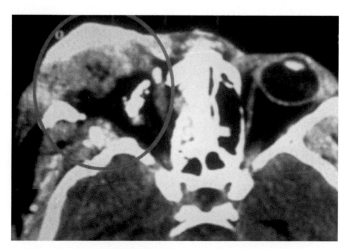

2.4E. CT scan showing destruction of the right eye with intraocular bone fragments and periorbital fractures.

2.5 Retrobulbar Hematoma

Commentary

Trauma to the globe can result in bleeding from retro-orbital vessels including the ophthalmic artery and vein. In addition, fractures of the orbit that communicate with paranasal sinuses can result in the accumulation of air in the retro-orbital space. If air or blood accumulates under sufficient pressure, ischemic necrosis of the optic nerve can occur. Clinical evidence of this condition includes proptosis, impaired extraocular movements, and progressive loss of vision. Tonometry will demonstrate elevated intraocular pressure.

Treatment of a symptomatic retrobulbar hematoma is by lateral canthotomy or by surgically perforating the floor of the orbit to allow decompression of the retrobulbar space. In a lateral canthotomy, the lateral canthal ligaments are grasped with a forceps and crushed. Iris scissors are then used to divide the ligament, allowing the globe to protrude forward. If done in a timely manner, normal vision can be restored once the globe is repositioned and the canthal ligament is repaired. Alternatively, a forceps can be introduced beneath the globe and the floor of the orbit fractured to allow drainage of the retro-orbital space.

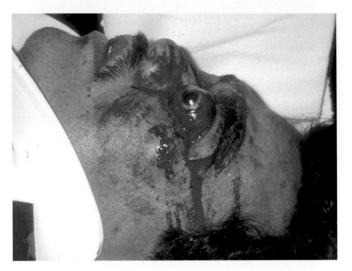

2.5B. Photograph showing increased proptosis of the eye after lateral canthotomy. Allowing the eye to protrude further decreases the retrobulbar pressure on the optic nerve.

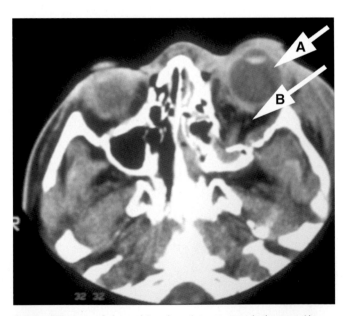

2.5C. CT scan of the orbits showing proptosis (arrow A), retro-orbital blood and air (arrow B), and a fracture of the posterior orbital wall.

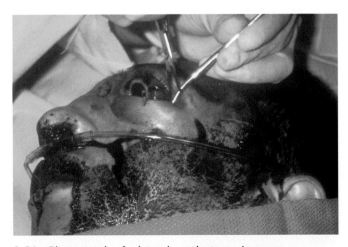

2.5A. Photograph of a lateral canthotomy in progress.

2.6 Periorbital Lacerations

Commentary

In addition to the globe itself, there are numerous structures in the adnexa of the eye that merit special consideration. The lacrimal system ensures that a constant flow of tears streams across the surface of the eye, maintaining lubrication to facilitate ocular motion, preventing desiccation, and clearing debris, including potential infectious agents. Lacerations involving the lacrimal apparatus, lid margins, and lacrimal duct must all be sought out and referred to an ophthalmologist for repair. Lacerations of the lid margins must be reapproximated exactly under microscopic vision to avoid a step-off that can result in constant dripping of tears onto the face. Injury to the lacrimal duct at the medial canthus of the eye is important to detect and repair, as scarring and stenosis of the duct can result in a similar problem. Delayed repair of a stenotic lacrimal duct is very difficult and yields suboptimal results in most cases.

Laceration of the eyebrow is common and can be repaired in the ED. Exact alignment is essential to preserve facial expression. Consequently, the eyebrows should never be shaved in preparation for suturing as the alignment landmarks will be lost. Repair of

each layer of tissue is done independently in a layered closure to preserve the mobility of the brow.

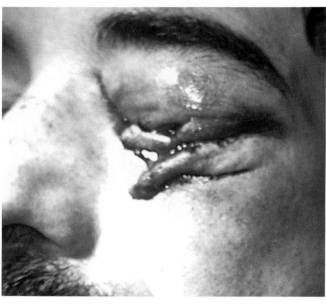

2.6A. Photograph of a complex laceration of the eyelid that involves the lid margins.

2.7 Orbital Blowout Fracture

Commentary

Blunt impact to the orbital area is common. The globe itself is usually spared when large objects strike the face because of the protection afforded by the malar prominence, nose, and superior orbital ridge. However, smaller objects can strike the globe directly, resulting in a massive rise in intraocular pressure. This pressure is transmitted to the bony orbit, often resulting in fracture at its weakest points, the orbital floor and the medial wall of the orbit (lamina papyracea). Fracture of the orbital floor by this means is called a blow-out

fracture. This injury typically occurs in certain sports activities such as racquetball, lacrosse, boxing, and baseball but may also be seen in blunt eye trauma of any type. The patient presents with enophthalmos and pain in the orbital area. A common complication of this injury is that the inferior rectus muscle becomes entrapped in the fracture fragments, resulting in restricted upward gaze and diplopia when the patient attempts to look upward. Consequently, it is essential that physical examination should verify that extraocular movements are intact. Finding an entrapped inferior rectus muscle mandates surgical repair.

Plain radiographs of the face seldom reveal the actual orbital floor fracture. The characteristic finding is opacification of the maxillary sinus caused by herniation of periorbital fat and blood into the sinus. CT scan reveals the herniation as well, and special reconstructions of the orbit may reveal the fracture in detail.

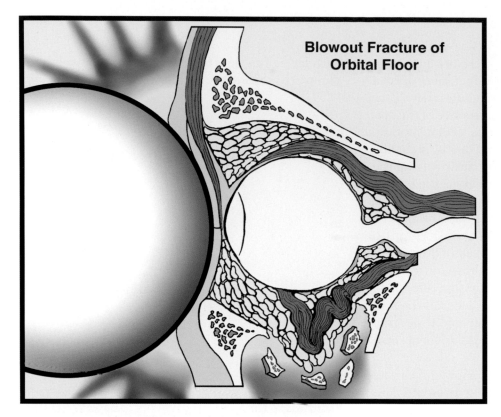

Blowout Fracture of Orbital Floor

2.7A. Illustration showing typical mechanism of injury that produces an orbital blowout fracture.

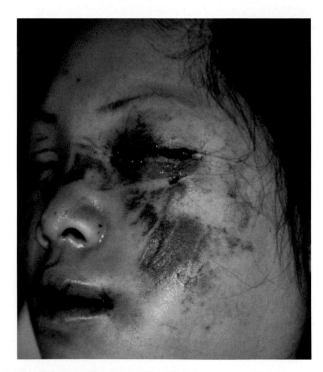

2.7B. Photograph of patient with blunt trauma to the orbital area from an airbag deployment, who proved to have an orbital blow-out fracture.

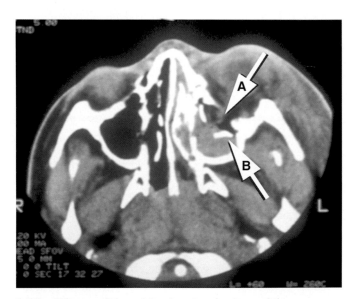

2.7C. CT scan of the orbits showing fracture of the posterior/inferior orbital wall (arrow A) with herniation of orbital contents into the maxillary sinus on the left (arrow B).

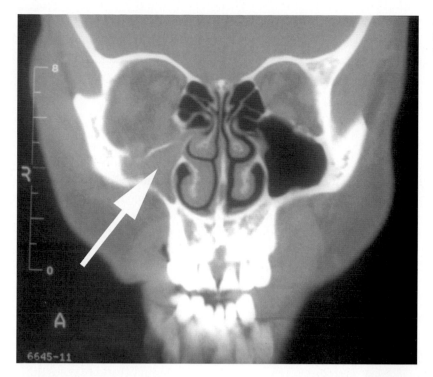

2.7D. CT scan showing fracture of the inferior orbital wall with opacification of the right maxillary sinus (arrow).

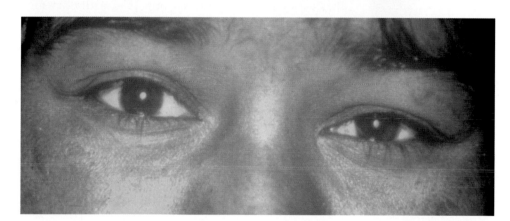

2.7E. Photograph of a patient with blow-out fracture showing enophthalmos of the left eye.

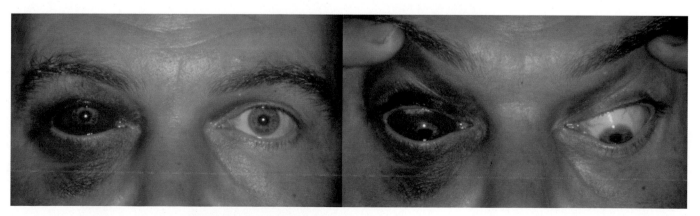

2.7F. Photographs of a patient with a blow-out fracture of the right eye and subconjunctival hemorrhage. There is no evidence of divergent gaze with the eyes in neutral position. Downward gaze reveals entrapment of the extraocular muscles of the right eye, resulting in a subtle divergent gaze.

2.8 Mandible Fracture

Commentary

Fractures of the mandible are common after blunt facial trauma. The most common etiologies are vehicular-related trauma and assaults. Fractures are distributed almost equally between the condyles, angle, and body of the mandible. Clinically, patients present with

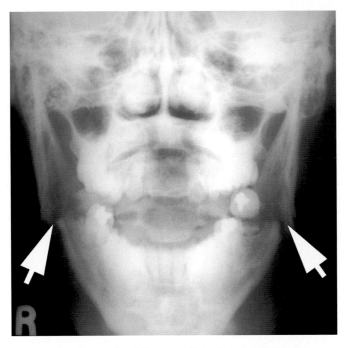

2.8A. AP radiograph of the mandible showing bilateral displaced fractures of the angles of the mandible (arrows).

swelling and tenderness over the fracture site. Dysarthria and drooling are common because any movement of the jaw is painful. Maximal incisor opening (normally 5 cm) is reduced, and the patient will note malocclusion of the teeth if the fracture fragments are displaced. At times bony crepitus can be elicited by examination or with voluntary movement of the mandible. Inspection of the mouth often reveals that the fracture is open, with gingival laceration overlying the fracture site. Airway obstruction can occur in unconscious patients with bilateral mandibular rami fractures, as the tongue is unsupported and falls back into the posterior pharynx. Trauma to the temporomandibular joint is common and may result in dislocation of the joint or chronic pain with chewing.

Plain films are usually adequate to reveal a mandibular fracture, particularly if it is displaced. However a Panorex view of the jaw is more accurate and should be used if available. Treatment is operative, with wiring or plating of the fracture fragments into anatomic position. Open fractures of the mandible should be treated with antibiotics that are active against mouth flora (e.g., penicillin or clindamycin) because osteomyelitis and abscess formation can occur.

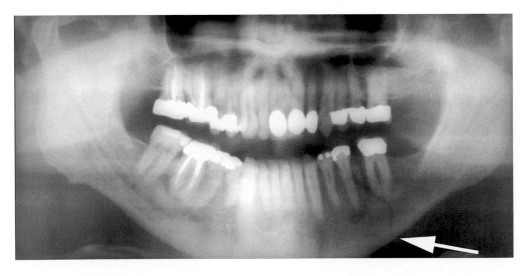

2.8B. Panorex view of the mandible showing an undisplaced fracture of the left mandibular ramus (arrow).

2.9 Zygoma Fractures

Commentary

The zygoma provides the bony support to the cheek and thus is commonly implicated in blunt trauma to the face. Because of its arched structure, comminuted fractures are typically seen. Associated injury to the infraorbital nerve should be sought out. The patient typically presents with loss of the malar prominence on the affected side. In the acute phase, however, swelling may mask this finding, so careful palpation of the facial bones to detect pain, a bony step-off, and crepitus of the zygoma should be routine. Injury to the infraorbital nerve may occur and results in anesthesia of the upper lip. Impingement of the zygoma onto the coronoid process of the mandible may result in limited excursion of the mandible. Diagnosis is made by plain radiographs. The submentovertex view (or "bucket handle" view) clearly demonstrates fractures of the zygoma and should be ordered if this fracture is suspected clinically. Treatment of displaced zygoma fractures is surgical elevation of the fragments to restore a normal facial contour.

A more complex zygoma fracture is the tripod fracture that involves fractures at the origins of the zygoma, resulting in a large triangular fragment. The fractures occur at the zygomaticofacial and zygomaticofrontal sutures and through the inferior orbital foramen. The result is a free-floating fragment of bone that often requires surgical repair.

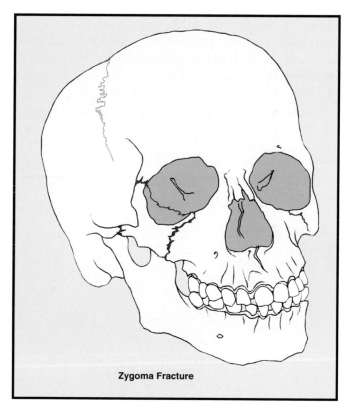

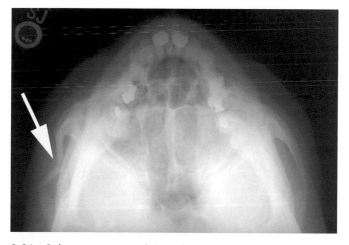

2.9A. Submentovertex plain radiograph showing a depressed right zygomatic arch fracture (arrow).

2.9B. Illustration outlining a tripod fracture of the zygoma (see 2.10E as well).

2.10 Le Fort Fractures

Commentary

Le Fort fractures result from high-energy facial trauma and are classified according to their location. Le Fort II and III fractures are potentially life-threatening injuries in that they are commonly associated with airway compromise, massive bleeding, basilar skull fracture, and intracranial injury. Nasal intubation and nasogastric tubes must be avoided in these patients, as fatal intracranial insertion may result. Patients often have combinations of injuries, such as a Le Fort II on one side with a Le Fort I on the other.

Le Fort I This fracture separates the upper alveolar ridge from the face and extends into the nasal fossa. Clinically, the patient will have mobility of the upper teeth when they are grasped and pulled forward. Airway compromise is rarely associated with this fracture.

Le Fort II The Le Fort II fracture separates the midface from the skull, resulting in a pyramid-shaped large fragment of the central maxilla and nasal bones.

Pulling on the upper teeth demonstrates mobility of the entire midface. Radiographs reveal fracture lines through both maxillae extending upward to include the nasal bones. Associated basilar skull fracture is common, and CSF rhinorrhea can occur. Massive epistaxis may require nasal packing or surgery to control the bleeding.

Le Fort III The most severe form of Le Fort fracture results in complete craniofacial dissociation due to fractures of both maxillae, zygomas, nasal bones, ethmoids, and vomer, as well as bones at the base of the skull. Examination reveals mobility of the entire face, as it can be pulled forward from the skull. Complications such as intracranial injury, airway compromise, basilar skull fracture, CSF rhinorrhea, and massive epistaxis are common. Nasal intubation and nasogastric tubes should be avoided.

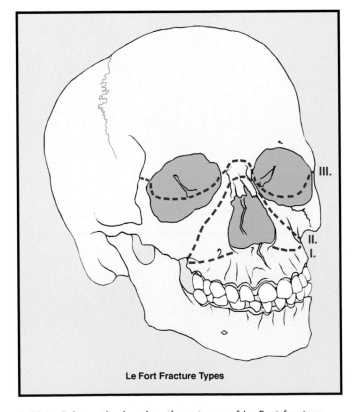

Le Fort Fracture Types

2.10A. Schematic showing three types of Le Fort fracture.

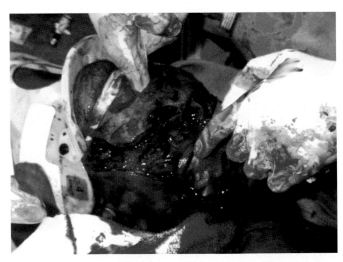

2.10B. Photograph of a car accident patient with Le Fort III fracture demonstrating the method of examining for craniofacial dissociation.

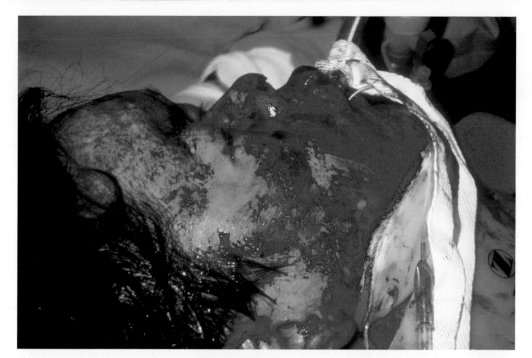

2.10C. Photograph of a patient who had a garage door crush his face. The abnormal concavity of the face ("dish face") is characteristic of a Le Fort III fracture.

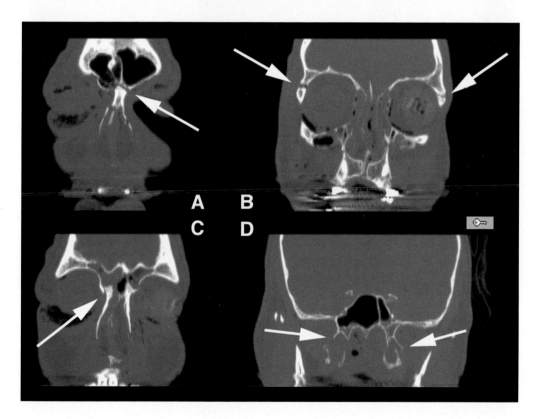

| A | B |
| C | D |

2.10D. CT scan of the face showing Le Fort III fracture: (a) anterior ethmoid fracture (arrow); (b) midethmoid and lateral orbit fractures (arrows); (c) frontal sinus fracture (arrow); (d) Pterygoid fractures (arrow).

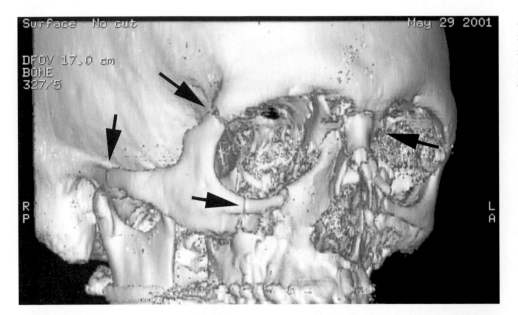

2.10E. 3-D reconstruction CT scan of a Le Fort III fracture showing multiple fractures, including a tripod fracture of the zygoma (arrows).

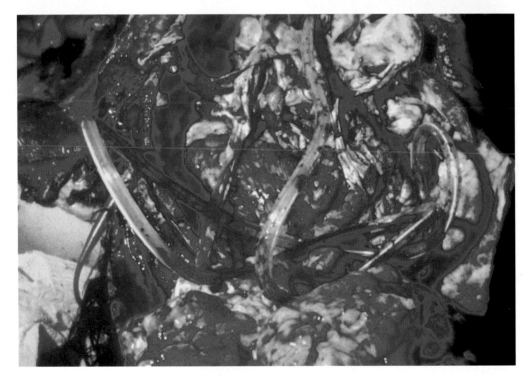

2.10F. Photograph at autopsy of nasogastric tube coiled intracranially.

2.11 Nasal Injuries

Commentary

Superficial lacerations of the nose are common and easily repaired, but several serious injuries merit discussion. Laceration extending through nasal cartilage must be repaired in separate layers using absorbable sutures for the cartilage repair. Avulsed cartilage should be preserved in saline if repair can be done urgently or in a subcutaneous pocket if repair is delayed. Reconstruction of the nose can be done in delayed fashion, but finding appropriate cartilage for reconstruction is difficult.

Nasal fractures may be treated conservatively if undisplaced. Deviation of the septum or impairment of nasal breathing is an indication for repair within the first week after injury. Open fractures should be treated with antibiotics. The nasal septum should be inspected for the presence of a septal hematoma, which appears as a swollen, ecchymotic area separating the nasal mucosa from underlying cartilage. The septal hematoma must be drained and the nose packed to avoid reaccumulation of the hematoma. Because the blood supply to the cartilage depends on the nasal mucosa, increasing the distance for diffusion causes ischemic necrosis of the cartilage, and eventually a saddle-nose deformity results.

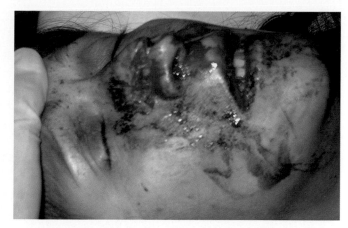

2.11A. Photograph of a laceration through the nasal cartilage.

2.12 Complex Facial Lacerations

Commentary

Massive facial injury can result from blunt force trauma or penetrating injury from gunshot or shotgun wounds. The primary initial challenge in these cases is to secure an airway. Massive facial injury can result in airway obstruction either by loss of the supporting bony framework of the face or by accumulation of blood, debris such as fractured teeth, edema, or tissue flaps that occlude the larynx. Immediate restoration of a patent airway is the highest priority in trauma management. Initially, simple airway maneuvers such as chin lift, suctioning blood and secretions, and placement of an oral airway should be attempted. If these are unsuccessful in restoring air flow, a definitive airway must be obtained rapidly. Orotracheal intubation is difficult because of massive bleeding and edema, distorted anatomic landmarks, and debris, including avulsed teeth, fragments of bone, and bullet fragments. Use of paralytic agents for orotracheal intubation may cause loss of voluntary muscle maintenance of a patent airway, but on the other hand will facilitate intubation in a struggling, hypoxic patient. Attempted awake orotracheal intubation, although often recommended in these cases, is similarly

extremely difficult and usually unsuccessful. Consequently, use of a cricothyrotomy is often the only viable choice to establish a patent airway and should be employed early in the management.

Once the airway is secured, the spine is immobilized and the remainder of the primary survey and resuscitative interventions are completed. Massive facial injuries are dramatic and often distract clinicians from a systematic primary survey. Unless there is massive bleeding present, repair of the vast majority of facial injuries can be deferred until the patient is stable. Repair of facial lacerations can produce surprisingly good results, providing that tissue has not been avulsed and the arterial supply is intact. Debridement of tissue should be kept to a minimum, and tissues should be closed in layers, with individual muscle layers, subcutaneous tissues, and skin closed separately. Fine sutures with minimal inflammatory properties are used to close the skin. Revision of wounds should attempt to orient wounds parallel to the natural wrinkle lines of the face, as these scars will be less noticeable. Scars that are perpendicular to the natural wrinkle lines are much more apparent.

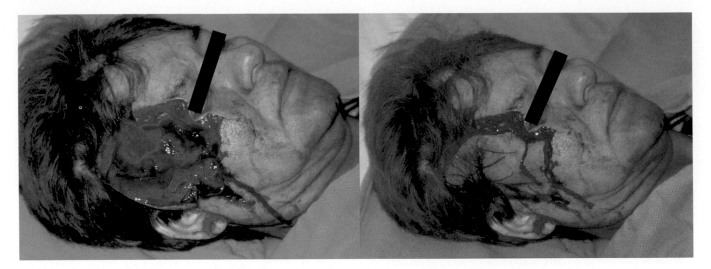

2.12A. Photograph of a large laceration of the temporal and malar area and the same laceration after placement of subcutaneous sutures as part of a multilayered closure. The ultimate cosmetic result was very acceptable.

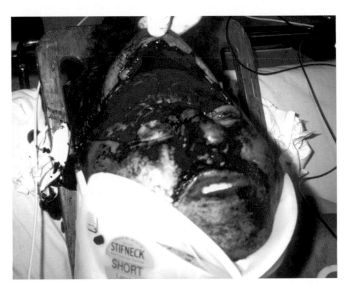

2.12B. Photograph of a patient with avulsion of the scalp.

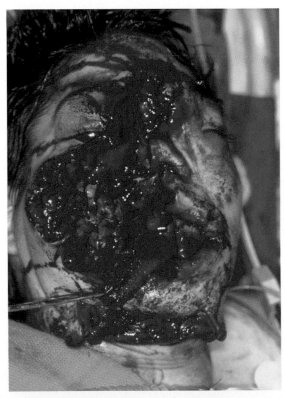

2.12C. Photograph of a patient with a shotgun wound of the face. Airway management is extremely difficult in these cases, as anatomic landmarks are severely distorted.

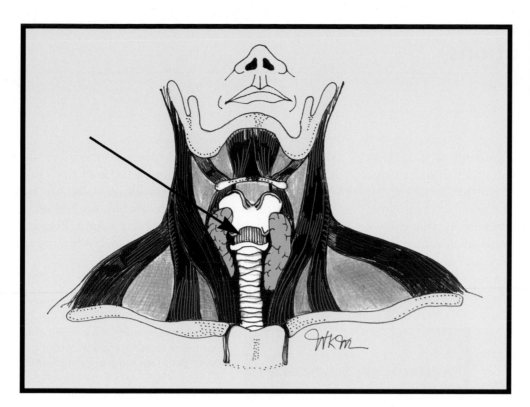

2.12D. Schematic showing the cricothyroid membrane (arrow) and its relationship to the thyroid cartilage (above) and the cricoid cartilage.

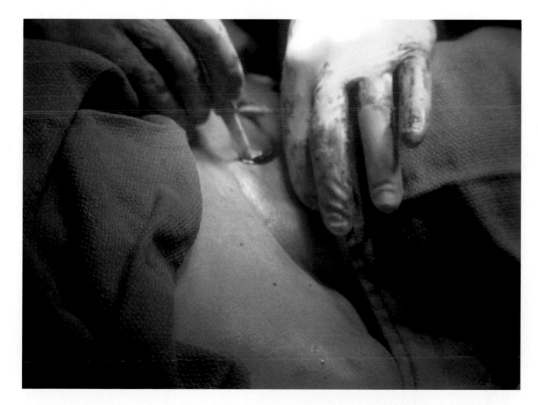

2.12E. Photograph of a cricothyrotomy in progress.

2.13 Oral Lacerations

Commentary

Lacerations of the lips occur commonly as the lip is crushed between a striking object and the underlying teeth. Because the blood supply to the lips is excellent, uncomplicated healing is the rule. However, care must be taken to properly align lacerations that transverse the vermilion border because even minor misalignment in this area is noticeable and disfiguring.

Intraoral lacerations should be repaired using soft, absorbable sutures. With through-and-through lacerations involving the skin and mucosal surfaces of the mouth, the mucosal laceration is repaired first, followed by skin closure. Lacerations of the tongue should be repaired using absorbable sutures after removal of clots and irrigation of the wound. Because of its rich vascularity, the tongue is capable of massive swelling, and delayed airway compromise is possible.

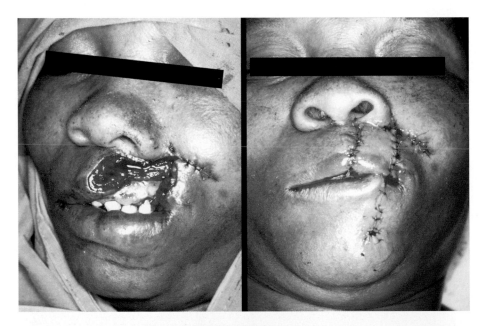

2.13A. Photographs of a patient with a complex facial laceration involving loss of tissue from the upper lip with avulsion of almost half the upper lip. After careful alignment of the vermilion border and restoration of the "cupid's bow," an acceptable cosmetic result is obtained.

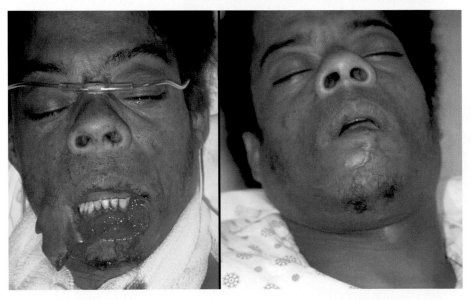

2.13B. Photograph before and after repair of a complex laceration of the lower lip caused by a human bite. An acceptable cosmetic result is obtained.

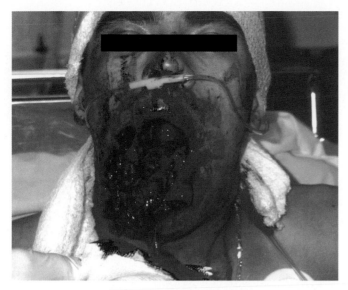

2.13C. Photograph of a patient with a close-range gunshot wound of the mouth and massive destruction of perioral tissue.

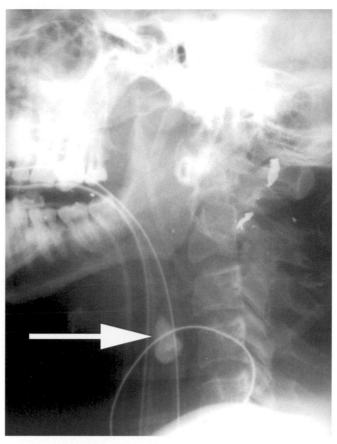

2.13E. Lateral radiograph of the soft tissues of the neck showing an aspirated tooth anterior to C4.

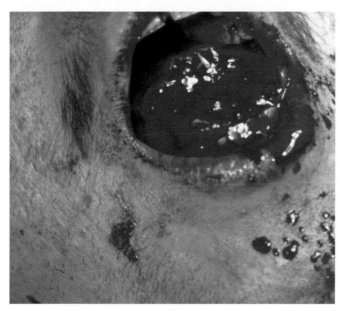

2.13D. Autoamputation of the distal tongue caused by a human bite from the patient's girlfriend.

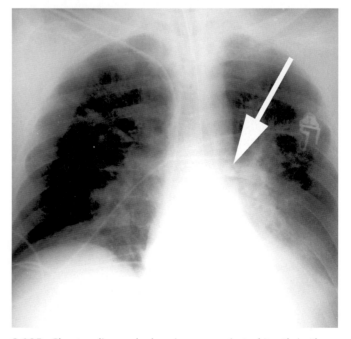

2.13F. Chest radiograph showing an aspirated tooth in the left main bronchus.

2.14 Facial Nerve Injury

Commentary

Facial nerve injury is most commonly idiopathic in etiology (Bell's palsy). However, penetrating facial trauma can occasionally result in transection of the facial nerve as it courses through the face. The facial nerve exits the base of the skull, enters the face just anterior to the tragus of the ear, and continues as a large trunk for approximately one centimeter before it subdivides extensively into smaller branches. Lacerations in the vicinity of the tragus should prompt care-ful examination of the muscles of facial expression because facial nerve injury is frequently missed during the initial examination of patients with multiple trauma. Injury of the smaller branches of the facial nerve may also merit exploration and surgical repair, depending on the severity of the deficit. Care should be taken to moisten the conjunctiva with artificial tears to avoid desiccation and ulceration of the cornea due to incomplete closure of the eyelid.

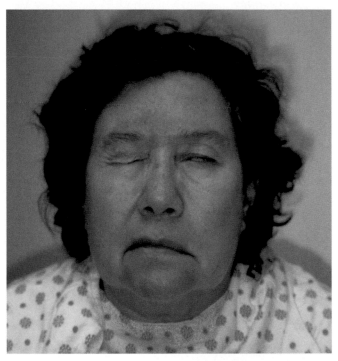

2.14A. Photograph of a patient with facial nerve injury on the left side showing loss of the left nasolabial fold, incomplete eyelid closure, and facial droop.

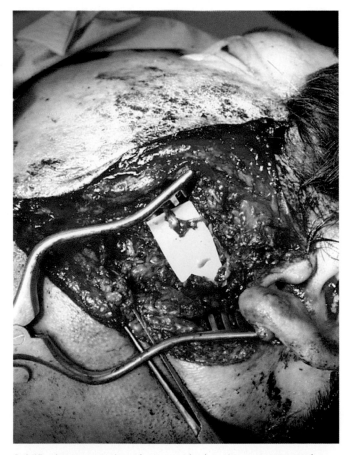

2.14B. Intraoperative photograph showing a transected facial nerve.

2.15 Facial Artery Injury

Commentary

The facial artery branches from the external carotid artery and courses deep to the angle of the mandible until it crosses under the middle of the mandibular ramus to run subcutaneously into the face. The transverse facial artery courses with the facial nerve before branching extensively in the face, and the maxillary artery branches from the external carotid deep to the coronoid process of the mandible.

Injury to any of the major arterial trunks supplying the face can result in massive bleeding and exsanguination. Accumulation of large hematomas may threaten the airway. Because they are located deep to bony structures of the face, they are often inaccessible for direct external compression and may require emergent surgical intervention to obtain vascular control. Lacerations of smaller arterial branches often heal without noticeable consequence because of the excellent collateral blood supply in the face. However, all of the recognized vascular complications including pseudoaneurysm, arteriovenous fistula, and delayed thrombosis can occur, and these often present weeks to months after the original injury.

Lacerations over the malar area can involve several other important structures. The parotid gland lies anterior to the tragus of the ear and extends to the midpupillary line external to the maxilla. Lacerations of the parotid gland may result in creation of a salivary fistula but generally heal uneventfully. Laceration of the parotid duct, however, commonly results in complications. The parotid duct courses through the parotid gland along a line drawn from the tragus to the upper lip and enters the mouth as Stensen's duct at the level of the second upper molar. Lacerations that cross this line proximal to the entry of the parotid duct into the mouth should be suspected of transecting the duct. Examination of the duct is performed by milking the parotid gland while examining Stensen's duct intraorally. Expression of saliva suggests that the duct is intact. Expression of blood or failure to express saliva suggests transection of the duct. If injury is suspected, Stensen's duct is probed retrograde, and the wound is examined for the probe. Alternately, a sialogram can be performed to determine the integrity of the duct. Careful surgical repair of the duct will prevent formation of a salivary-cutaneous fistula.

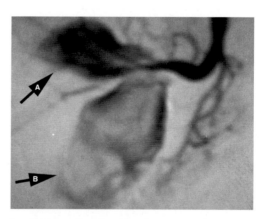

2.15A. Angiogram showing two large pseudoaneurysms of the facial artery (arrows A and B).

3 Neck Injury

Introduction

Neck injuries, especially penetrating ones, are considered difficult to evaluate and manage because of the dense concentration of so many vital structures in a small anatomical area and the difficult surgical access to many of these structures. However, very few patients with blunt trauma and only 15–20% of cases with penetrating trauma require operative treatment. The combination of a meticulous clinical examination and appropriate investigations can safely identify those patients requiring operative treatment. Advanced trauma life support (ATLS) principles should always be followed.

During the primary survey, the following life-threatening conditions in the neck should be identified and treated:

1. Airway obstruction due to laryngotracheal trauma or compression by external hematoma
2. Tension pneumothorax
3. Severe active bleeding, externally or in the thoracic cavity
4. Spinal cord injury or ischemic brain damage due to carotid artery occlusion

During the secondary survey, the following neck pathologies should be identified and managed:

1. Occult vascular injuries
2. Occult laryngotracheal injuries
3. Occult pharyngoesophageal injuries
4. Cranial or peripheral nerve injuries
5. Small hemopneumothoraces

Clinical Examination

Clinical examination according to a carefully written protocol is the cornerstone of the diagnosis and management. The examination should be systematic and evaluate the vessels, the aerodigestive tract, the spinal cord, the nerves, and the lungs:

1. Vascular structures: "Hard" signs and symptoms highly diagnostic of vascular trauma include active bleeding, shock not explained by other injuries, expanding or pulsatile hematoma, absent or significantly diminished peripheral pulses, and a bruit. "Soft" signs and symptoms suggestive but not diagnostic of vascular trauma include mild shock, moderate hematoma, and slow bleeding. This group of patients requires further investigation.

2. Aerodigestive tract: Hard signs or symptoms highly diagnostic of significant laryngotracheal trauma include respiratory distress, air bubbling through a neck wound, and massive hemoptysis. There are no hard signs diagnostic of esophageal trauma. Soft signs and symptoms suspicious of aerodigestive trauma include subcutaneous emphysema, hoarseness, odynophagia, and minor hemoptysis.

3. Nervous system: The examination should include Glasgow Coma Score, localizing signs, pupils, cranial nerves (VII, IX–XII), spinal cord, brachial plexus (median, ulnar, radial, axillary, musculocutaneous nerves), the phrenic nerve, and the sympathetic chain (Horner's syndrome).

Investigations in Neck Trauma

History and clinical examination will determine the need and type of investigations in the evaluation of neck trauma. Patients with hard signs of major vascular or laryngotracheal injuries should be operated on without any delay for ancillary investigations. These investigations should be considered only in stable patients.

1. Plain chest and neck films: Look for foreign bodies, fractures, pneumothorax, subcutaneous emphysema, and hematoma.

2. Angiography: Angiography should be reserved for selected cases with soft signs of vascular trauma when the color flow Doppler study is not

definitive or for cases where angiographic therapeutic intervention (embolization of a bleeding vessel or stenting) may be an option.

3. Color flow Doppler (CFD): CFD has largely replaced angiography. It is noninvasive, accurate, and cost-effective. The combination of a good physical examination and CFD can detect or highly suspect all vascular injuries, including minor ones. It has some limitations in the visualization of the proximal left subclavian artery in obese patients, the internal carotid artery near the base of the skull, and parts of the vertebral artery under the bony part of the vertebral canal.

4. Esophagogram: This should be considered in all patients with subcutaneous emphysema, odynophagia, or hematemesis. Very often it is supplemented by esophagoscopy.

5. Endoscopy: Esophagoscopy and laryngoscopy/tracheoscopy are indicated in patients with soft signs of aerodigestive trauma (subcutaneous emphysema, hemoptysis, hematemesis, hoarseness) or in patients who are clinically not evaluable (i.e., unconscious patients) and have penetrating injuries in proximity to the esophagus.

6. CT scan of the neck: CT is valuable in the evaluation of patients with gunshot wounds to the spine or suspected blunt trauma to the larynx.

General Management

In an urban environment, the "scoop and run" principle should be applied in penetrating neck injuries. Any external bleeding should be controlled by direct pressure. Protective C-spine collars should be applied loosely and with caution because of the risk of airway obstruction in patients with large neck hematomas. Neck collars are not necessary in knife injuries, and though gunshot wounds to the spine can cause fractures, they rarely are unstable.

Airway compromise may occur because of an external compressing hematoma, a laryngotracheal hematoma, or a major transection of the larynx or trachea. Orotracheal intubation can be a difficult and potentially dangerous task in the prehospital environment and should not be undertaken lightly.

The initial assessment in the emergency department should always follow ATLS guidelines. Approximately 10% of penetrating neck injuries present with airway compromise. Endotracheal intubation should be attempted only in the presence of a physician who can perform a cricothyroidotomy in case of intubation failure. In fairly stable patients with airway compromise, fiberoptic nasotracheal intubation should be attempted first. For attempted orotracheal intubation, muscle relaxants should be used only in selected cases and by experienced intubators, because of the risk of airway loss. On the other hand, intubation without pharmacological paralysis may aggravate bleeding and airway obstruction due to patient coughing and straining, and thus the optimal method of airway establishment should be individualized.

Any external bleeding is controlled by direct pressure or by balloon tamponade using a Foley catheter. In order to avoid air embolism, all patients with suspected venous injuries should be put in the Trendelenburg position. Intravenous lines should be avoided on the same side as the injury because of the possibility of a proximal venous injury.

Patients arriving in the emergency department with imminent or established cardiac arrest should have an emergency department thoracotomy performed. As part of the resuscitation efforts, the right ventricle of the heart should be aspirated for air embolism.

Following a careful initial physical examination and appropriate investigations, a decision should be made about operation or observation. Overall, only about 20% of penetrating neck injuries require surgical intervention. The selection of the type of management can safely be made on the basis of a good clinical examination and appropriate investigations.

Common Mistakes and Pitfalls

1. Pharmacological paralysis for emergency endotracheal intubation in the presence of a large neck hematoma without being ready or not having the skills for a cricothyroidotomy. The loss of airway may be lethal.

2. Attempts to insert a nasogastric tube in an awake patient in the presence of a large neck hematoma or suspected vascular injury. Straining and coughing may precipitate bleeding. If a nasogastric tube is needed, wait until the patient is anesthetized.

3. Insertion of an intravenous line in the arm on the same side as the neck injury. Any infused fluids may be extravasated from an injury to the axillary or subclavian vein. Always use the opposite side.

4. Failure to perform a clinical examination according to a written protocol (see Table 3.1). The inexperienced physician can easily miss important signs and symptoms.

3.1 Anatomical Zones of the Neck

Commentary

The description of penetrating neck injuries according to zones is useful in the evaluation and management of the patient. The incidence of significant injuries with zone I wounds is about 15%, in zone II 25%, and in zone III 25%. About 12% of patients with zone I injuries, 14% with zone II, and 5% with zone III injuries require surgical intervention. Also, vascular evaluation in zones I and III is more difficult than in zone II. The vessels in these areas are not easily accessible to color flow Doppler studies, and angiographic evaluation may be more appropriate.

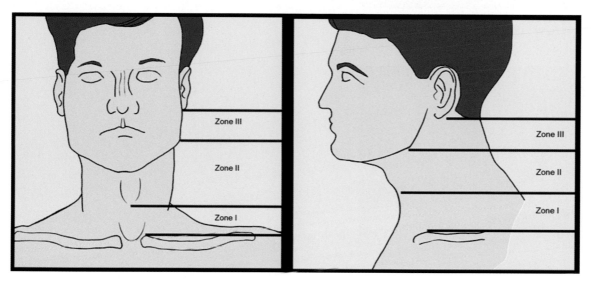

3.1A. Zone I is confined between the clavicle and the cricoid cartilage, zone II between the cricoid and the angle of the mandible, and zone III between the angle of the mandible and the base of the skull.

3.2 Epidemiology of Penetrating Neck Trauma

Commentary

Overall, about 35% of all gunshot wounds and 20% of stab wounds to the neck result in significant injuries to vital structures. Transcervical gunshot wounds are associated with the highest incidence (73%) of significant injuries. The most commonly injured structures are the vessels (22% of patients), followed by the spinal cord, aerodigestive tract, and nerves (about 7% each).

Overall, only about 20% of gunshot wounds and 10% of stab wounds require operation. The remaining patients can be managed nonoperatively. The selection of patients for operation or observation can safely be made by physical examination and special investigations such as radiography, color flow Doppler studies, angiography, CT scan, endoscopy, and contrast swallow studies.

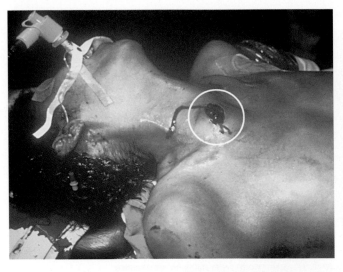

3.2A. Photograph of a zone I penetrating neck injury.

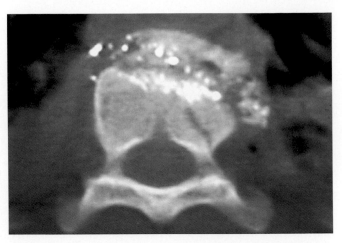

3.2C. CT scan of a transcervical gunshot wound with spinal fracture.

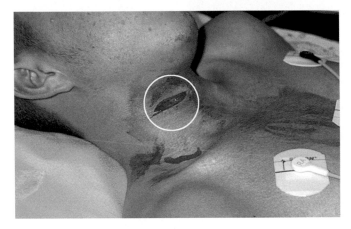

3.2B. Photograph of a zone II penetrating neck injury.

3.3 Physical Examination of Penetrating Injuries of the Neck

Commentary

Physical examination is very reliable in diagnosing or highly suspecting significant injuries requiring surgical repair. In order to avoid missing significant signs or symptoms, the physician is strongly recommended to perform the examination according to a written protocol. A careful examination in penetrating neck trauma is more important than in any other anatomical region.

Hard signs diagnostic of vascular trauma include severe bleeding, unexplained severe shock, absent or diminished peripheral pulses, bruits, and large, expanding hematomas. Soft signs suggestive but not diagnostic of vascular trauma include stable hematomas, mild hypotension responsive to small amounts of fluid resuscitation, abnormal ankle-brachial index (ABI), and proximity injuries. Only about 22% of patients with soft signs have significant vascular injuries. These patients need further investigation by means of color flow Doppler or angiography.

Hard signs diagnostic of aerodigestive tract trauma include respiratory distress, air bubbling through the wound, and major hemoptysis. These patients need an operation without any special investigations. Soft signs suggestive but not diagnostic of aerodigestive injuries include subcutaneous emphysema, minor hemoptysis, hoarseness, subcutaneous emphysema, and odynophagia. Only about 15% of these patients have significant aerodigestive injuries. These patients require further investigation by means of endoscopy and/or contrast swallow studies.

Asymptomatic patients are highly unlikely to have any significant trauma requiring surgical treatment.

Table 3.1. Physical Examination Protocol for Penetrating Injuries of the Neck

A. URGENT PRIORITIES
1. Control any active bleeding (pressure, packing, Foley's catheter).
2. If active bleeding: Trendelenburg position to prevent air embolism.
3. Secure airway.
4. IV fluids (no IV line on the side of the injury).

B. SYSTEMIC EXAMINATION
1. Dyspnea: ☐ yes ☐ no
2. Blood pressure:
3. Pulse:
4. Color: ☐ pale ☐ normal

C. LOCAL EXAMINATION
Vascular structures
1. Active bleeding: ☐ minor ☐ severe ☐ nil
2. Expanding hematoma: ☐ small ☐ large ☐ nil
3. Pulsatile hematoma: ☐ yes ☐ no
4. Peripheral pulses (compare with normal side, Doppler?):
☐ normal ☐ diminished ☐ absent
5. Bruit: ☐ yes ☐ no

D. LARYNX-TRACHEA-ESOPHAGUS
1. Hemoptysis: ☐ yes ☐ no
2. Air bubbling through wound (ask patient to cough):
☐ yes ☐ no
3. Subcutaneous emphysema: ☐ yes ☐ no
4. Pain on swallowing sputum: ☐ yes ☐ no

E. NERVOUS SYSTEM
1. Glasgow Coma Scale (GCS):
2. Localizing signs:
3. Cranial nerves:
■ Facial nerve: ☐ yes ☐ no
■ Glossopharyngeal nerve: ☐ yes ☐ no
■ Recurrent laryngeal nerve: ☐ yes ☐ no
■ Accessory nerve: ☐ yes ☐ no
4. Spinal cord: ☐ normal ☐ abnormal
5. Brachial plexus injury:
■ Median nerve: ☐ yes ☐ no
■ Ulnar nerve: ☐ yes ☐ no
■ Radial nerve: ☐ yes ☐ no
■ Musculocutaneous nerve: ☐ yes ☐ no
■ Axillary nerve: ☐ yes ☐ no
■ Horner's syndrome: ☐ yes ☐ no

F. INVESTIGATIONS (Only in fairly stable patients)
Chest x-ray (erect), neck x-ray:
☐ hemopneumothorax
☐ subcutaneous emphysema
☐ widened upper mediastinum
☐ retained knife blade or missile

Depending on the findings of clinical examination, further investigations such as color flow Doppler or angiography may be indicated.

3.4 Horner's Syndrome

Commentary

Horner's syndrome consists of ptosis of the upper eyelid, miosis of the ipsilateral eye, and anhidrosis of the ipsilateral side of the face. It is the result of injury of the stellate ganglion (on the neck of the first rib) of the sympathetic chain.

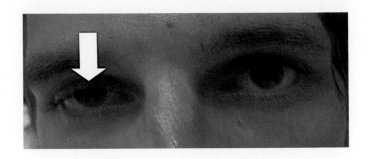

3.4A. Right Horner's syndrome following a knife injury to zone I of the neck.

3.5 Protocol for Initial Evaluation and Management of Penetrating Injuries to the Neck

Commentary

Clinical examination according to a written protocol remains the cornerstone for the selection of the appropriate treatment and investigation of a patient with penetrating neck trauma.

The selection of investigation (e.g., angiography versus color flow Doppler) should also take into consideration the experience and facilities of the particular trauma center.

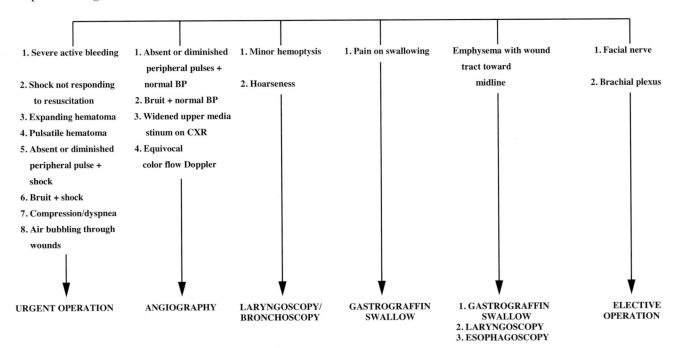

1. Severe active bleeding	1. Absent or diminished peripheral pulses + normal BP	1. Minor hemoptysis	1. Pain on swallowing	Emphysema with wound tract toward midline	1. Facial nerve
2. Shock not responding to resuscitation	2. Bruit + normal BP	2. Hoarseness			2. Brachial plexus
3. Expanding hematoma	3. Widened upper mediastinum on CXR				
4. Pulsatile hematoma	4. Equivocal color flow Doppler				
5. Absent or diminished peripheral pulse + shock					
6. Bruit + shock					
7. Compression/dyspnea					
8. Air bubbling through wounds					
↓	↓	↓	↓	↓	↓
URGENT OPERATION	ANGIOGRAPHY	LARYNGOSCOPY/ BRONCHOSCOPY	GASTROGRAFFIN SWALLOW	1. GASTROGRAFFIN SWALLOW 2. LARYNGOSCOPY 3. ESOPHAGOSCOPY	ELECTIVE OPERATION

3.5A. Algorithm for indications for emergency operation, nonoperative management, and selection of investigations in penetrating neck trauma.

3.6 Plain Radiography in Penetrating Neck Trauma

Commentary

Anteroposterior and lateral films of the neck should be obtained for all patients with penetrating neck trauma who are hemodynamically stable. Important radiological findings include hematoma, subcutaneous emphysema, fractures, and foreign bodies. A chest film is also recommended in all stable patients. In about 15% of patients with penetrating neck trauma, there is an associated pneumothorax or hemothorax. A widened upper mediastinum is suggestive of a hematoma secondary to a vascular injury, and an elevated diaphragm may be due to a phrenic nerve injury.

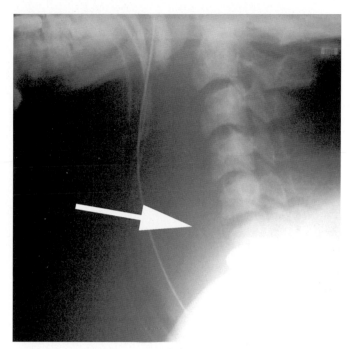

3.6B. Plain film of the neck shows a prevertebral hematoma and deviation of the nasogastric tube.

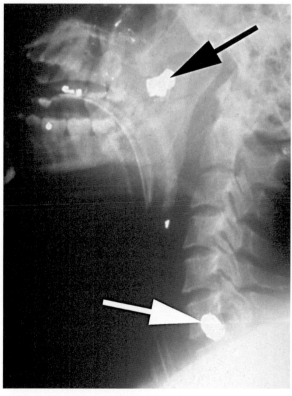

3.6A. Plain film of the neck showing two missiles, one in zone I and another in zone III.

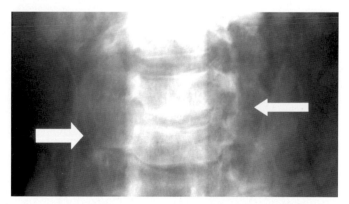

3.6C. AP neck film showing subcutaneous emphysema secondary to tracheal injury.

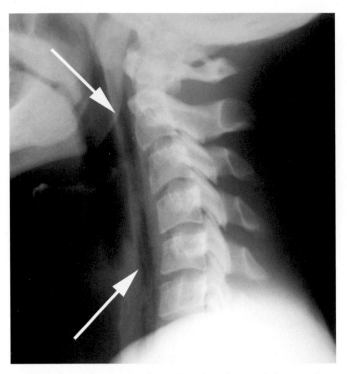

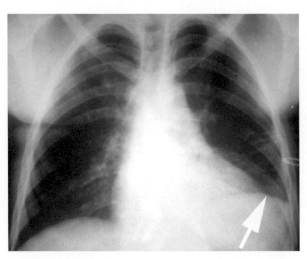

3.6F. CXR showing elevated left hemidiaphragm secondary to phrenic nerve injury.

3.6D. Prevertebral air on lateral neck radiograph in a patient with a stab wound to the neck.

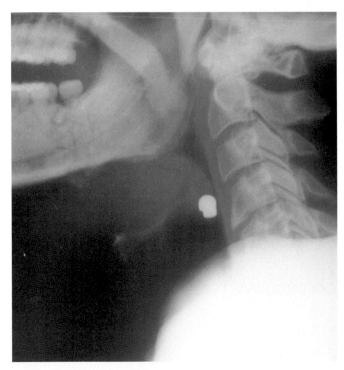

3.6E. Markedly narrow airway seen on lateral x-ray of a patient with a gunshot wound to the neck.

3.7 CT Scan in Penetrating Neck Trauma

Commentary

A cervical CT scan is indicated in patients with gunshot wounds who are hemodynamically stable and have neurological deficits or a transcervical injury. The CT may provide information about the site and nature of any fracture, involvement of the spinal cord, the presence of fragments in the spinal canal, and the presence of any hematomas compressing the cord. In addition, the direction of the bullet tract may help the physician determine the need for angiography, endoscopy, or contrast swallow studies.

A brain CT scan may be helpful in patients with penetrating neck trauma and unexplained neurological deficits. It may identify an anemic infarction or brain edema secondary to a carotid artery injury or an associated direct brain injury due to a missile.

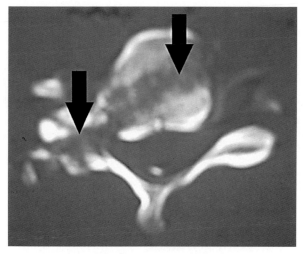

3.7A. CT scan of the cervical spine following a gunshot wound shows a vertebral fracture.

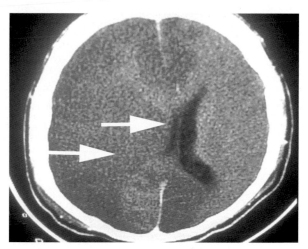

3.7C. Head CT scan of a patient with a penetrating injury of the internal carotid artery, presenting with hemiplegia, showing an anemic brain infarction of the right hemisphere with midline shift.

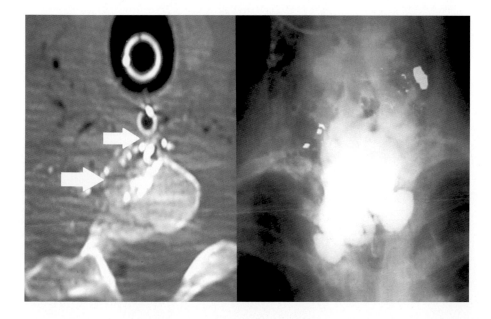

3.7B. CT scan shows a gunshot wound tract to be near the esophagus (left side). A contrast swallow study demonstrates an esophageal injury (right side).

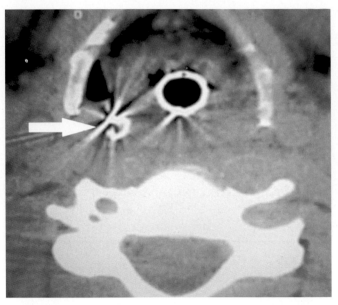

3.7D. Gunshot wound to the neck. CT shows hematoma with compression and deviation of the nasogastric tube.

3.8 Evaluation of Vascular Structures in the Neck

Commentary

Asymptomatic patients are highly unlikely to have significant vascular injuries requiring surgical intervention or angiographic embolization. However, in about 8% of asymptomatic patients investigated by angiography, there is a vascular injury not requiring any type of treatment.

Patients with soft signs of vascular trauma need evaluation by color flow Doppler and, in appropriate cases, angiography. The combination of physical examination and color flow Doppler will detect almost all vascular injuries.

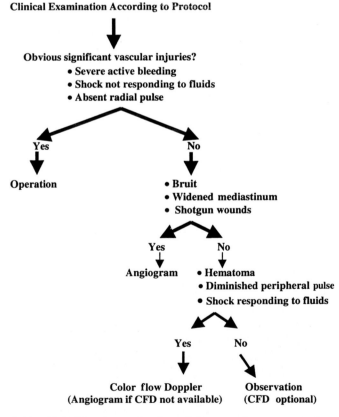

3.8A. Algorithm for evaluation of the vascular structures in the neck.

3.9 Vascular Trauma—Zone I

Commentary

The presence of a peripheral pulse does not preclude a significant proximal arterial injury. It is essential that the pulse is compared with the contralateral one. In addition, the ABI should be measured. An index >0.90 is unlikely to be associated with significant arterial injury. It is recommended that all asymptomatic penetrating injuries in proximity of major vessels be evaluated routinely by ABI and color flow Doppler studies.

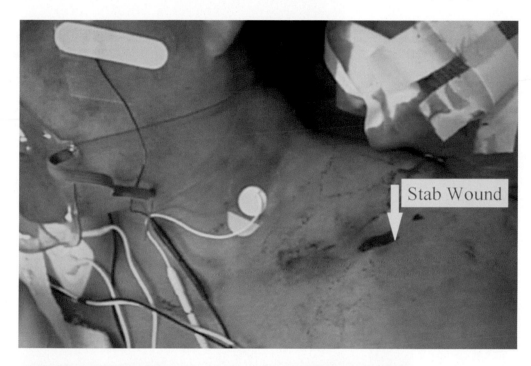

3.9A. Photo of a stab wound in zone I of the neck. The victim has peripheral pulse present on the left arm.

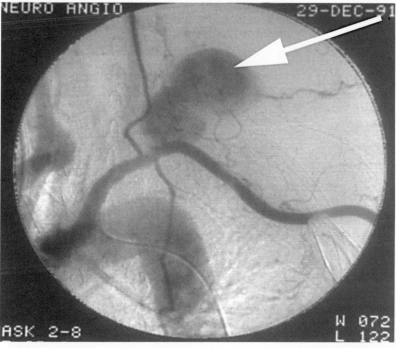

3.9B. Angiography reveals a significant subclavian artery false aneurysm.

3.10 Vascular Trauma—Zone III

Commentary

Failure to perform a meticulous physical examination and the appropriate investigations may result in missing significant injuries and serious complications. Auscultation is an important part of physical examination in penetrating neck trauma.

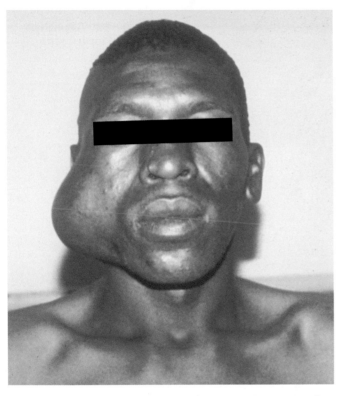

3.10A. Photograph of a patient with penetrating trauma in zone III of the neck, presenting many days after the injury. There is a pulsatile mass and a bruit.

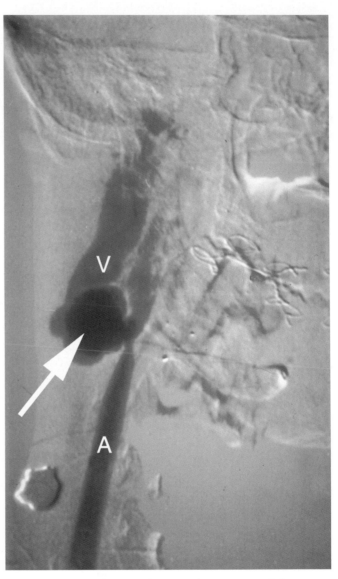

3.10B. Angiography reveals a pseudoaneurysm of the internal carotid artery and communication with the internal jugular vein (A–V fistula).

3.11 Color Flow Doppler (CFD)

Commentary

CFD should be the first line of investigation for suspected vascular trauma in most patients who are hemodynamically stable. The combination of physical examination and CFD imaging is a safe and cost-effective alternative to routine contrast angiography. It is noninvasive, can be performed at the bedside, has a high sensitivity and specificity, and is relatively inexpensive. However, it is operator dependent and has some limitations in the visualization of the internal carotid artery near the base of the skull, sections of the vertebral artery directly underneath the bony part of the vertebral canal, and the proximal subclavian vessels, especially on the left side and in obese patients. In patients where the CFD is inconclusive, an arteriogram should be considered.

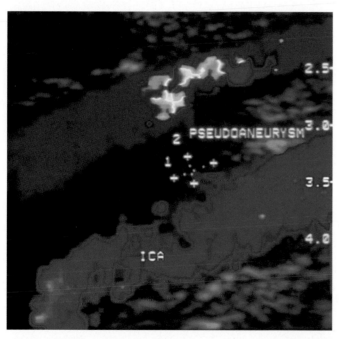

3.11A. CFD demonstrates a false aneurysm of the internal carotid artery.

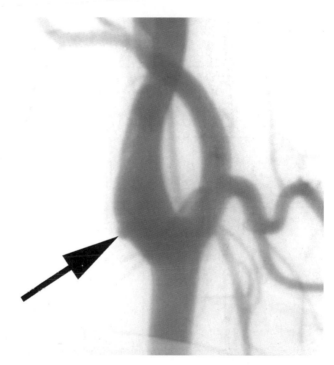

3.11B. Angiographic confirmation of the aneurysm in same patient.

3.12 Angiography for Penetrating Injuries of the Neck

Commentary

Angiography may be used for diagnostic or therapeutic purposes in penetrating neck trauma.

Diagnostic indications: (a) inconclusive color flow Doppler, (b) hematoma in zone III of the neck, (c) a widened upper mediastinum on chest film, (d) gunshot wound involving the transverse foramen of the cervical spine, (e) shotgun injuries, and (f) embedded knife blades before blade removal.

Therapeutic indications for stenting or embolization: (a) bruit; (b) diminished upper extremity pulse; (c) ongoing, slow, continuous bleeding from suspected vertebral artery injury; and (d) continuous bleeding following a gunshot wound to the face.

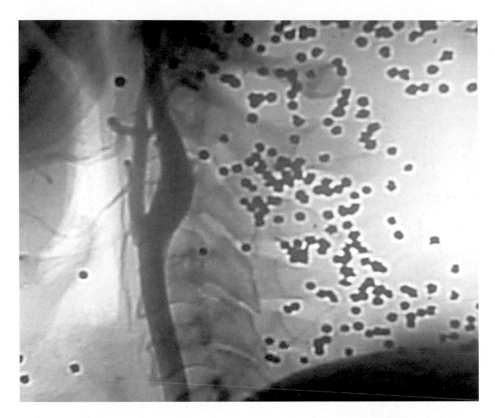

3.12A and B. Shotgun injuries of the neck. Angiography reveals two false aneurysms.

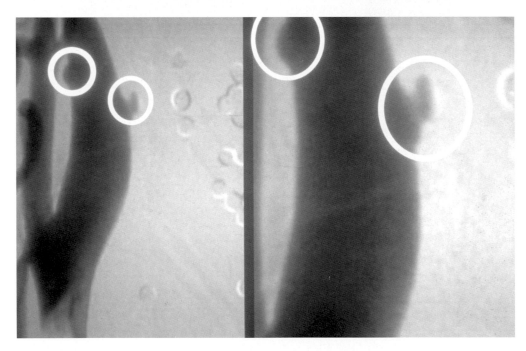

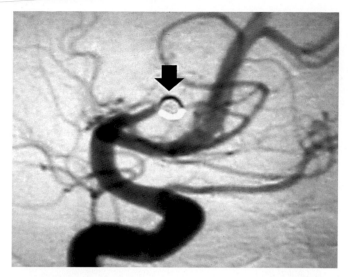

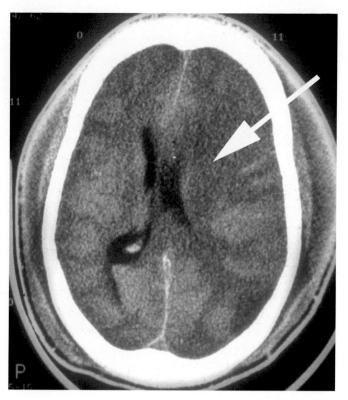

3.12C. Pellet embolization of the middle cerebral artery.

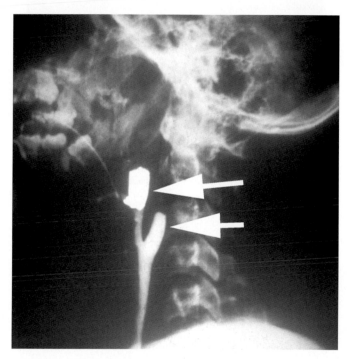

3.12E. CT head of the same patient shows anemic infarction and edema of the left hemisphere.

3.12D. Gunshot injury to zone III of the neck. The patient had a neck hematoma and contralateral hemiplegia. Angiogram reveals thrombosis of the internal and external carotid arteries.

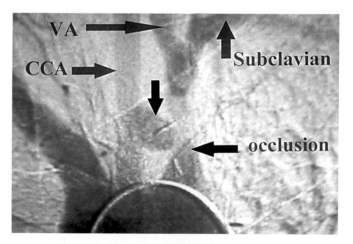

3.12F. Multiple gunshot wounds to the neck, with a large neck hematoma and no peripheral radial pulse. Angiogram shows a false aneurysm at the origin of the common carotid artery (middle arrow), complete occlusion of the left subclavian artery, and reconstitution of the distal subclavian artery from the vertebral artery (steal syndrome).

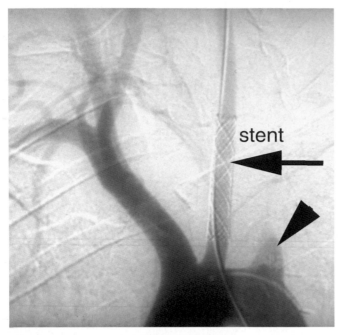

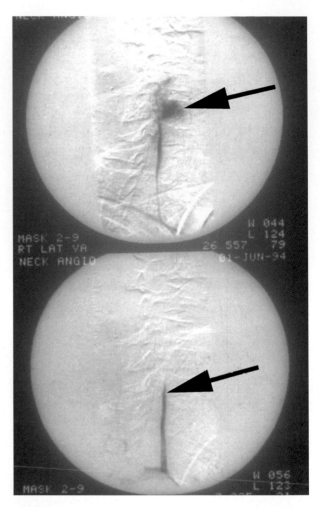

3.12G. Because of other associated injuries, a carotid stent was successfully placed angiographically in the same patient. The subclavian artery is still occluded (lower arrow).

3.12I. False aneurysm of the vertebral artery, before (top) and after embolization (below).

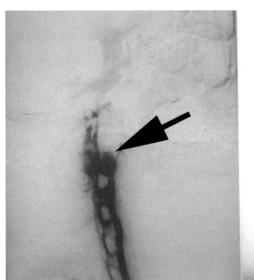

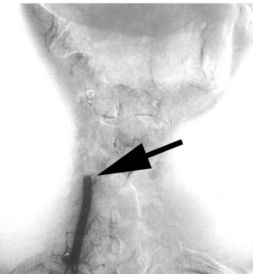

3.12H. Gunshot wound with a neck hematoma and a bruit. Angiograms shows an arteriovenous fistula between the vertebral artery and veins, before (left side) and after embolization (right side).

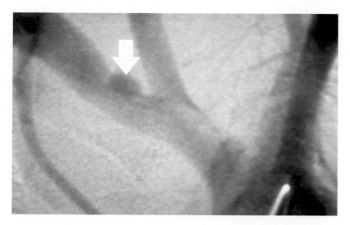

3.12J. False aneurysm of the origin of the right subclavian artery. The peripheral pulse was present.

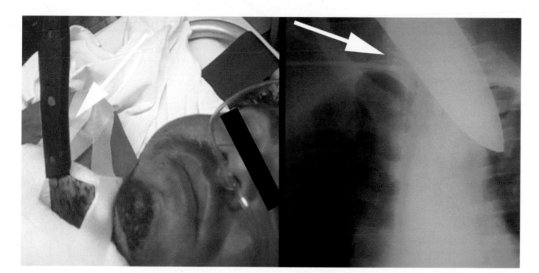

3.12K and L. Cases with knives embedded in the neck. In the second case, the angiography was normal and the blade was removed.

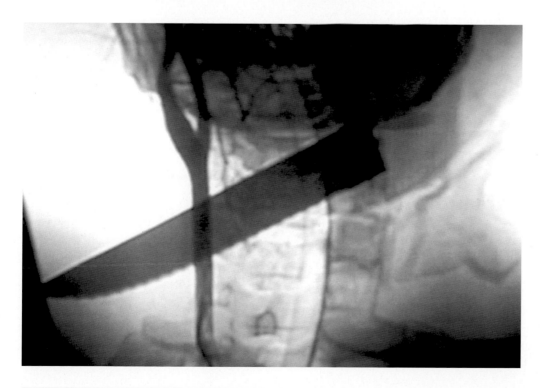

3.13 Evaluation of the Aerodigestive Tract in the Neck

Commentary

Asymptomatic patients are highly unlikely to have a significant injury requiring surgical management. Unevaluable patients or patients with soft symptoms of aerodigestive injuries need investigation by endoscopy and contrast swallow studies.

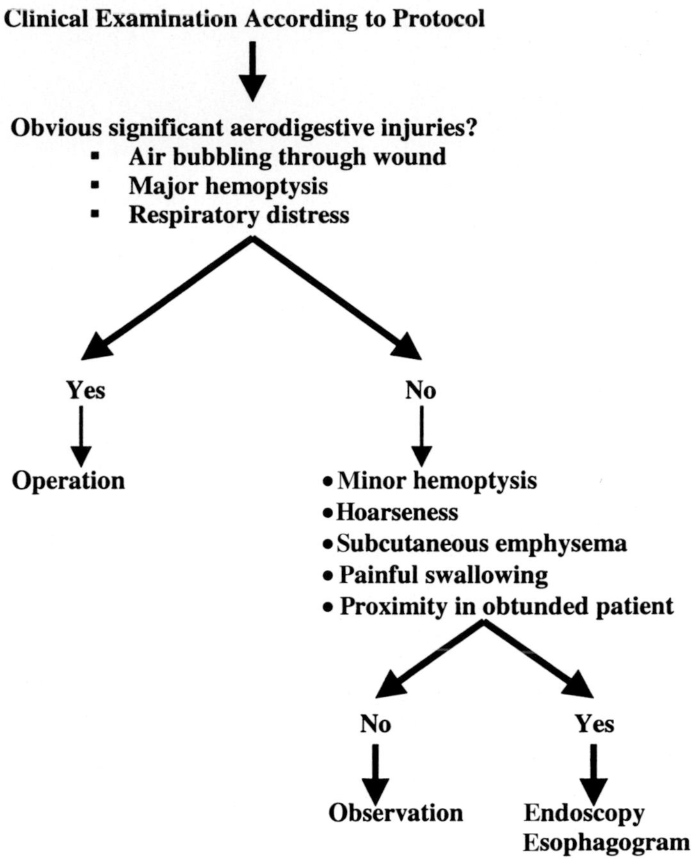

Clinical Examination According to Protocol

Obvious significant aerodigestive injuries?
- Air bubbling through wound
- Major hemoptysis
- Respiratory distress

Yes → **Operation**

No →
- Minor hemoptysis
- Hoarseness
- Subcutaneous emphysema
- Painful swallowing
- Proximity in obtunded patient

No → **Observation**

Yes → **Endoscopy Esophagogram**

3.13A. Algorithm for the evaluation of the aerodigestive tract in the neck.

3.14 Esophageal Trauma

Commentary

The esophagus can be evaluated by means of esophagography or endoscopy. The combination of the two investigations has a sensitivity of 100%. Rigid esophagoscopy is superior to flexible esophagoscopy in evaluating the upper esophagus; however, rigid endoscopy can be performed only under general anesthesia. Thus this investigation is best reserved for patients undergoing anesthesia for another reason.

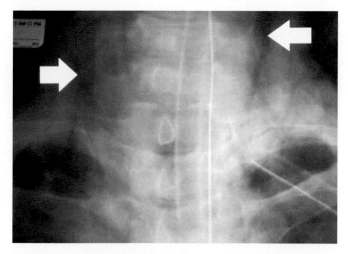

3.14A. Subcutaneous emphysema following a gunshot wound to the neck. This finding is an absolute indication for evaluation of the aerodigestive tract.

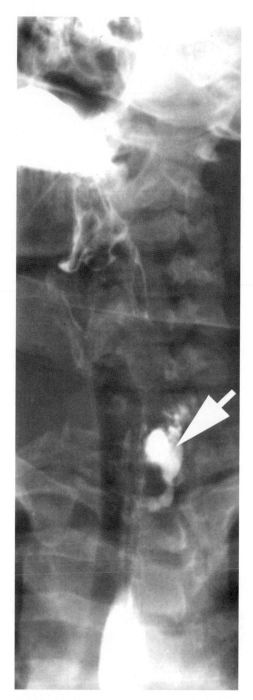

3.14B. Gastrograffin swallow shows a perforation of the cervical esophagus.

3.15 Airway Establishment in the Presence of a Neck Hematoma

Commentary

About 10% of patients with penetrating neck trauma present with airway compromise due to direct trauma to the larynx or trachea or to external compression by a large hematoma. Airway establishment in the emergency department or the operating room in the presence of a large neck hematoma can be a difficult and potentially dangerous procedure. Pharmacological paralysis for endotracheal intubation should always be performed in the presence of an experienced physician ready to perform a cricothyroidotomy if the intubator cannot visualize the cords. Orotracheal intubation without pharmacological paralysis should be avoided because patient straining may precipitate massive hemorrhage. (For the same reason, insertion of a nasogastric tube should be avoided in the awake patient.) In addition, in the presence of a neck hematoma due to penetrating trauma, a cervical collar should be applied loosely because it may precipitate or aggravate an airway obstruction. The best approach is fiberoptic nasotracheal intubation under light sedation and local anesthesia. It must be remembered that in the presence of a large neck hematoma a cricothyroidotomy may be a difficult and bloody procedure.

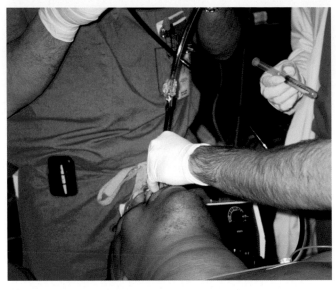

3.15B. Photograph of an awake, fiberoptic intubation of a patient with a large neck hematoma, following a gunshot wound.

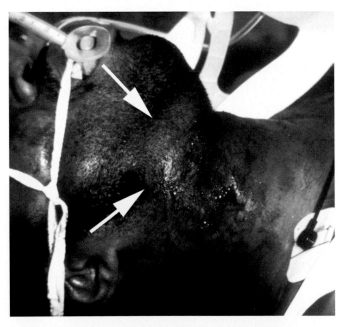

3.15A. Photograph of a large right neck hematoma in a patient with a zone II stab wound.

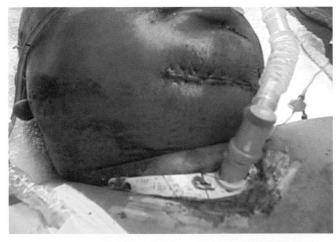

3.15C. Photograph of an emergency cricothyroidotomy on a patient with failed orotracheal intubation in the presence of a large neck hematoma.

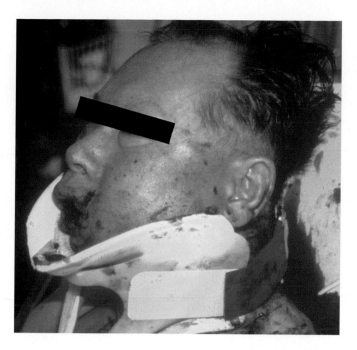

3.15D. Photograph of a patient with a stab wound to the neck. Note the left neck and facial swelling. In the presence of a neck hematoma, a cervical collar should be used with caution because it may aggravate airway compromise.

3.16 Bleeding Control in the Emergency Department

Commentary

In most cases, the bleeding may be controlled by direct pressure over the wound. However, in some cases, especially in zones I and III, direct pressure is not effective. In these situations, insertion of the tip of a Foley catheter into the wound and inflation of the balloon with sterile water may control the bleeding.

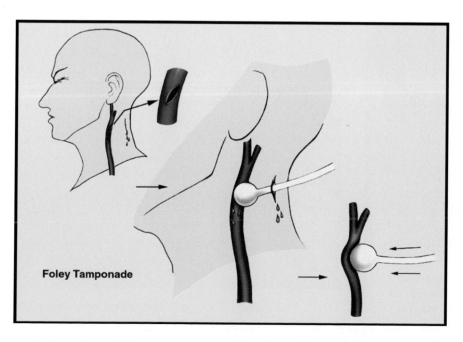

Foley Tamponade

3.16A. Illustration of balloon tamponade of severe bleeding in zone III of the neck.

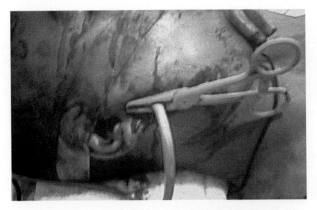

3.16B. Photograph of balloon tamponade in a stab wound victim.

3.17 Operative Approaches

Commentary

Most patients with penetrating injuries to the neck do not require surgical intervention. Only about 15–20% of all patients will require an operation. The selection of patients for operation or observation can safely be made on the basis of a careful physical examination and appropriate investigations. Even in transcervical gunshot wounds, where the incidence of injury to vital structures is about 75%, only 20% require an operation.

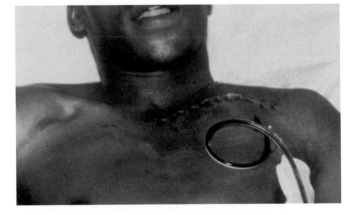

3.17B. Photograph of the clavicular incision for exposure of the distal subclavian axillary vessels.

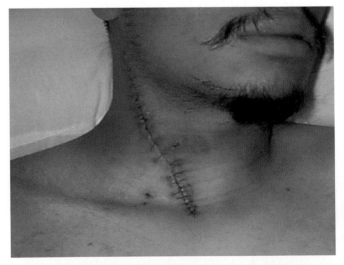

3.17A. Photograph of the surgical exposure of carotid sheath structures and the aerodigestive tract through an incision along the anterior border of the sternomastoid muscle.

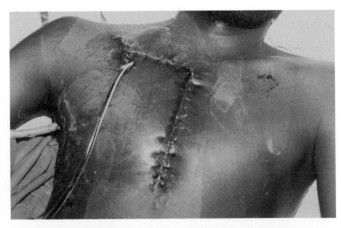

3.17C. Photograph of the clavicular incision combined with a median sternotomy for proximal subclavian injuries.

3.18 Penetrating Trauma to the Carotid Artery

Commentary

Traumatic thrombosis of the common or internal carotid artery may result in ipsilateral anemic infarction and brain edema, although in some cases this may be well tolerated. Early revascularization, ideally within the first 2–4 hours, is associated with good results. Delayed revascularization after the establishment of an anemic infarction may worsen the brain edema or lead to a hemorrhagic infarction. Early surgical reconstruction remains the mainstay of management of penetrating carotid injuries. In selected cases such as in high internal carotid injuries, where surgical exposure is difficult, angiographic stenting may be a good alternative.

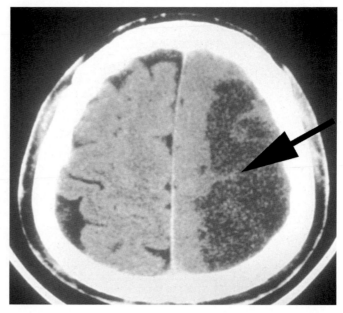

3.18B. CT of the brain with severe anemic infarction and brain edema following thrombosis of the internal carotid artery due to a gunshot wound.

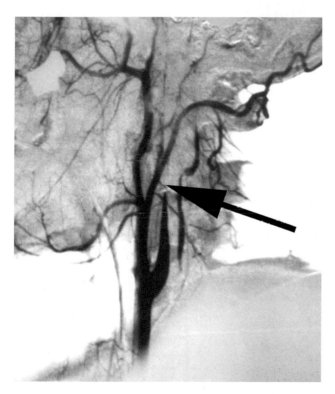

3.18A. Angiogram showing gunshot wound–related occlusion of the internal carotid artery.

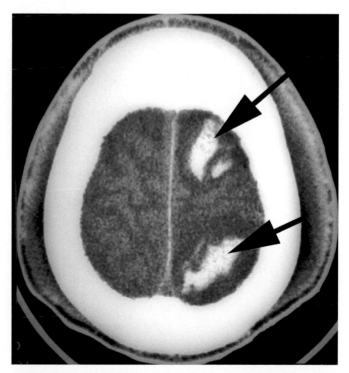

3.18C. CT of the brain showing hemorrhagic infarction following delayed revascularization of a thrombosed carotid artery.

3.19 Penetrating Injuries to the Vertebral Artery

Commentary

Occlusion of a vertebral artery is tolerated very well, and there is no need to attempt revascularization. The majority of vertebral artery injuries can be managed by observation or angiographic embolization (see 3.12H and I). Surgical intervention is indicated only in the presence of severe active bleeding or in cases where angiographic embolization has failed.

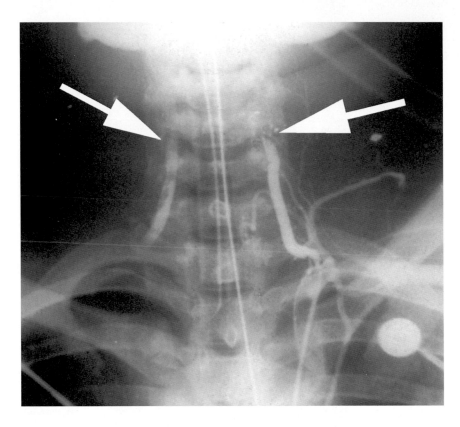

3.19A. Angiogram showing thrombosis of both vertebral arteries following a gunshot wound. The patient had no neurological signs.

3.20 Blunt Carotid Injury

Commentary

Blunt trauma to the carotid artery occurs in about 0.3% of all severe blunt trauma cases. The usual mechanism is overextension of the neck, although overflexion of the head or direct trauma to the neck may result in such injuries as well. The clinical picture may vary from a seatbelt mark sign or neck hematoma to severe neurological deficits such as hemiparesis or hemiplegia. The usual site of carotid injury is at the bifurcation of the common carotid or high at the internal carotid. The diagnosis is suspected from the mechanism of injury and the hematoma or seatbelt mark sign at the neck or the presence of unexplained central neurological findings. Confirmation is established by color flow Doppler or angiography.

The treatment depends on the site of carotid injury and the experience of the surgeon. In low lesions that are surgically accessible, an operation with reestablishment of the blood flow by means of a homologous venous graft is recommended. In high internal carotid lesions that are not easily amenable to surgical repair, angiographically placed stents or anticoagulation may be the best alternatives.

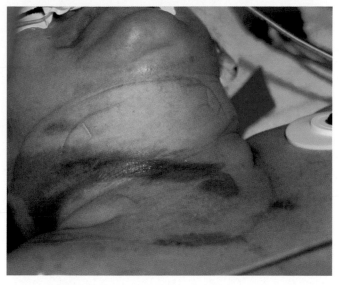

3.20A. Photograph of a seatbelt mark sign on the right side of the neck.

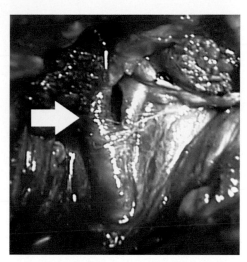

3.20B. Intraoperative appearance of "bruised" carotid artery.

3.21 Blunt Laryngotracheal Trauma

Commentary

Blunt trauma to the larynx or trachea may occur as a result of direct trauma to the neck or anteroposterior crush trauma to the chest, which causes intratracheal high pressures while the glottis is closed. Also, deceleration injuries may cause shearing injuries at fixed points, such as the cricoid or the carina. These injuries may vary from submucosal hematomas to complete transection.

The patient often complains of pain in the neck, dyspnea, hemoptysis, or hoarseness. Physical examination usually reveals subcutaneous emphysema. The diagnosis is confirmed by CT scan of the larynx and endoscopy.

About 28% of patients with blunt laryngotracheal trauma require emergency airway control. Depending on the severity of the injury and the condition of the patient, the airway can be established by orotracheal intubation, fiberoptic intubation, or surgical airway. Many patients with no airway problem and with no major disruption of the laryngotracheal structures may be managed nonoperatively. Perforation of the larynx or trachea or major fractures of the thyroid or arytenoid cartilages or the hyoid bone often need surgical intervention.

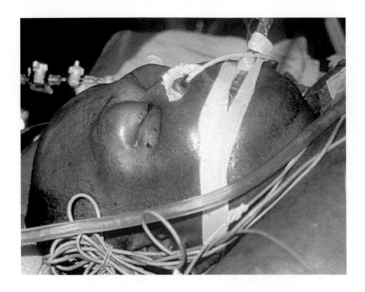

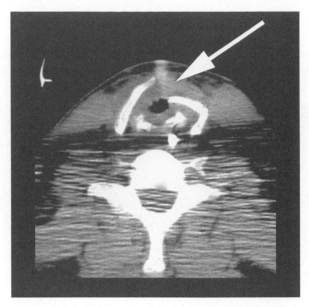

3.21A. Photograph showing subcutaneous emphysema following blunt trauma to the neck and laryngeal fracture.

3.21B. CT scan of the neck confirms fracture of the thyroid cartilage.

Thoracic Injury

Introduction

Chest trauma is estimated to be the primary cause of death in 25% of traumatic mortalities and a contributing factor in another 25% of deaths. Good understanding of the pathophysiology of chest trauma and timely selection of the appropriate investigations and treatment are all critical components for optimal outcome.

Clinical Examination

Advanced trauma life support (ATLS) principles are particularly important in the initial evaluation and management of the chest trauma patient.

During the primary survey, there are six life-threatening conditions that need to be identified and treated:

1. Airway obstruction
2. Tension pneumothorax
3. Open pneumothorax with a "sucking wound"
4. Flail chest
5. Massive hemothorax
6. Cardiac tamponade

During the secondary survey, there are another six potentially lethal chest injuries that should be identified and treated. The diagnosis of these conditions may need more complex and time-consuming investigations.

1. Lung contusion
2. Myocardial contusion
3. Aortic rupture
4. Diaphragmatic rupture
5. Tracheobronchial rupture
6. Esophageal injury

Investigations

History and clinical examination will determine the type and timing of investigations necessary for the safe and efficient evaluation of the chest trauma patient. Very often, in unstable patients, therapeutic interventions such as thoracostomy tube insertion or thoracotomy may be initiated without any investigations.

Investigations are necessary in fairly stable patients when the diagnosis is uncertain. The following investigations may be useful in chest trauma:

1. Chest x-ray: Ideally it should be taken during deep expiration and erect position for more accurate detection of small pneumothoraces, small hemothoraces, and mediastinal abnormalities. In many cases this is not possible because of associated hemodynamic instability, depressed level of consciousness, or concern about spinal injury. The following radiological findings should be sought: pneumothorax, hemothorax, lung contusion, subcutaneous or mediastinal emphysema, fractures, mediastinal widening, enlarged cardiac shadow, pneumopericardium, elevated diaphragm or suspicious shadows suggestive of diaphragmatic hernia, free air under the diaphragm, and foreign bodies.

2. Electrocardiogram (ECG): ECG should be performed in most blunt chest trauma patients and selected penetrating injuries. It is essential in the diagnosis of blunt cardiac trauma or myocardial infarction.

3. Trauma ultrasound: This is a very important investigation and should be available in the emergency department. Emergency physicians and trauma surgeons should be trained in its use, as it allows early diagnosis of cardiac tamponade or hemoperitoneum at the bedside.

4. Pericardiocentesis: This diagnostic procedure has little or no value in the evaluation of suspected cardiac trauma in a modern trauma center as it is

associated with an unacceptably high incidence of false-negative results because of clot formation in the pericardium. In addition, it is a potentially dangerous procedure because of the risk of myocardial or coronary vessel perforation, especially if performed in the absence of hemopericardium.

5. Subxiphoid pericardial window: This major invasive procedure has been used by many surgeons to diagnose cardiac tamponade. With bedside echocardiography to evaluate the pericardium, it has very little or no place in a modern trauma center.

6. Chest computed tomography (CT): CT is very valuable in blunt trauma in the evaluation of the mediastinum, the thoracic spine, and suspected lung contusions. All stable blunt trauma patients with a suspicious mechanism of injury (high-speed accidents, falls from height) or those with an abnormal mediastinum on chest films should be evaluated by spiral CT scan for aortic rupture. Spiral CT scan is highly sensitive and specific in detecting aortic rupture and has replaced aortography to a great extent. CT scan is also useful in the evaluation of suspected lung contusions or persistent opacifications on chest x-ray following insertion of a thoracostomy tube. In these cases, the differential diagnosis between atelectasis, contusion, and residual hemothorax may be difficult or impossible on the basis of clinical examination and chest x-ray.

   CT scan also has a definitive role in the evaluation of selected patients with penetrating chest trauma. In patients with transmediastinal gunshot wounds who are hemodynamically stable, a spiral CT scan with thin cuts may be useful in identifying the bullet track and in determining the need for further investigations such as aortography or endoscopy. If the direction of the bullet track is away from the aorta, esophagus, and other important mediastinal structures, no further investigations are necessary.

7. Angiography: Aortography is still used by many centers as the standard investigation for suspected aortic injuries. In some trauma centers, it has largely been replaced by spiral CT scan, and aortography is reserved for cases with indeterminate CT scan findings.

   Angiography also has a role for selected penetrating injuries of the thoracic inlet with suspected innominate or subclavian vascular injuries. In some of these cases with subclavian false aneurysms or arteriovenous fistulae, angiographically placed stents may provide the definitive management of the injury.

8. Color flow Doppler: Color flow Doppler ultrasound is a very good noninvasive vascular study that can reliably evaluate the subclavian and neck vessels and is recommended for hemodynamically stable patients with thoracic inlet penetrating injuries. Its major weaknesses are its operator-dependent accuracy and inability to visualize the left proximal subclavian vessels, especially in obese patients.

9. Endoscopy: Esophagoscopy and bronchoscopy may be necessary for suspected aerodigestive tract injuries, usually as a result of mediastinal penetrating trauma.

10. Laparoscopy: Laparoscopy has a definitive role in the evaluation of the diaphragm in asymptomatic patients with left thoracoabdominal or right anterior thoracoabdominal penetrating injuries. Failure to recognize and repair a diaphragmatic injury may result in a diaphragmatic hernia at a later stage. Right posterior thoracoabdominal injuries do not need evaluation and repair of any diaphragmatic laceration because the presence of the liver protects against herniation of intra-abdominal organs. The procedure may be performed under general anesthesia or under sedation and local anesthesia.

11. Thoracoscopy: Thoracoscopy is used in the evaluation of diaphragmatic injuries, especially in the posterior region. It is particularly useful in cases with residual hemothorax that can be evacuated through the port. It has the disadvantage of needing double lumen intubation and lung collapse, which may be technically demanding and sometimes not well tolerated by the patient.

12. Troponin levels: Serial troponin measurements have replaced cardiac enzymes (e.g., CPK-MB) for monitoring in suspected myocardial contusion. Though routinely used, troponin levels do not correlate with the severity of the myocardial trauma.

13. Arterial blood gas: Arterial blood gases are indicated in all severe chest trauma cases in order to assess severity, plan treatment, and monitor progress of treatment.

General Management

In an urban environment, there is no place for prehospital attempts to stabilize patients with severe chest trauma, and the principle of "scoop and run" should be applied. The patient should be placed on a spinal board, receive oxygen by mask, and be transferred without any delay to the nearest trauma hospital. Intravenous access should be attempted in the ambulance en route. In patients with severe respiratory distress and clinical suspicion of tension pneumothorax, a needle thoracostomy may be attempted. Open sucking wounds should be covered with a clean square gauze taped only on three sides to avoid a tension pneumothorax. Patients with respiratory failure or a depressed level of consciousness will need prehospital intubation or bag valve mask ventilation en route. In the emergency department, the primary survey will determine the need and type of immediate treatment. Patients with imminent or established cardiac arrest should be managed with an emergency department resuscitative thoracotomy. Any bleeding is controlled by sutures or clamping. Aortic cross-clamping is performed, and cardiac massage is initiated. Transfusions with O negative blood, cardiac drugs, and defibrillation are administered as necessary. If cardiac activity returns, the operation is completed in the operating room.

Patients with severe hypotension and suspicion of cardiovascular trauma should be taken directly to the operating room with minimal investigations. A trauma ultrasound is very valuable in determining the source of hypotension in patients with multiple injuries as it can evaluate the pericardial, pleural, and peritoneal spaces.

Hemodynamically stable patients are examined carefully, and further investigations are performed as indicated. Thoracostomy tubes, analgesia, intubation, and mechanical ventilation may be necessary.

Elderly patients with multiple rib fractures despite a normal respiratory status on initial examination should be admitted to the intensive care unit for close monitoring, as these patients are prone to deteriorate a few hours after admission. Adequate analgesia by means of epidural or patient-controlled analgesia are critical components of the management of these cases.

Indications for Thoracotomy

Fewer than 10% of blunt chest traumas, about 15% of stab wounds, and about 20% of gunshot wounds require thoracotomy. The majority of patients with chest trauma can safely be managed with a thoracostomy tube and other supportive treatment. The indications for emergency thoracotomy are generally the following:

- Cardiac arrest or imminent cardiac arrest
- Evidence of cardiovascular injury, such as severe hypotension or severe active external or internal bleeding
- Immediate blood loss in the thoracostomy tube more than 1,000–1,200 ml
- Diagnosis of aortic rupture or esophageal or tracheobronchial injury

Semielective thoracotomies are indicated for large residual hemothoraces or persistent major air leaks.

Common Mistakes and Pitfalls

1. Elderly patients with multiple rib fractures may seem stable on admission, but rapid respiratory deterioration may occur a few hours later. Close monitoring in an ICU environment is critical.
2. Patients with flail chest may seem stable on admission. Decompensation with severe respiratory failure may occur during prolonged radiological investigation with potentially catastrophic consequences. Liberal early intubation is recommended before these patients are transferred to the radiology suite.
3. A widened mediastinum following a traffic accident or a fall from height may be due to rupture of the thoracic aorta or to fractures of the thoracic spine.
4. Many diaphragmatic injuries may be asymptomatic, and the chest films may be normal or nondiagnostic. For left thoracoabdominal or anterior right thoracoabdominal penetrating injuries, routine laparoscopy should be performed on all asymptomatic patients.

4.1 Chest Wall Seatbelt Mark

Commentary

Seatbelt marks on the thoracic wall are indicators of severe trauma, and 20% of these patients have significant intrathoracic injuries. These patients should have routine evaluation for lung contusion, myocardial contusion, aortic rupture, and hemopneumothorax.

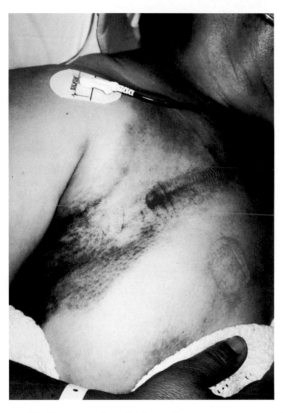

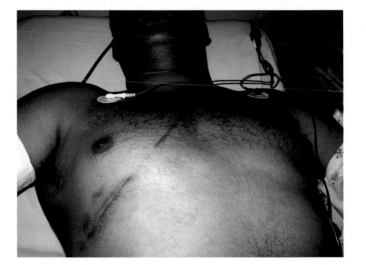

4.1A and B. Photographs of skin ecchymoses corresponding to the seatbelt.

4.2 Fractures of the Upper (First or Second) Ribs

Commentary

Fractures of the upper ribs, especially the first rib, are associated with a high incidence of subclavian vascular injuries. A color flow Doppler evaluation of the vessels will help exclude this injury. The force required to fracture an upper rib is severe, and thus mediastinal structures, including the aorta, are also at high risk with this mechanism. Children have a much more compliant chest wall, and thus any rib fractures are significant.

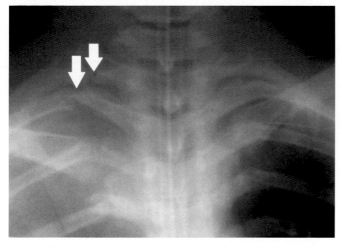

4.2A. CXR with fractures of the upper ribs.

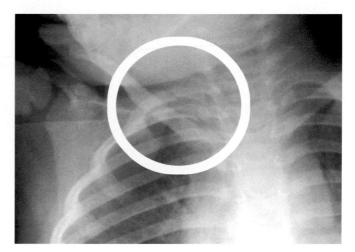

4.2B. CXR showing upper rib fractures in a small child.

4.3 Fractures of Middle (Third to Eighth) Ribs

Commentary

Rib fractures are diagnosed clinically (pain aggravated by breathing or coughing, pain on anteroposterior chest compression) or radiologically. Fractures at the costochondral junction may not show on x-rays. Associated injuries include hemopneumothorax, lung contusion, cardiac trauma, and diaphragmatic tear. Pain relief is extremely important, especially in elderly patients with multiple rib fractures, in order to prevent atelectasis and pneumonia. Patient-controlled analgesia (PCA) or epidural anesthesia should be used in multiple fractures.

Rib fractures in children are uncommon and signify severe impact to the chest wall, and there is a high incidence of underlying lung contusion.

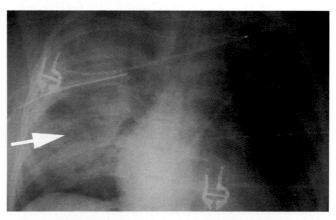

4.3A. Plain radiograph of multiple rib fractures with underlying lung contusion.

4.4 Fractures of the Lower (Ninth to Twelfth) Ribs

Commentary

Fractures of the lower ribs are often associated with injuries to the kidneys, liver, or spleen. Liberal use of abdominal CT scan is highly recommended.

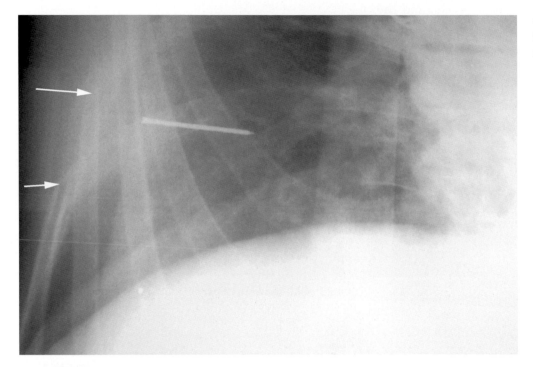

4.4A. Radiograph showing fractures of the right lower ribs.

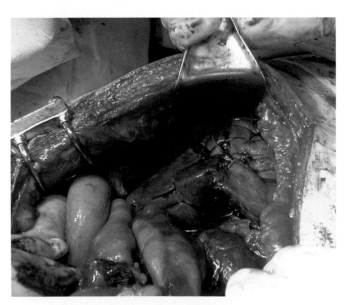

4.4B. Intraoperative photograph of the associated liver injury in the same patient.

4.5 Flail Chest

Commentary

Flail chest is the result of anterior or lateral double fractures of at least three adjacent ribs. In most cases there is an underlying lung contusion. Clinically the flail segment moves paradoxically to normal chest wall motion, and the patient may be in respiratory distress. All patients with flail chest should have a thoracostomy tube inserted and be monitored in an ICU setting with serial blood gases and continuous pulse oximetry. Analgesia by means of patient-controlled or epidural anesthesia should always be used. Mechanical ventilation is necessary for respiratory failure or imminent failure. Internal, operative fracture fixation has been used in selected cases without underlying lung contusion and in patients having difficulty weaning off mechanical ventilation.

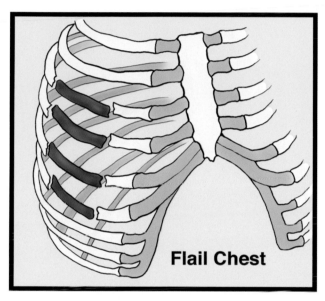

4.5A. Illustration of flail chest. Double fractures of at least three adjacent ribs are required in order to produce a flail chest.

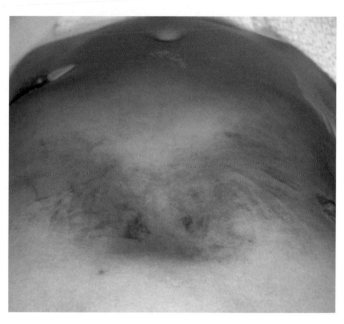

4.5C. Photograph of a flail sternal segment. Note the midsternal depression.

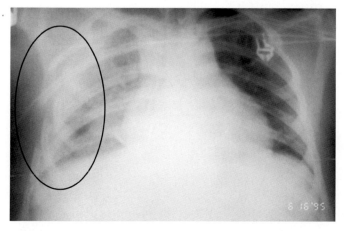

4.5B. CXR showing a flail chest with underlying lung contusion.

4.6 Pneumothorax

Commentary

A pneumothorax may be due to blunt or penetrating trauma. Small pneumothoraces are usually asymptomatic and can safely be managed nonoperatively, provided the patient does not need mechanical ventilation or air transportation. In these cases, any size pneumothorax should be treated with a thoracostomy tube to avoid the creation of tension pneumothorax. Large pneumothoraces may cause respiratory distress, and tension pneumothoraces can cause cardiorespiratory failure. The diagnosis of simple pneumothorax is usually made by plain chest film. An erect chest x-ray in deep expiration is the most suitable film to identify small pneumothoraces.

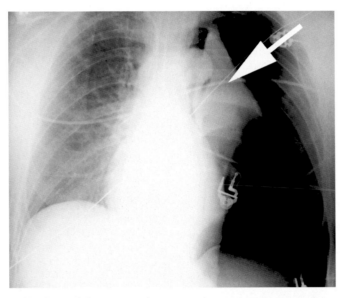

4.6A. Large left pneumothorax on chest x-ray. Arrow points to collapsed lung.

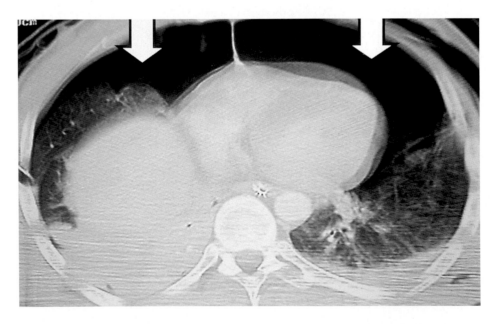

4.6B. Bilateral pneumothoraces on CT scan. Arrows point to pneumothorax.

4.7 Tension Pneumothorax

Commentary

In tension pneumothorax, air leaks into the pleural cavity with no escape avenue on account of a one-way valve effect. It is a life-threatening condition because of the severe cardiorespiratory failure that ensues. The patient is panicky and has dyspnea, cyanosis, shock, and distended neck veins. The trachea is shifted to the opposite side, there are no breath sounds in the affected hemithorax, and there is hyperresonance on percussion. Immediate lifesaving therapy is needle decompression of the chest, followed by formal thoracostomy tube insertion. The mere suspicion of a tension pneumothorax is an absolute indication for a needle decompression whenever a thoracostomy tube cannot be inserted immediately (prehospital stage, areas outside the emergency department or operative room). A thoracostomy tube should be subsequently inserted as soon as possible.

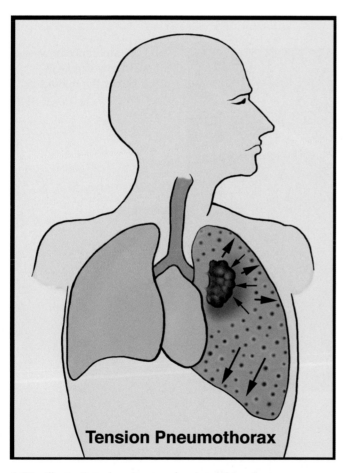

Tension Pneumothorax

4.7A. Illustration showing mechanism of tension pneumothorax: Air under tension collapses the lung, expands the hemithorax, depresses the diaphragm, and pushes the heart toward the opposite side. These changes cause acute cardiorespiratory failure.

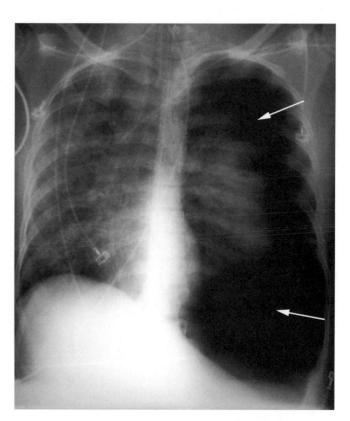

4.7B. CXR showing a large tension pneumothorax on the left side, mediastinal shift to the opposite side, and downward displacement of the left hemidiaphragm.

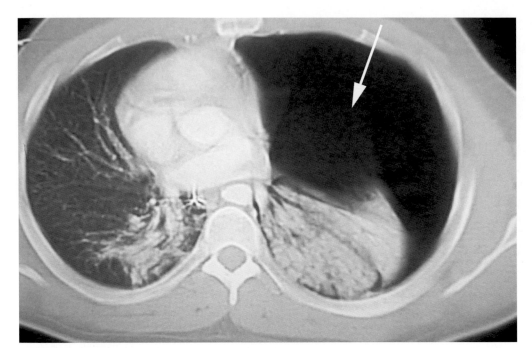

4.7C. Tension pneumothorax on CT scan.

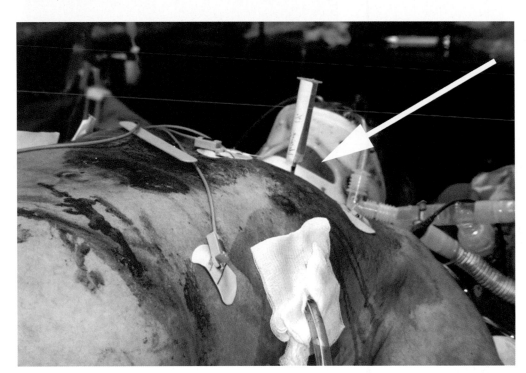

4.7D. Photograph showing a thoracostomy needle in place, below the middle of the clavicle.

4.8 Hemothorax

Commentary

A hemothorax can be due to blunt or penetrating trauma. Large hemothoraces may present with hypovolemia or dyspnea, but small hemothoraces can be asymptomatic. On physical examination, the breath sounds are diminished, there is dullness on percussion, and the affected hemithorax moves poorly. A chest x-ray, preferably in the erect position, confirms the diagnosis, although many times it cannot distinguish between a hemothorax and intrapulmonary hematoma, contusion, or atelectasis.

The treatment of significant hemothoraces is thoracostomy tube insertion through the fourth or fifth intercostal space, in the midaxillary line. A thoracotomy should be considered if the initial thoracostomy tube output exceeds 1,000–1,500 ml of blood, or if the patient is hemodynamically unstable.

Significant residual hemothorax following thoracostomy tube insertion should be evaluated by means of CT scan and evacuated within 3–5 days. Early evacuation is easy and can be performed with thoracoscopy or a small anterolateral thoracotomy. Thrombolytic agents, such as streptokinase or urokinase may be effective in some cases and should be the first line of treatment before an operative approach is attempted. Delayed evacuation is difficult because of clot organization and inflammation, and it requires a thoracotomy with decortication.

An undrained significant hemothorax is associated with increased risk of empyema and may cause respiratory compromise due to fibrosis.

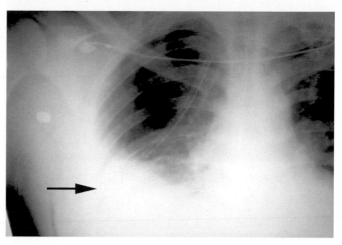

4.8B. Gunshot wound to the right chest with a suspected "residual hemothorax" on CXR two days after injury.

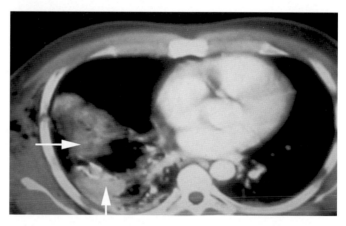

4.8C. Chest CT scan of the same patient shows intrapulmonary hematomas and parenchymal lacerations.

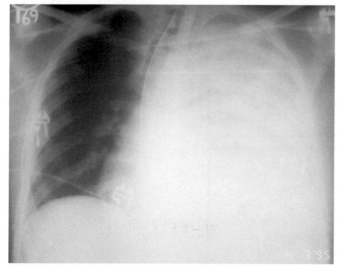

4.8A. Chest radiograph with extensive opacification of left hemithorax due to massive hemothorax with mediastinal shift to the opposite site.

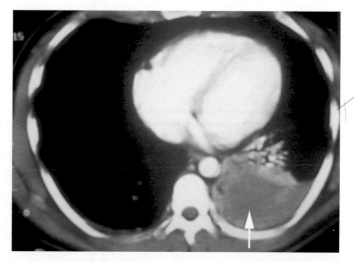

4.8D. Residual hemothorax suspected on chest radiography and confirmed by CT scan of the chest.

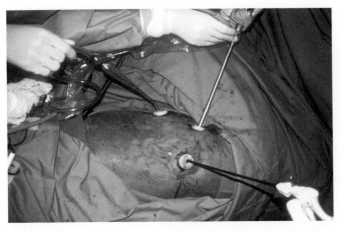

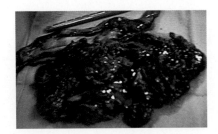

4.8F. Photograph of material removed during decortication. Delayed evacuation of a clotted hemothorax is difficult and requires thoracotomy and decortication.

4.8E. Thoracoscopy for residual hemothorax.

4.9 Thoracostomy Tube Insertion

Commentary

The site and technique of the insertion of the thoracostomy tube are the same for both hemothorax and pneumothorax. With the patient in the supine position and the arm abducted at 90 degrees, a 1.5–2 cm incision is made in the fourth to fifth intercostal space, midaxillary line. A Kelly forceps is inserted into the pleural cavity. Finger exploration should be per-formed in all patients with previous chest trauma or infection in order to evaluate for adhesions and avoid the risk of intrapulmonary placement of the tube. Standard thoracostomy tube sizes are adult male, 34–36; adult female, 32–34; newborn, 10; 4 years, 16–20; 8 years, 20–24; and 12 years, 24–28.

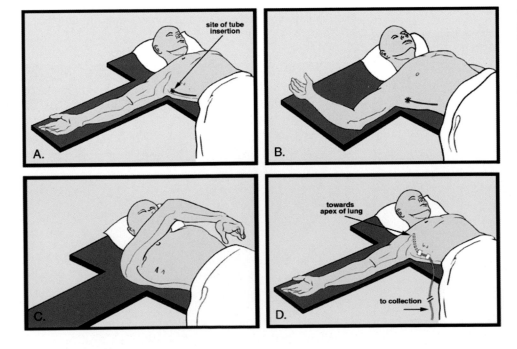

4.9A. Illustration showing the sequence of chest tube insertion: The patient is in the supine position, and the arm is abducted at 90 degrees (A or B). Abduction and internal rotation of the arm is a suboptimal position because of the interposition of the latissimus dorsi muscle. (C) The insertion site should be in the midaxillary line, fourth to fifth intercostal space. The tube is directed posteriorly toward the apex (D).

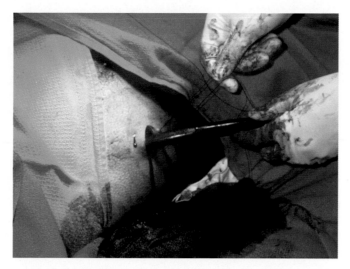

4.9B. Photograph showing thoracostomy tube being secured in place.

4.10 Autotransfusion of Blood in Chest Trauma

Commentary

Blood autotransfusion following chest trauma is easy, safe, and cheap. The system is recommended for use in all patients with suspected large hemothoraces. Anticoagulant (citrate) is advisable but not necessary.

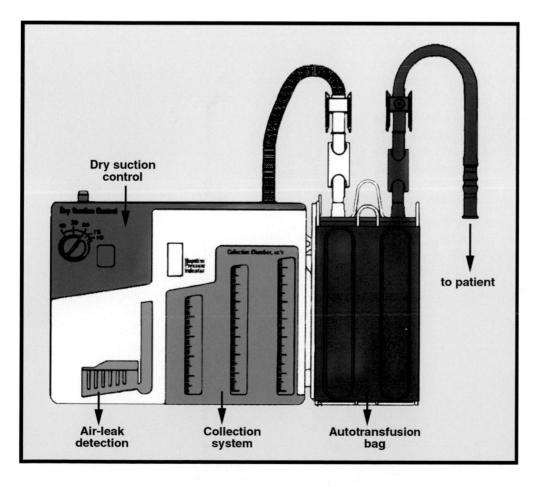

4.10A. Illustration of autotransfusion apparatus: The autotransfusion bag to the right is detachable from the rest of the system. The tube to the right (red) is connected to the thoracostomy tube, and the one to the left (black) is connected to the standard collection system. About 60 ml of citrate per 600 ml of blood may be added to the bag. When the container fills up, it is detached from the rest of the collection system and transfused through a standard blood filter. Overflowing blood is collected in the standard collection system. The next chamber has an air-escape valve with an air-leak detection system, and part of the last chamber controls negative suction.

Dry suction control

to patient

Air-leak detection

Collection system

Autotransfusion bag

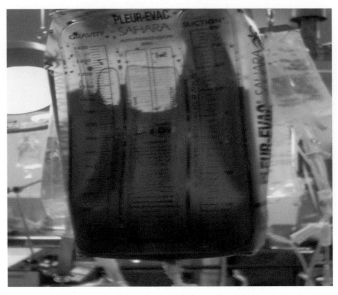

4.10B. Photograph of blood collected with the autotransfusion technique ready for transfusion.

4.11 Lung Contusion

Commentary

Lung contusion may occur after blunt trauma to the chest, rapid deceleration injuries, or gunshot wounds to the lung. Associated rib fractures are a common finding in adults but unusual in children. The symptoms vary from minor chest discomfort or hemoptysis to severe dyspnea, massive hemoptysis, and respiratory failure. The treatment is symptomatic, and mechanical ventilation may be necessary. Independent lung ventilation may be necessary in patients who do not respond to conventional ventilation.

The radiological diagnosis of a lung contusion is not always easy with plain chest radiography because it has a similar appearance to hemothorax or pneumonia. CT scan delineates lung parenchyma well and provides an accurate diagnosis.

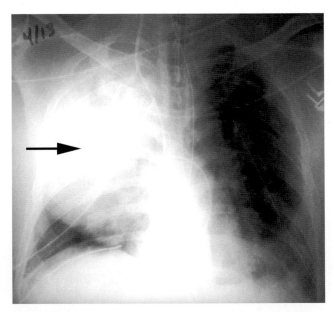

4.11A. Chest x-ray with large opacification in the right lung, highly suspicious of lung contusion.

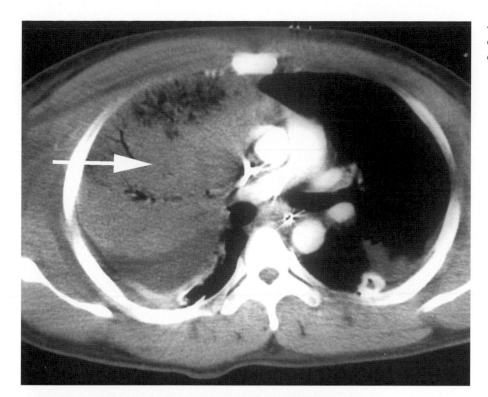

4.11B. Chest CT scan in above case confirms the presence of lung contusion.

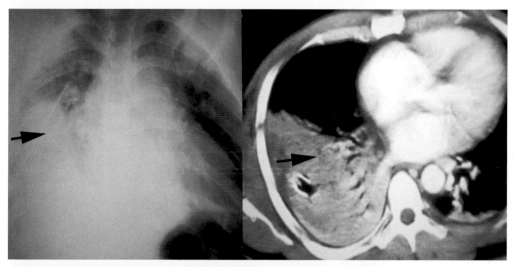

4.11C. Gunshot wound to the right chest. The chest film cannot distinguish between a hemothorax and a lung contusion. The CT scan clearly demonstrates a large contusion without any significant hemothorax.

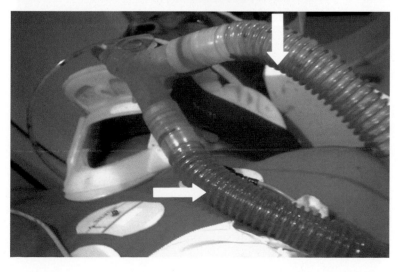

4.11D. Photograph showing bronchial bleeding in respiratory tubing in severe lung contusion.

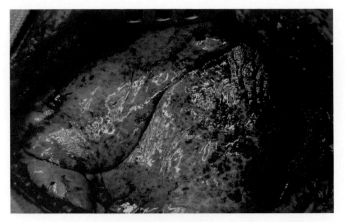

4.11E. Intraoperative photograph of a lung contusion.

4.12 Subcutaneous Emphysema

Commentary

Subcutaneous emphysema may be secondary to a pneumothorax or aerodigestive tract perforation. Inappropriately placed thoracostomy tubes with a fenestration outside the pleural cavity may also result in extensive emphysema. The first step in evaluating the cause of the emphysema is to check the position of any thoracostomy tube. For massive, unexplained emphysema, endoscopy and esophagography should be performed to evaluate the aerodigestive tract. Subcutaneous emphysema rarely causes symptoms, and the treatment is directed toward the underlying cause.

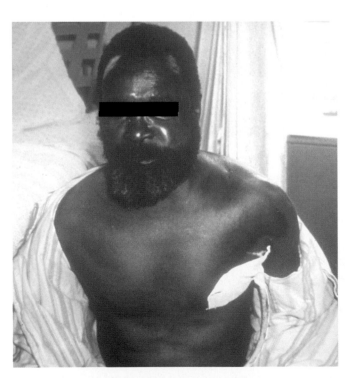

4.12A. Photograph showing extensive subcutaneous emphysema involving the chest, neck, and face.

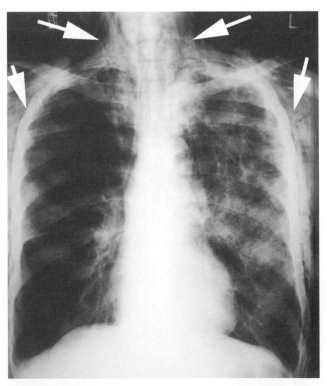

4.12B. Chest x-ray showing extensive subcutaneous emphysema.

4.13 Penetrating Cardiac Injury

Commentary

More than 80% of patients with penetrating cardiac injuries do not reach the hospital alive. For those who reach the hospital alive, early diagnosis and operation are critical factors for survival.

Clinically the patient is restless, and the inexperienced physician often mistakes it for alcohol or drug intoxication. The victim is almost always in shock, although in cases with small cardiac wounds and short prehospital times, the initial blood pressure may be normal. Beck's triad (hypotension, distant cardiac sounds, distended neck veins) is found in about 90% of cases with tamponade.

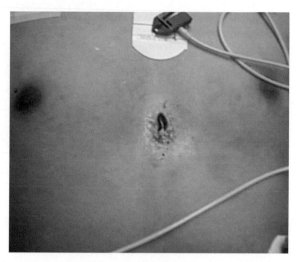

4.13A. Photograph of a precordial penetrating wound with injury to the right ventricle of the heart. Every penetrating trauma to the chest, especially in the presence of hypotension, should be considered a cardiac injury until proven otherwise.

4.14 Mechanisms of Penetrating Cardiac Injury

Commentary

Stab wounds usually involve the right ventricle, and the prognosis is fairly good, with a hospital survival of about 65%. Bullet injuries usually involve multiple cardiac chambers and the prognosis is poor, with an overall hospital survival of about 15%. High-velocity bullets cause massive injury and are always fatal.

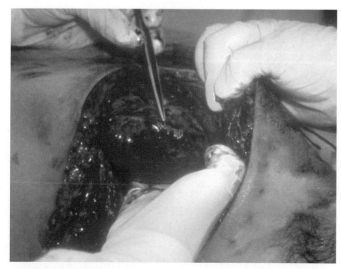

4.14A. Photograph of a stab wound to the heart (stapled during an emergency department thoracotomy).

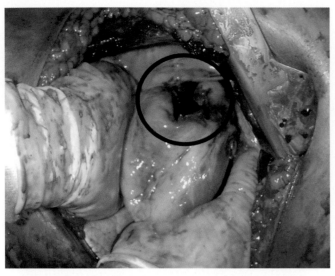

4.14B. Photograph of a low-velocity bullet injury to the heart.

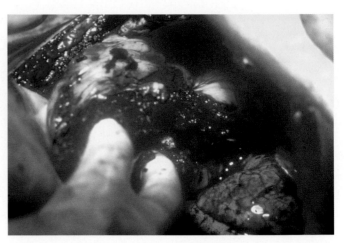

4.14D. Photograph of a massive trauma to the heart from a high-velocity bullet injury.

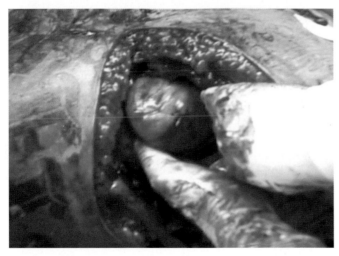

4.14C. Photograph of a low-velocity bullet injury to the heart.

4.15 Survival Factors in Penetrating Cardiac Injuries

Commentary

The outcome of penetrating cardiac trauma depends on many factors: Short prehospital times, an experienced trauma team, low-velocity injuries, right ventricular injuries, and the presence of cardiac tamponade are favorable factors for survival.

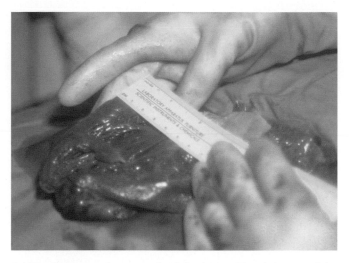

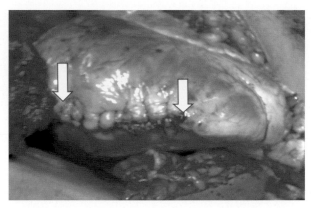

4.15B. Photograph of the heart during thoracotomy with repair of a 6-cm-long laceration following a gunshot wound. Such injuries are usually fatal.

4.15A. Autopsy photograph of the heart. The right ventricle has a relatively thick wall (4 mm) with relatively low pressures. This is an optimal combination for survival. The left ventricle has a thick wall (12 mm) but high pressures, which result in a tense tamponade or rapid exsanguination, and thus the prognosis is poor.

4.16 Diagnosis of Cardiac Injury

Commentary

The diagnosis of penetrating cardiac injury is usually clinical and can be confirmed by trauma ultrasound performed in the emergency department by emergency physicians or surgeons, and thus it should be part of the standard primary survey. A chest film may be helpful in about half the cases with cardiac trauma. Radiological signs suggestive of cardiac trauma include an enlarged cardiac shadow, a widened upper mediastinum (due to a dilated superior vena cava), and pneumopericardium.

An ECG may be diagnostic in about 30% of cases. It may show low-voltage QRS complexes, elevated ST segments, inverted T waves, electrical alternans, and other nonspecific findings. Subxiphoid windows are major invasive procedures and have a diminished role, and pericardiocentesis has almost no role in a modern trauma center. The blood in the pericardial sac usually clots, and this results in high incidence of false-negative pericardiocentesis.

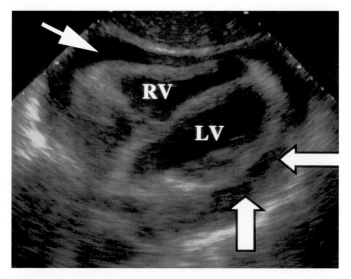

4.16A. Trauma ultrasound showing a circumferential pericardial effusion.

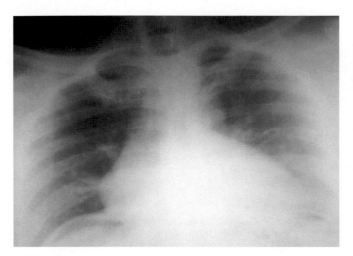

4.16B. Chest x-ray showing enlargement of the cardiac shadow suggestive of cardiac tamponade. Free air is also noted below the diaphragm bilaterally.

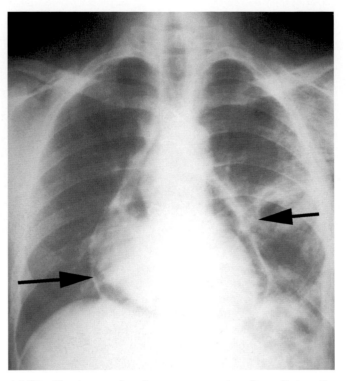

4.16D. Chest x-ray showing pneumopericardium diagnostic of pericardial violation.

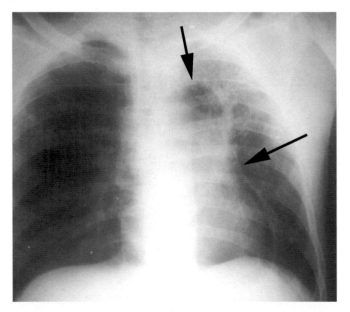

4.16C. Chest x-ray showing a widened upper mediastinum and pneumopericardium suggestive of cardiac tamponade.

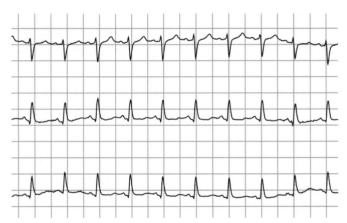

4.16E. ECG with sinus tachycardia and low-voltage QRS complexes suggestive of cardiac tamponade.

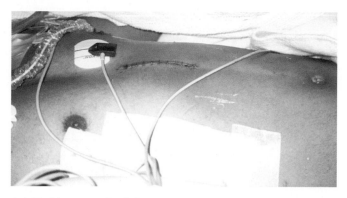

4.16F. Photograph of the incision for subxiphoid window.

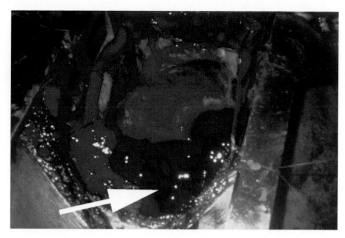

4.16G. Photograph of a clot within the pericardial sac. A pericardiocentesis would have been falsely negative.

4.17 Retained Cardiac Missiles

Commentary

The diagnosis of retained cardiac missile is suspected on the chest x-ray and confirmed by echocardiogram or CT scan. All missiles diagnosed at the acute stage should be removed because of the risk of delayed hemorrhage, embolization, false aneurysm, and endocarditis. Retained missiles that have been diagnosed long after the injury and are asymptomatic do not need removal.

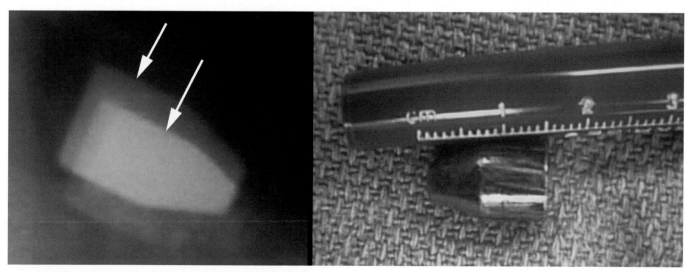

4.17A. Chest x-ray of a retained bullet. The double shadow of the bullet is due to movement of the heart and is diagnostic of contact with the beating heart (left side). Removed bullet postoperatively (right side).

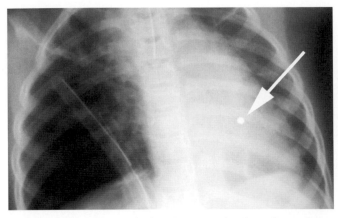

4.17B. Chest radiograph showing a retained cardiac pellet.

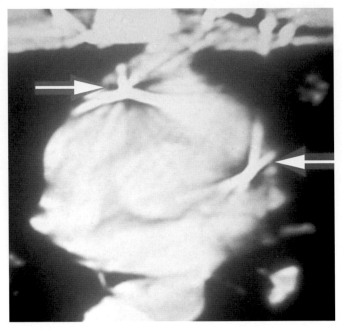

4.17C. Chest CT scan showing two pellets in the myocardium.

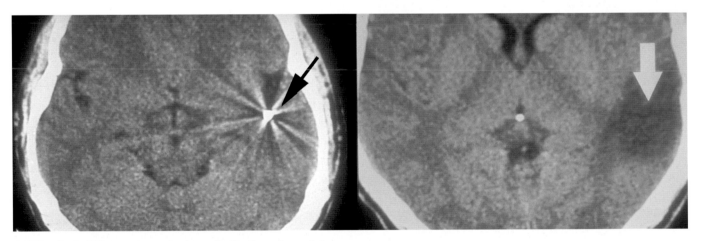

4.17D. Brain CT scan shows brain embolization of a pellet and anemic infarction following a shotgun injury to the heart.

4.18 Emergency Department Thoracotomy for Cardiac Trauma

Commentary

Patients with cardiac arrest or imminent cardiac arrest in the emergency department should be managed with an immediate left anterolateral thoracotomy. The pericardium is opened longitudinally to avoid injury to the phrenic nerve, and the clot is evacuated. The cardiac wound is repaired by suturing or stapling. A

Foley catheter balloon may be useful in achieving temporary control of bleeding. In the presence of cardiac arrest, the aorta is cross-clamped just above the diaphragm, and direct cardiac massage is performed. Adrenaline or defibrillation may be administered when the heart is full, and their use in an empty heart reduces the chances of successful resuscitation. Internal cardiac pacing may be useful in cases that do not respond to conventional treatment. If cardiac activity returns, the operation is completed in the operating room. The survival rate for emergency department thoracotomy is about 10%.

Indications of emergency department thoracotomy include cardiac arrest or imminent cardiac arrest due to both penetrating and blunt trauma, excluding fatal head injuries. Some of the survivors suffer brain death, but they may become useful organ donors.

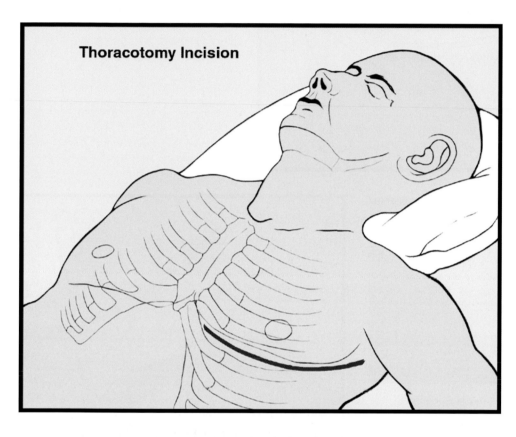

4.18A. Illustration of the incision for an emergency department left anterolateral thoracotomy.

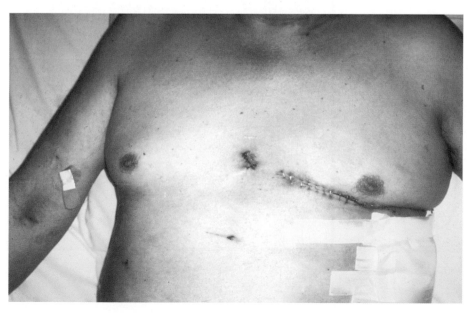

4.18B. Photograph of a healing emergency department thoracotomy incision just below the nipple.

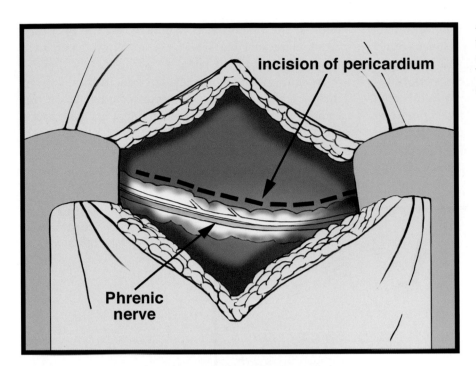

4.18C. Illustration of the pericardium at thoracotomy. The phrenic nerve is seen on the lateral aspect of the pericardium. The pericardium should be opened above the nerve.

incision of pericardium

Phrenic nerve

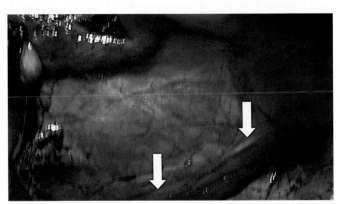

4.18D. Thoracotomy photograph of the phrenic nerve.

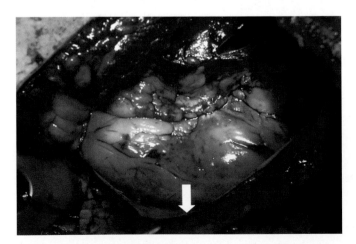

4.18E. Photograph at thoracotomy. The pericardium is opened and the heart exposed.

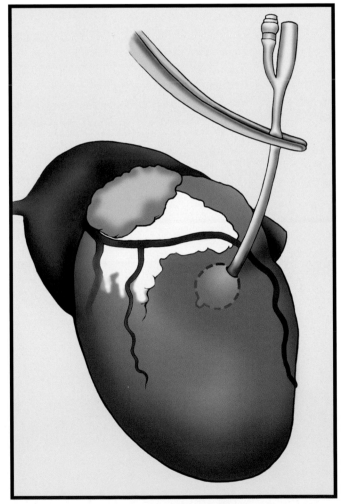

4.18F. Illustration of Foley tamponade in the heart. Inflated Foley catheter balloon may provide temporary bleeding control of a penetrating wound.

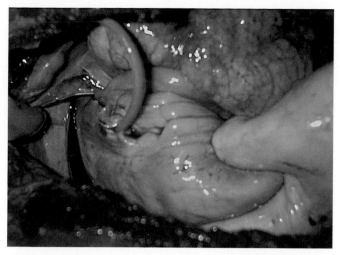

4.18G. Photograph of Foley inflation and occlusion of a cardiac wound.

4.18H. Photograph of a cross-clamping of the aorta.

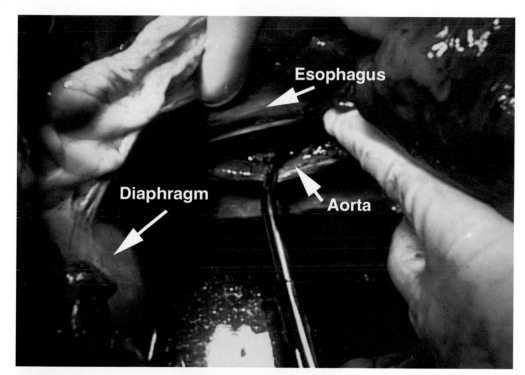

Esophagus

Diaphragm

Aorta

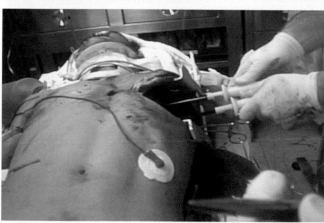

4.18I. Photograph of internal cardiac defibrillation.

4.19 Late Sequelae of Penetrating Cardiac Injuries

Commentary

Late post-traumatic cardiac sequelae include anatomical defects (pericardial effusion, atrial or ventricular septal defects, valvular or papillary muscle lesions) and functional abnormalities (dyskinesia, hypokinesia). All survivors should be evaluated early and late postoperatively, clinically and by means of ECG and echocardiography. Many abnormalities may not manifest early, and a late cardiac evaluation performed about one month postinjury is essential.

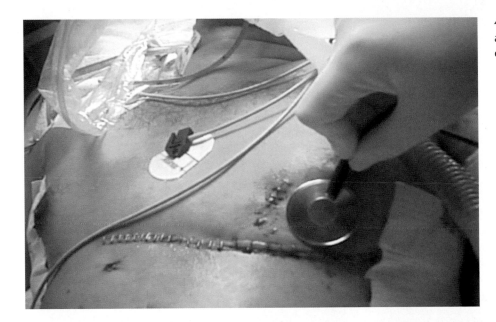

4.19A. Postcardiac repair clinical auscultation examination reveals a cardiac murmur.

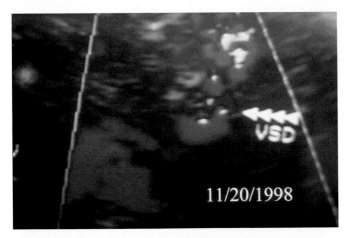

4.19B. Echocardiogram demonstrates a ventricular septal defect (VSD).

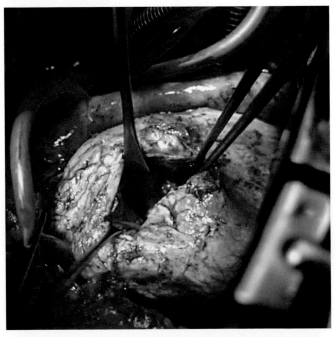

4.19C. Intraoperative photograph of a post-traumatic VSD.

4.20 Blunt Cardiac Trauma

Commentary

There are no uniform criteria for the diagnosis of blunt cardiac trauma. Many patients are asymptomatic with only ECG changes or cardiac enzyme or troponin elevations. Others may present with tachycardia, arrhythmia, or cardiogenic shock. All patients with a suspicious mechanism of injury or fractured sternum or anterior ribs should have routine ECG, troponin levels, and a trauma echocardiogram performed. If these tests are normal, no further investigation is needed. If the ECG is abnormal or the troponin levels are elevated, the patient should be monitored closely and evaluated with formal echocardiogram. Symptomatic patients may need inotropes or antiarrhythmic treatment. Cardiac rupture may result from major anteroposterior chest compression, rapid deceleration, perforation by fractured ribs or sternum, or massive sudden crushing forces on the abdomen. Patients with blunt cardiac rupture rarely reach the hospital alive. These patients are in severe shock, and the diagnosis can be confirmed by trauma ultrasound or during an emergency department thoracotomy. Most ruptures involve the right heart. In these cases, immediate thoracotomy with cardiac repair should be performed.

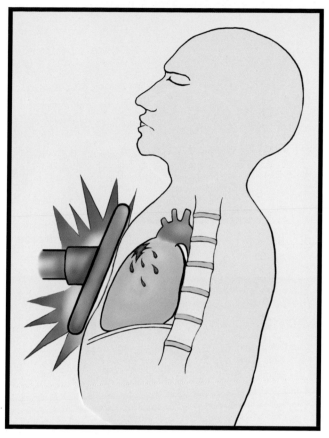

4.20B. Illustration of the mechanism of blunt cardiac injury from steering wheel trauma.

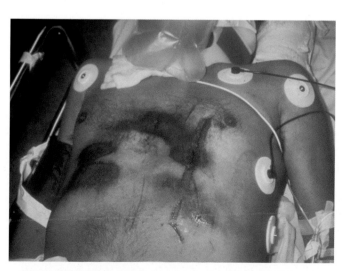

4.20A. Photograph of blunt chest trauma to the anterior chest from a steering wheel injury. This patient arrived in ventricular tachycardia.

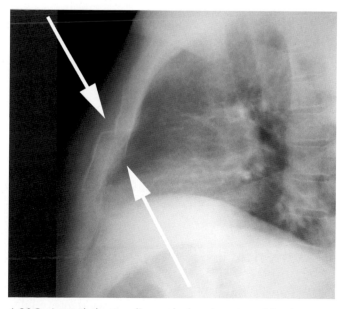

4.20C. Lateral chest radiograph showing sternal fracture. Blunt trauma with sternal fracture is often associated with cardiac trauma. These patients should be evaluated by ECG and troponin levels.

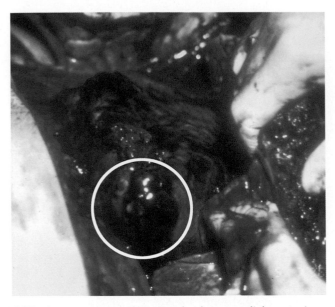

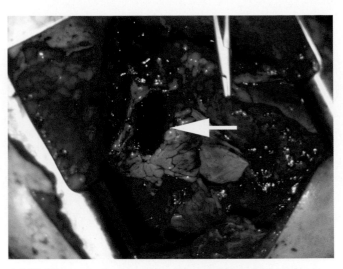

4.20F. Photograph of cardiac rupture (right atrium) due to blunt trauma.

4.20D. Intraoperative photograph of myocardial contusion.

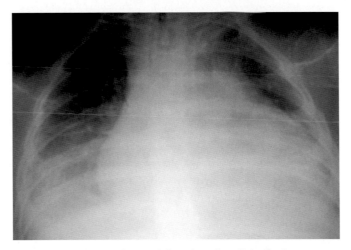

4.20E. Chest x-ray shows delayed pericardial effusion following myocardial contusion.

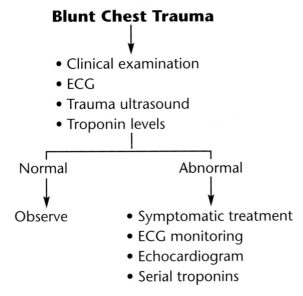

Blunt Chest Trauma

↓

- Clinical examination
- ECG
- Trauma ultrasound
- Troponin levels

Normal → Observe

Abnormal →
- Symptomatic treatment
- ECG monitoring
- Echocardiogram
- Serial troponins

4.20G. Algorithm for the evaluation of suspected cardiac trauma.

4.21 Blunt Thoracic Aortic Injury

Commentary

Blunt thoracic aortic injury usually occurs after deceleration injuries, such as high-speed traffic accidents or falls from heights. In about 93% of cases, the rupture occurs just distal to the left subclavian artery and in about 7% the rupture occurs in the ascending aorta. Most of the victims die at the scene, with only about 15% reaching the hospital alive. The diagnosis is based on the history of the injury and suspicious chest x-ray findings. Radiological findings suggestive of aortic rupture include a widened mediastinum, left apical pleural cap, obliteration of the aortic knob, and deviation of the nasogastric tube or the left main bronchus to the right. However, in many cases of aortic rupture, the chest x-ray may be normal. All patients with a suspicious mechanism of injury should be evaluated by means of helical CT scan after stabilization. Aortography should be reserved for patients requiring angiography for another reason (e.g., pelvic fracture) or cases when the CT scan is not definitive. The treatment of aortic rupture is surgical repair. While preparing for the operation, the systolic blood pressure should be kept low, at 90–100 mm Hg. Nitroprusside or beta-blockers should be used for this purpose. Angiographically placed stents may be used in poor-risk patients. There is some evidence that multi-trauma elderly patients with minor aortic injuries can safely be managed nonoperatively.

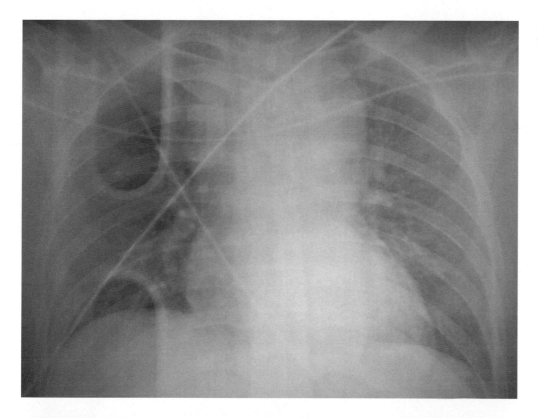

4.21A. Chest x-ray shows a widened mediastinum.

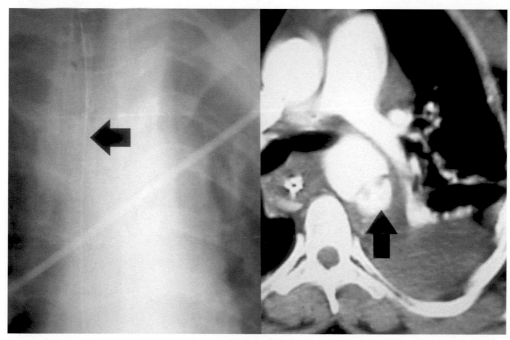

4.21B. Chest x-ray shows a widened mediastinum with deviation of the nasogastric tube (left side), and helical CT scan confirms aortic rupture (right side).

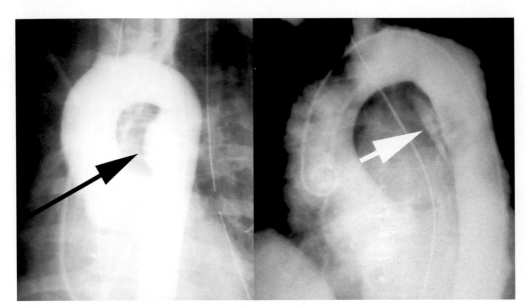

4.21C. Aortograms of traumatic aortic ruptures.

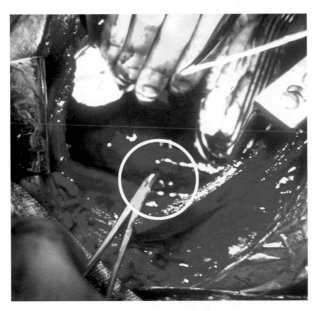

4.21D. Intraoperative photograph of aortic rupture with a large hematoma, distal to the left subclavian artery.

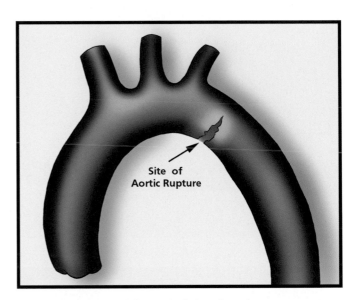

4.21E. Illustration of the typical site of aortic rupture.

Site of
Aortic Rupture

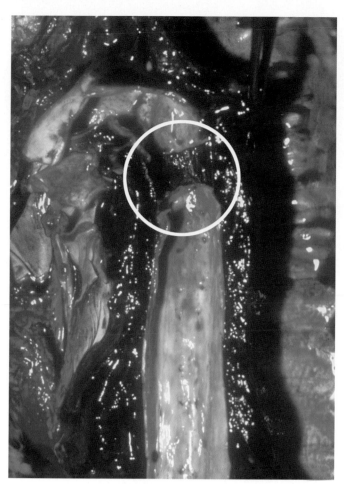

4.21F. Autopsy photograph of aortic rupture illustrating classic rupture site and hematoma.

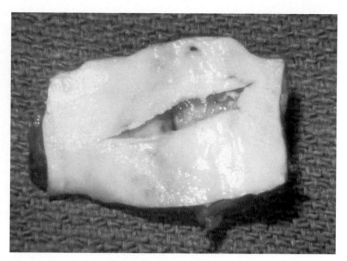

4.21G. Operative photograph of contained aortic rupture.

4.22 Penetrating Thoracic Outlet Injuries

Commentary

The most important structures of the thoracic outlet are the aortic arch with its major branches (innominate artery, origin of left carotid artery, and left subclavian artery), the superior vena cava, the innominate vein, and the subclavian veins.

Hemodynamically stable patients with penetrating injuries in this anatomical area should be investigated for vascular injuries. Color flow Doppler is an excellent investigation for suspected subclavian vascular injuries. Angiography should be reserved for cases when the color flow Doppler evaluation is not definitive or endovascular stent is a possibility. Injuries to the branches of the aortic arch require surgical repair, though angiographically placed endovascular stents can be used in selected cases.

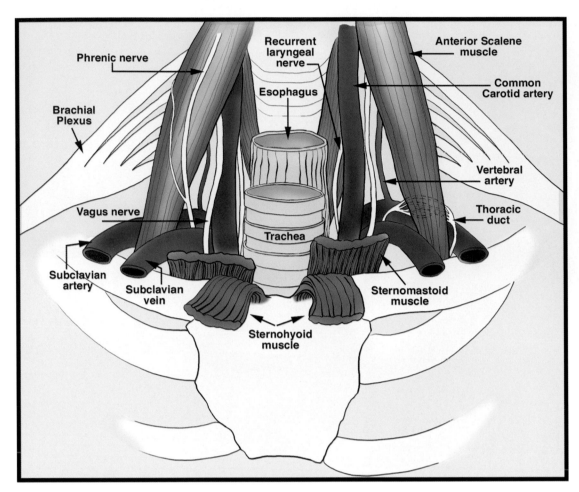

4.22A. Illustration of the anatomy of vital structures in the thoracic outlet.

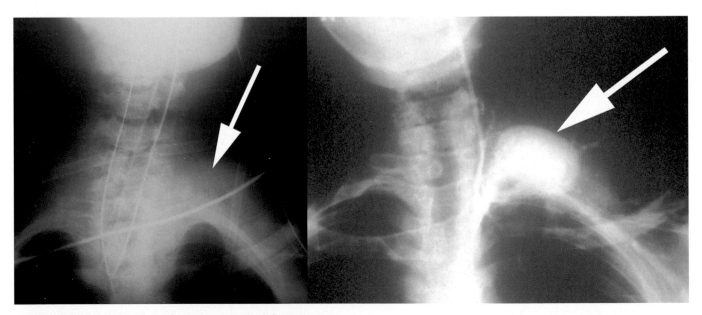

4.22B. Chest x-ray showing a hematoma in the left upper mediastinum suggestive of significant vascular injury (left side). Clinically the hematoma was pulsating. Arteriography shows a false aneurysm of the left subclavian artery (right side).

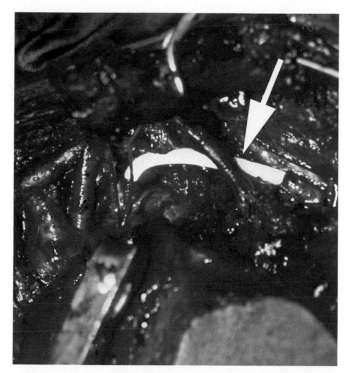

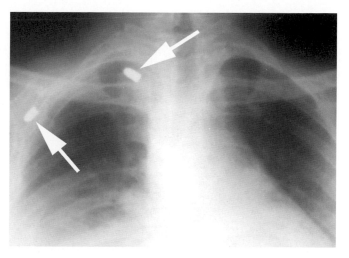

4.22D. CXR of a patient with two gunshot wounds in the right clavicular region who presented with hard signs of vascular injury, including a decreased peripheral pulse and a bruit below the clavicle.

4.22C. Photograph of the same patient showing operative repair of the left subclavian artery with prosthetic graft.

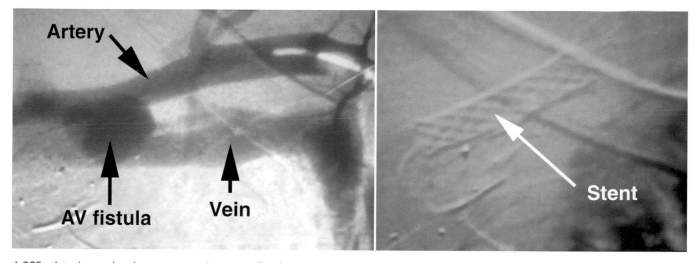

4.22E. Arteriography shows an arteriovenous fistula between the subclavian artery and vein. Right image shows successful angiographic stenting of the lesion.

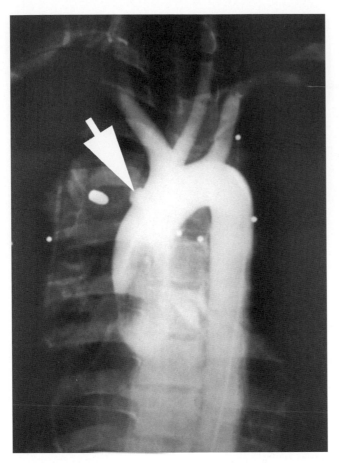

4.22F. Gunshot wound of the upper mediastinum. Aortography shows a small aneurysm of the ascending aorta.

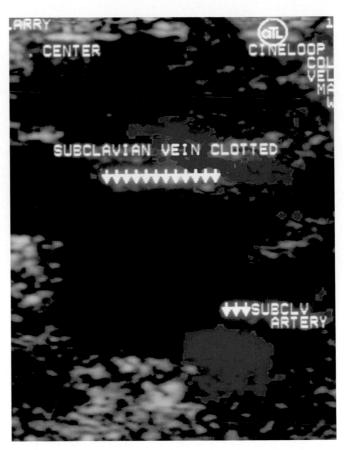

4.22G. Color flow Doppler showing thrombosis of the subclavian vein.

4.23 Transmediastinal Gunshot Wounds

Commentary

Transmediastinal gunshot wounds are associated with a high incidence of major injuries to mediastinal structures. Hemodynamically unstable patients should have an emergency operation. About 70% of hemodynamically stable patients do not have significant injuries. These patients need evaluation of the mediastinal structures (heart, aorta, esophagus, tracheobronchial tree). Besides the routine trauma ultrasound and ECG for the evaluation of the heart, aortography and esophagography/esophagoscopy are extensively used. Chest CT scan may be used to select patients who might benefit from aortography or esophageal studies. Patients with bullet tracks toward the aorta or the esophagus are candidates for further studies.

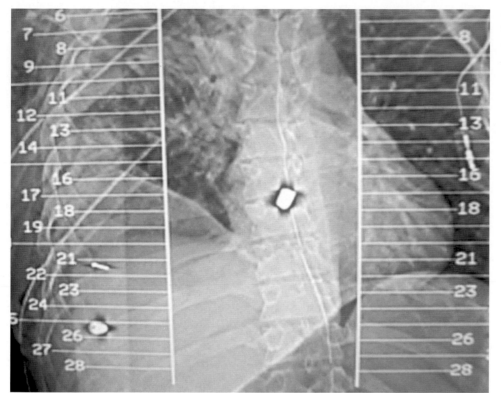

4.23A. Chest x-ray of a patient with a gunshot wound to the chest. The bullet entry is in the right lateral chest, and the missile is located in the mediastinum.

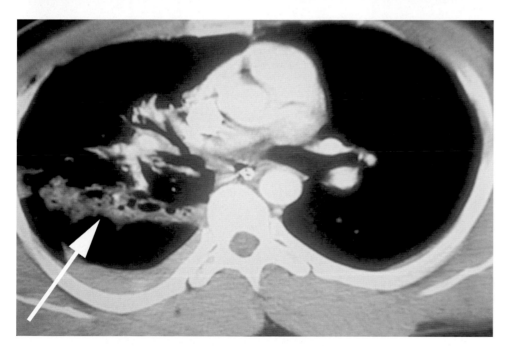

4.23B. The mediastinal CT scan shows a bullet track away from major mediastinal structures (aorta, esophagus). There is no need for further investigations.

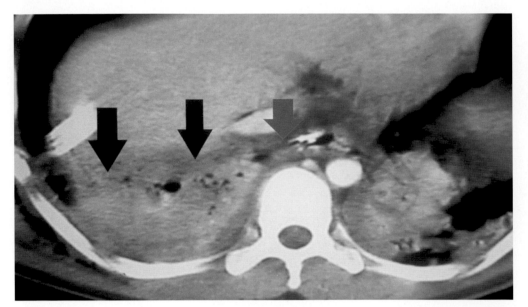

4.23C. Mediastinal gunshot wound. The CT scan shows a bullet track near the esophagus. This patient required further esophageal evaluation, and the esophagogram showed an esophageal leak.

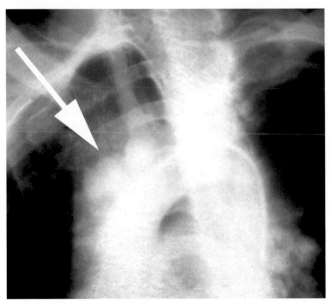

4.23D. Angiogram showing innominate arteriovenous fistula following a transmediastinal gunshot wound.

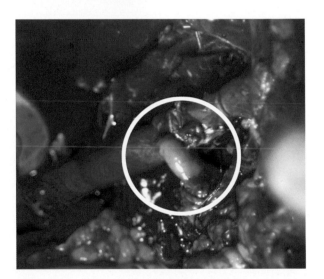

4.23E. Photograph of a gunshot wound to the descending thoracic aorta.

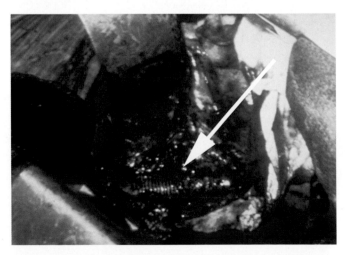

4.23F. Intraoperative photograph showing repair of thoracic aorta with prosthetic graft.

4.24 Penetrating Diaphragmatic Injuries

Commentary

About 60% of all gunshot wounds and 30% of all stab wounds to the left thoracoabdominal area (the area between the nipple and costal margin anteriorly and the tip of the scapula and lower ribs posteriorly) are associated with diaphragmatic injuries. About 13% of gunshot wounds and 26% of stab wounds to this area with no abdominal symptoms have diaphragmatic injuries. Unrecognized diaphragmatic injuries may result in diaphragmatic hernias that may manifest long after the injury. To prevent late diaphragmatic hernias, early diagnosis and repair of left diaphragmatic perforations is essential. Right diaphragmatic injuries, with the exception of anterior injuries, rarely result in hernias because of the protective presence of the liver.

The diagnosis of penetrating diaphragmatic injury should be suspected from the presence of a wound over the thoracoabdominal area. The chest x-ray is normal in the majority of patients with uncomplicated diaphragmatic perforations. An elevated hemidiaphragm is suspicious but not diagnostic of diaphragmatic injury. (Conditions that may be associated with an elevated diaphragm include atelectasis, hepatic or splenic hematoma, gastric dilatation, fractures of the lower ribs, and phrenic nerve injury.) CT scan and MRI are usually not diagnostic in small, uncomplicated diaphragmatic injuries. The most reliable way to diagnose uncomplicated diaphragmatic injuries is routine laparoscopy for all asymptomatic patients with suspicious penetrating wounds in the left thoracoabdominal or anterior right thoracoabdominal regions. In the presence of a diaphragmatic hernia, the chest x-ray, CT scan, or MRI is diagnostic or highly suggestive.

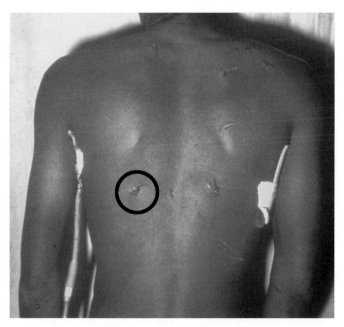

4.24A. Photograph of stab wounds to the back. Penetrating trauma to the left lower chest is highly suspicious for diaphragmatic injury requiring surgical repair.

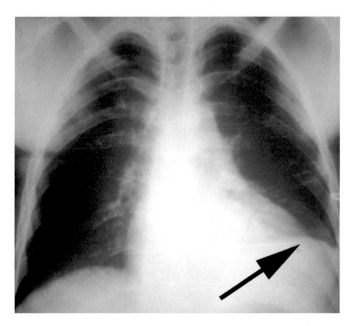

4.24B. Chest x-ray shows an elevated left diaphragm, which is suspicious for diaphragmatic injury.

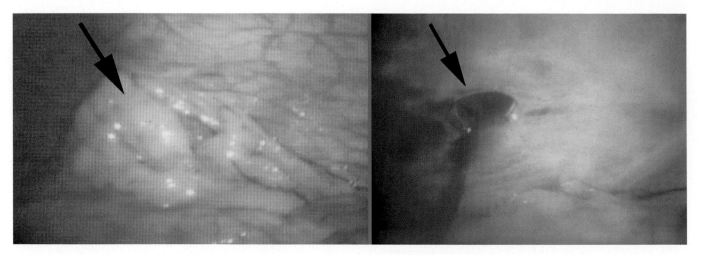

4.24C. Laparoscopy shows a diaphragmatic perforation with omentum herniating through it (left side) and diaphragmatic tear after reduction of the herniating omentum (right side).

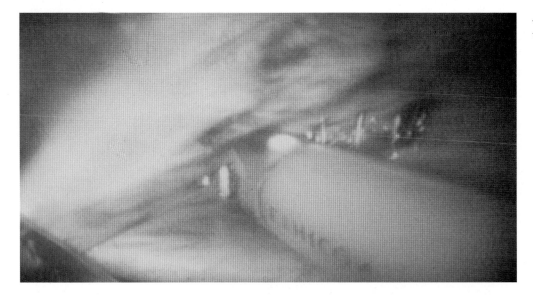

4.24D. Laparoscopic repair of the diaphragmatic injury.

4.25 Blunt Diaphragmatic Injuries

Commentary

Rupture of the diaphragm is found in about 7% of all laparotomies for blunt trauma. The left diaphragm is involved in about 70% of the cases and the right diaphragm in about 30%. In 3% of cases, both diaphragms are ruptured. The tear is about 7–10 cm long as compared with 2–3 cm in penetrating trauma. Blunt abdominal trauma with a sudden increase of the intra-abdominal pressure (usually in belted car occupants) is the most common mechanism of diaphragmatic rupture, though fractured ribs may also cause tears. Deceleration injuries may cause detachment of the diaphragm from the ribs.

The chest x-ray, CT scan, or MRI are usually more diagnostic than in penetrating trauma because of the large size of the diaphragmatic tear in blunt trauma. In most patients there are major associated intra-abdominal injuries, and the diagnosis of diaphragmatic injuries is made intraoperatively. However, in many cases there is no associated abdominal trauma, and in the absence of herniation the diagnosis of diaphragmatic tear may be missed. Laparoscopy in suspected cases remains the most reliable investigation.

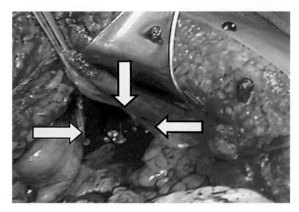

4.25A. Emergency department thoracotomy following a traffic accident. Photograph of left diaphragmatic rupture with cardiac rupture and omentum, stomach, and colon in the chest.

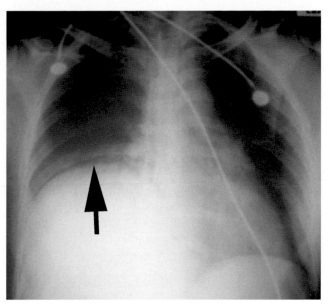

4.25C. Chest x-ray of a traffic accident victim shows an elevated right diaphragm.

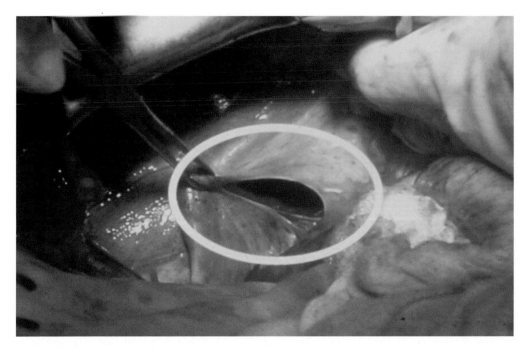

4.25B. Photograph of blunt diaphragm injury at laparotomy.

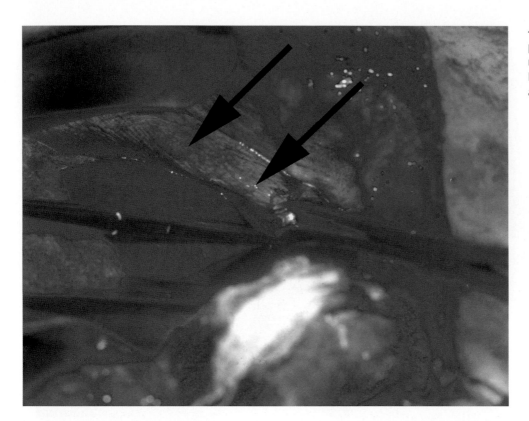

4.25D. Intraoperative photograph shows there was rupture of the right diaphragm. Note lung protruding through a large diaphragmatic tear.

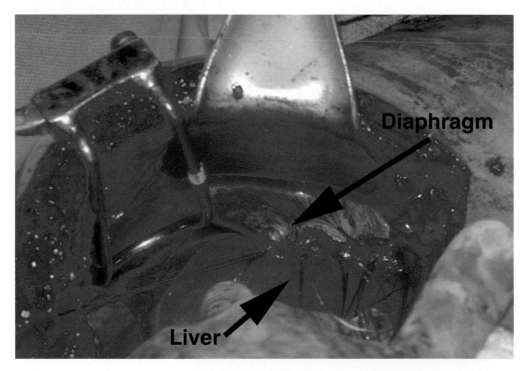

4.25E. Intraoperative photograph shows repair of the same rupture with heavy suture.

Diaphragm

Liver

4.26 Traumatic Diaphragmatic Hernias

Commentary

Traumatic diaphragmatic hernias may appear within minutes, hours, days, weeks, or many years after injury to the diaphragm. In the vast majority of cases, the hernia is found in the left hemidiaphragm, although right diaphragmatic hernias may occur as well. The most commonly herniating viscera are the omentum, stomach, and colon, followed by spleen, small bowel, liver, and tail of pancreas.

Many hernias remain asymptomatic and are discovered during routine chest x-rays. Other patients present with signs of gastrointestinal obstruction, respiratory distress, and sepsis due to a gangrenous viscus. The diagnosis is suspected from the chest x-ray and history of previous trauma and confirmed by CT scan, MRI, or contrast studies. A nasogastric tube may be seen curling into the left chest on x-ray and is pathognomonic of gastric herniation. The radiological appearance of a diaphragmatic hernia may be confused with many other pathologies such as lung laceration, bronchopneumonia, residual hemothorax, phrenic nerve injury, intrapulmonary abscess, and diaphragmatic eventration. The history of trauma and high index of suspicion remain the cornerstone of early diagnosis. Delayed diagnosis of a complicated diaphragmatic hernia

(obstruction, ischemia or necrosis, or cardiorespiratory complication due to compression) is associated with high mortality. All diaphragmatic hernias require surgical repair through a laparotomy or laparoscopically.

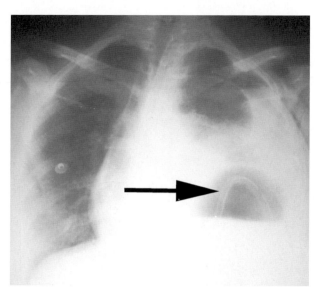

4.26B. Chest x-ray shows the nasogastric tube curling into the left chest, pathognomonic of gastric herniation.

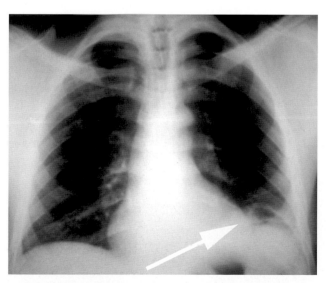

4.26A. Chest x-ray with a suspicious shadow at the base of the left hemithorax, following a stab wound many months earlier. Further investigations showed gastric herniation into the chest.

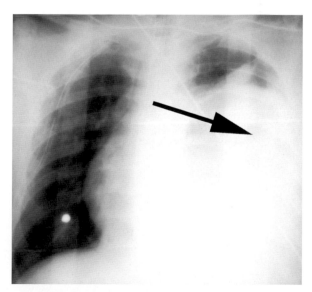

4.26C. Chest x-ray shows a tension diaphragmatic hernia a few weeks after a stab wound to the left lower chest. At operation, the stomach, spleen, and colon were found in the chest.

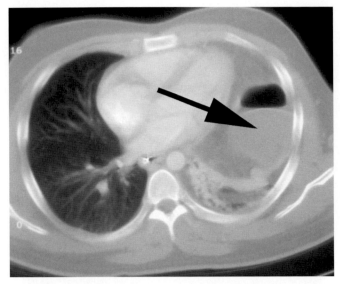

4.26D. CT scan with colon in the chest.

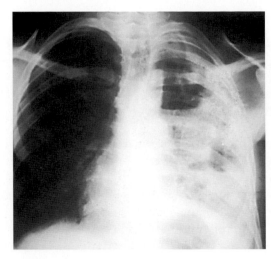

4.26G. Chest x-ray of a large diaphragmatic hernia containing stomach, colon, and small bowel, initially diagnosed as bronchopneumonia.

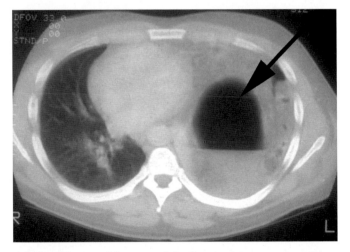

4.26E. CT scan with stomach in the chest many years after a car accident.

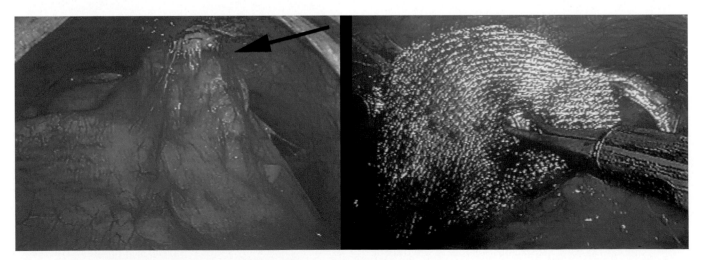

4.26F. Laparoscopic appearance of the stomach and omentum herniating into the chest (left side) and successful repair with a mesh (right side).

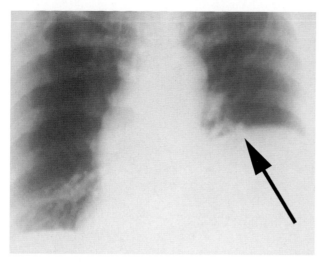

4.26H. Chest x-ray of a patient with diaphragmatic eventration. The differential diagnosis from a diaphragmatic hernia is difficult and can be done only with laparoscopy.

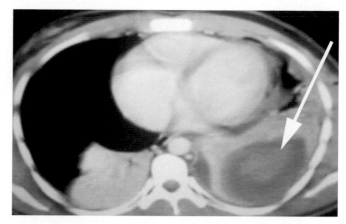

4.26I. CT scan of a post-traumatic infected pulmonary hematoma, which may be confused with a diaphragmatic hernia.

4.27 Esophageal Injuries

Commentary

Esophageal injuries should be suspected in all penetrating proximity injuries, especially if the x-ray shows mediastinal or subcutaneous emphysema in the neck. In suspected cases, esophagography and/or esophagoscopy should be performed. The combination of both investigations is highly sensitive in the identification of esophageal injuries. Early diagnosis and surgical repair are critical for good outcome. Delayed diagnosis is associated with a high incidence of sepsis and mortality.

4.27A. Penetrating upper mediastinal injury with extensive neck and mediastinal emphysema. Gastrograffin swallow shows an esophageal perforation.

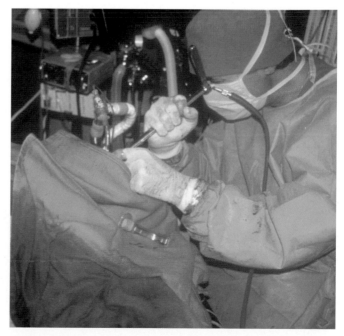

4.27B. Photograph of rigid esophagoscopy for suspected esophageal injury.

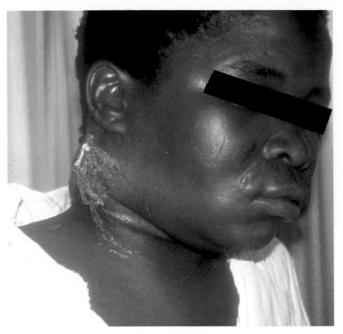

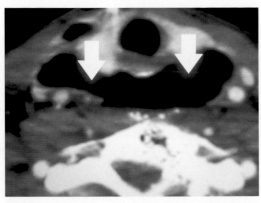

4.27D. CT scan demonstrates a large neck abscess.

4.27C. Photograph of a neck abscess following missed cervical esophageal injury.

4.28 Thoracic Duct Injury

Commentary

Rupture of the thoracic duct is usually due to penetrating trauma and rarely due to blunt deceleration trauma. The diagnosis should be suspected in the presence of milky fluid in the pleural cavities. Sometimes in patients who did not receive any oral feeding for a few days, the fluid may be clear or blood-stained. The diagnosis is confirmed by the presence of many lymphocytes and the high concentration of lipids in the fluid.

Most thoracic duct leaks heal nonoperatively with a low-fat oral diet or TPN. In patients with high output (more than 500 ml per day) persisting for more than 2–3 weeks without any sign of improvement, a thoracotomy or thoracoscopy with thoracic duct ligation may be necessary.

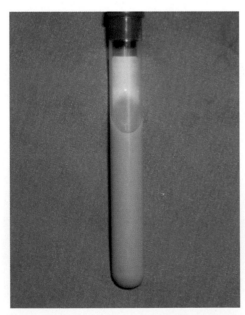

4.28A. Photograph of chylothorax following penetrating chest trauma. Note the milky appearance of the thoracic collection.

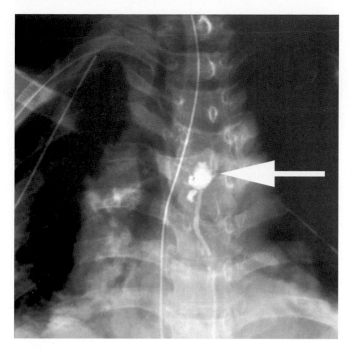

4.28B. Lymphangiogram shows a significant leak from the thoracic duct.

4.29 Traumatic Asphyxia

Commentary

Traumatic asphyxia is the result of severe crush injury to the chest. Because of the sudden increase of pressure in the venous and capillary systems, the victim develops extensive petechiae in the skin and conjunctivae. Similar microhemorrhages may develop in the brain and lungs, and the patient may present with central nervous or respiratory problems. The treatment is symptomatic.

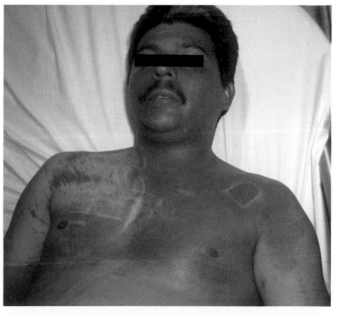

4.29A. Photograph of a patient with crush trauma to the chest and traumatic asphyxia. Note the extensive petechiae on the face and chest.

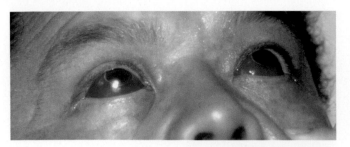
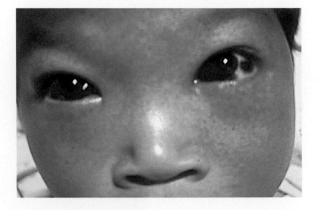

4.29B and C. Photographs of extensive petechiae on the face and conjunctival hemorrhages in an adult and a child with traumatic asphyxia.

5 Abdominal Injury

Blunt Abdominal Trauma

Introduction

Traffic accidents, followed by falls, are by far the most common causes of severe blunt abdominal trauma. Solid organs, usually the spleen and liver, are the most commonly injured organs. Hollow viscus perforations are fairly uncommon, and they are usually associated with seatbelts or high-speed deceleration.

There are five main mechanisms of injury with blunt trauma:

1. Direct crushing of organs between the anterior and posterior abdominal walls.

2. Avulsion injuries from deceleration forces, as in high-speed accidents or falls from heights.

3. Transient formation of closed bowel loop with high intraluminal pressure and rupture of the hollow viscus.

4. Lacerations by bony fragments (e.g., pelvis, lower ribs).

5. Sudden and massive elevation of the intra-abdominal pressure (usually seatbelted individuals involved in high-speed accidents) may cause diaphragmatic or even cardiac rupture.

Clinical Examination

The clinical evaluation of blunt abdominal trauma is often complicated by associated soft tissue contusion, fractures of the lower ribs or pelvis, head injuries with depressed level of consciousness, and spinal injuries. These conditions make clinical examination difficult and unreliable, and significant hollow viscus injuries may be missed with potentially lethal consequences. Most preventable deaths due to trauma are the result of delayed diagnosis of intra-abdominal injuries. Despite its limitations, physical examination remains the cornerstone of abdominal evaluation. Of particular importance is the "seatbelt sign" on the abdominal wall. Its presence is associated with a high incidence (about 20%) of significant intra-abdominal injuries.

Investigations

1. Chest and pelvic x-rays should be obtained in all major trauma cases. Thoracic trauma is a commonly associated problem. Fractures of the lower ribs, an elevated diaphragm, and free intraperitoneal air are important radiological signs suggestive of intra-abdominal trauma.

2. Trauma ultrasound: Portable ultrasound or bedside ultrasound has become one of the most valuable emergency department investigations in the evaluation of abdominal trauma or the multitrauma patient. The ultrasound should be performed by emergency physicians or trauma surgeons. The study determines the presence or absence of free intraperitoneal fluid, mainly in the hepatorenal, splenorenal, and suprapubic spaces. It is quick, noninvasive, safe, portable, and accurate. Its most important weaknesses are the inability to identify the source of free intraperitoneal fluid or to detect injuries to the bowel, retroperitoneum, and diaphragm. The presence of free fluid on ultrasound in a hemodynamically unstable patient is an indication for urgent laparotomy. However, in hemodynamically stable patients, an abdominal CT scan is the most appropriate next step.

3. Diagnostic peritoneal lavage (DPL): DPL has largely been replaced by the trauma ultrasound. It still has an important role in the evaluation of the abdomen in a hemodynamically unstable patient, if the ultrasound is not definitive or not available. The procedure can be performed with the open or percutaneous closed technique; the closed one is faster and less invasive. The aspiration of gross blood has major significance and is a strong indication for laparotomy in the hemodynamically unstable multitrauma patient. The role of microscopically positive DPL is of much lower importance.

4. CT scan: CT scan has become the most important and useful investigation in the evaluation of sus-

pected blunt abdominal trauma. It is very sensitive in diagnosing solid organ injuries. In addition to the site and size of solid organ injury, it may give valuable information about the presence of active bleeding or false aneurysms, provided intravenous contrast has been administered. The role of CT scan in the diagnosis of hollow viscus perforation is rather limited, and up to 30–40% of injuries may be missed. CT scan findings suggesting bowel injury include pneumoperitoneum, thickened bowel wall, extravasation of oral contrast, and free intraperitoneal fluid in the absence of solid organ injury.

5. Intravenous pyelogram (IVP): One-shot IVP in the emergency department has little or no role in the evaluation of abdominal trauma. Formal IVP has largely been replaced by contrast CT scan, though it may still have a role in suspected ureteric injuries.

6. Angiography: This is an important diagnostic and therapeutic tool in selected cases of abdominal trauma, such as in suspected bleeding from pelvic fractures or complex liver injuries.

7. Magnetic resonance cholangiopancreatography (MRCP): This is a good test for evaluation of the integrity of the pancreatic duct in suspected pancreatic trauma.

8. Urinalysis: All fairly stable patients should be evaluated for hematuria. Gross or symptomatic microscopic hematuria should be evaluated by means of contrast CT scan and cystogram. Asymptomatic microscopic hematuria does not need further evaluation.

9. Serum amylase: This may be a useful laboratory test for suspected pancreaticoduodenal trauma, although its sensitivity and specificity are fairly low. Normal levels do not reliably exclude pancreatic trauma, and it is elevated in only about 70% of cases with proven pancreatic trauma. Serial measurements are more useful than the initial values.

General Management

The initial evaluation and management should follow the standard ATLS guidelines. Trauma ultrasound studies should be part of the standard evaluation of all suspected abdominal blunt trauma. Hemodynamically unstable patients or those with signs of peritonitis should be taken to the operating room with no delay. Time-consuming investigations should be reserved only for the patient who is hemodynamically stable and whose diagnosis is uncertain.

In the multitrauma patient, there is often combined abdominal and head trauma. The timing of evaluation and management of the injuries of these anatomical areas is important and can have a major effect on outcome. In the presence of hemodynamic instability, the abdomen should be evaluated by trauma ultrasound or DPL. If there is evidence of free intraperitoneal fluid, the patient should have a laparotomy first and a head CT scan postoperatively. If there are localizing neurological signs, burr holes should be considered during laparotomy before CT evaluation. In the hemodynamically stable patient with peritonitis and GCS ≤12 or localizing signs, a CT scan of the head should precede laparotomy, under close monitoring. It is rare that both a laparotomy and a craniotomy are required simultaneously.

Many carefully selected patients with solid organ injury (liver, spleen, kidney) can safely be managed nonoperatively, provided that they are hemodynamically stable and have no signs of peritonitis. Overall, about 70% of blunt liver injuries, about 80% of splenic injuries, and about 90% of renal injuries can be managed nonoperatively.

Common Mistakes and Pitfalls

1. Delayed diagnosis of hollow viscus perforation in a clinically unevaluable patient (e.g., associated head injury, spinal cord injury, or intoxication) is a common problem. The presence of a seatbelt sign should raise the index of suspicion. Look for subtle CT scan findings, such as bowel edema, intraperitoneal gas, and free intraperitoneal fluid in the absence of a solid organ injury. They are highly suspicious findings, and exploratory laparotomy should be considered. Repeat abdominal CT scan or DPL should be considered in suspicious cases.

2. Missed pancreaticoduodenal injuries are notorious for their fairly silent clinical presentation. The initial CT scan may miss the injury, and the serum amylase may be normal. In suspicious cases, repeat the CT scan 6–10 hours later and perform serial amylase determinations.

Penetrating Abdominal Trauma

Introduction

The initial evaluation of penetrating abdominal trauma is usually very different from evaluation of blunt trauma. Penetrating trauma, especially gunshot wounds, is much more likely to be associated with life-threatening major vascular injuries than blunt trauma.

Knife injuries to the anterior abdomen are associated with significant intra-abdominal injuries in about

50% of patients. In gunshot wounds, about 80% of cases have major injuries requiring surgical repair.

Clinical Examination

Physical examination is usually reliable in identifying patients with significant intra-abdominal injuries. The physician must remember that patients with a short prehospital time may seem hemodynamically stable despite severe active intra-abdominal bleeding, and thus serial examinations are critical in the initially asymptomatic patient. Tachycardia and elevated diastolic pressure are suspicious markers of bleeding, and these patients should be reevaluated every few minutes during admission. Of note, the presence of hemoperitoneum in the absence of hollow viscus perforation very often does not produce peritoneal signs.

Investigations

Very few investigations are needed in the evaluation of penetrating abdominal trauma. Radiological studies should be reserved for fairly stable patients.

1. Chest x-ray should be obtained in selected patients with stab wounds or gunshot wounds with suspected thoracic involvement. The x-ray may show hemopneumothoraces, an elevated diaphragm, free air under the diaphragm, and foreign bodies.

2. Abdominal x-rays have no role in stab wounds to the abdomen, and they should not be obtained. However, they may be useful in gunshot wounds with no exit or suspected spinal or pelvic fractures.

3. CT scan studies may be useful in evaluating patients with gunshot wounds who are hemodynamically stable and have a soft abdomen. The CT scan may show a bullet track away from any major structures and avoid an unnecessary operation. Some trauma centers practice nonoperative management of gunshot wounds to the liver or kidney in carefully selected patients who are hemodynamically stable and have a soft abdomen. CT scanning of these patients can demonstrate the extent of the solid organ injury and may identify false aneurysms or active bleeding.

4. Bedside ultrasound can identify patients with surgical amounts of hemoperitoneum. This can be useful in deciding which patients are stable candidates for further evaluation by CT. In addition, the pericardium can be examined in patients with proximity wounds.

5. Angiography may play an important diagnostic and therapeutic role in patients with liver or kidney injuries when the CT scan is suspicious for false aneurysms, arteriovenous fistula, or active bleeding. Similarly, in patients who have undergone damage control operations for severe liver injuries, angiographic embolization of any remaining bleeding vessels may be life saving.

6. Diagnostic laparoscopy has a definitive role in the evaluation of suspected diaphragmatic injuries (see Chapter 4).

General Management

One of the most important goals in managing penetrating abdominal injuries is to avoid nontherapeutic laparotomies and yet not miss any significant injuries. Patients presenting with hemodynamic instability or signs of peritonitis require an emergency operation without any delay. Patients with minimal or equivocal abdominal signs should be monitored with serial clinical examinations and continuous hemodynamic recordings. Further investigations, such as CT scanning or diagnostic laparoscopy, should be performed in appropriate cases. If the patient develops hemodynamic instability or signs of peritonitis, an exploratory laparotomy should be performed. Patients who remain asymptomatic are discharged after 48–72 hours of observation. The selective nonoperative management policy can be applied in both stab wounds and gunshot wounds, provided the patient is clinically evaluable.

Common Mistakes and Pitfalls

1. Patients with short prehospital times may seem hemodynamically stable on admission, despite significant active intra-abdominal bleeding. Once a decision for laparotomy has been made, no time should be wasted for further investigations.

2. Penetrating injuries to the diaphragm are usually clinically and radiologically silent. All patients with left or anterior right thoracoabdominal injuries who are asymptomatic should be evaluated by diagnostic laparoscopy.

3. Patients with associated severe head or spinal cord injuries and those undergoing general anesthesia for an extra-abdominal operation cannot be evaluated clinically. In these groups of patients, the presence of a deep penetrating abdominal wound should be an indication for laparotomy, irrespective of signs or symptoms.

4. Patients selected for observation and nonoperative management should not receive analgesics or prophylactic antibiotics because of the risk of masking important signs and symptoms.

5.1 Mechanism of Injury in Blunt Abdominal Trauma

Commentary

Intra-abdominal injuries may occur by three mechanisms:

1. Crushing of an organ against the spine, pelvis, or ribs and the abdominal wall

2. Deceleration, such as high-speed accidents or falls from heights

3. Sudden increase of the intraluminal pressure and bursting of a hollow viscus, commonly seen with seatbelt injuries

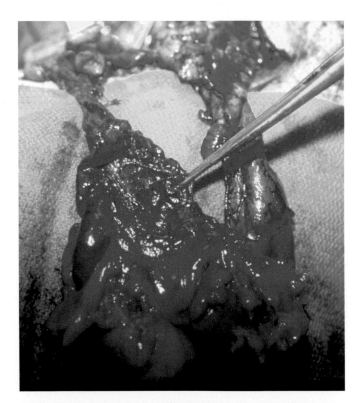

5.1A. Photograph of a splenic injury due to direct crushing.

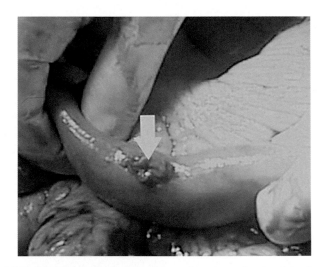

5.1C. Photograph of a small-bowel rupture due to closed loop and increased intraluminal pressure.

5.1B. Photograph of an avulsion and transverse colon mesenteric tear due to deceleration injury.

5.2 Seatbelt Sign

Commentary

Seatbelts have significantly decreased deaths in motor vehicle accidents. Although the incidence of intra-abdominal injuries has not changed with the use of seatbelts, the nature of the injuries has changed: Seatbelt wearers are more likely to suffer hollow viscus perforation.

The presence of seatbelt marks on the abdominal wall is an important physical finding because of the high incidence of associated intra-abdominal injuries (22% with seatbelt marks versus 3% in patients wearing seatbelts but without a seatbelt mark).

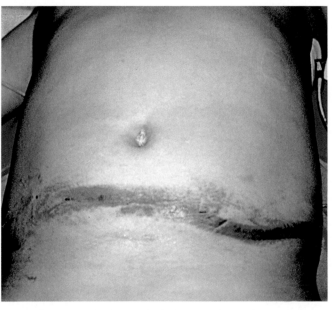

5.2A. Photograph of a seatbelt sign on the abdominal wall.

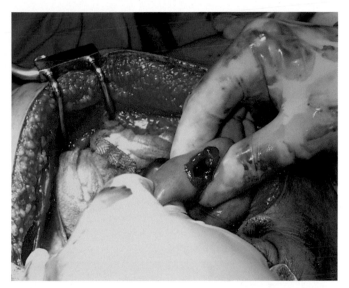

5.2B. Intraoperative photograph of a rupture of the small bowel associated with the seatbelt mark sign shown in the previous picture.

5.3 Diagnosis of Hemoperitoneum

Commentary

Hemoperitoneum in itself does not always give peritoneal signs. Thus, the clinical diagnosis, especially in the presence of multitrauma, can be difficult. Trauma ultrasound, performed in the emergency department by emergency physicians or surgeons, is a fast, reliable, and noninvasive method of detecting intraperitoneal bleeding. The hepatorenal, splenorenal, and suprapubic spaces are the usual areas examined for free fluid during the trauma ultrasound exam. However, ultrasound does not identify the source of the bleeding and cannot evaluate the retroperitoneum, hollow viscera, and the diaphragm.

DPL has largely been replaced by ultrasound, although it still has a definitive role in the evaluation of an unstable patient when the ultrasound is not diagnostic or not available. It can be performed with the open technique or the closed guide-wire technique.

CT scan should be considered in hemodynamically stable patients. Under these circumstances, it is the most valuable investigation. It can also identify the source of the bleeding and visualize the retroperitoneum.

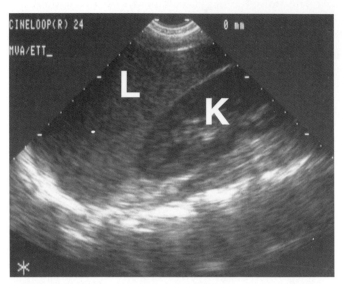

5.3A. Normal trauma ultrasound depicts the liver and the right kidney with no free fluid between the two organs (K = kidney, L = liver).

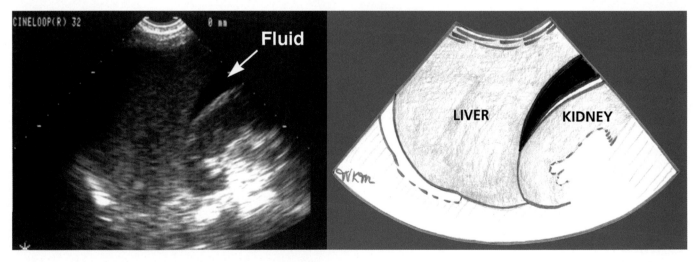

5.3B. Trauma ultrasound shows fluid (blood) between the liver and the kidney.

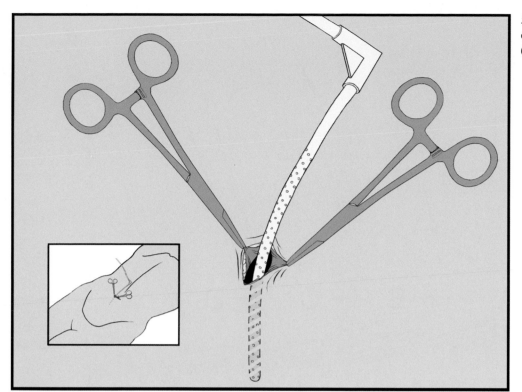

5.3C. Illustration of open diagnostic peritoneal lavage (DPL) technique.

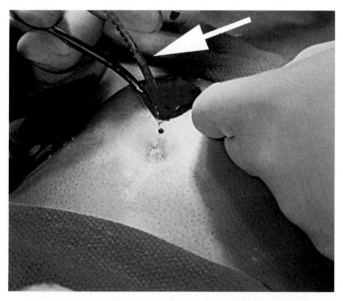

5.3D. Photograph of the introduction of the DPL catheter under direct vision, using the open technique.

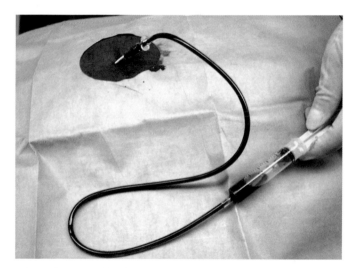

5.3E. Photograph of gross blood aspirated from DPL catheter.

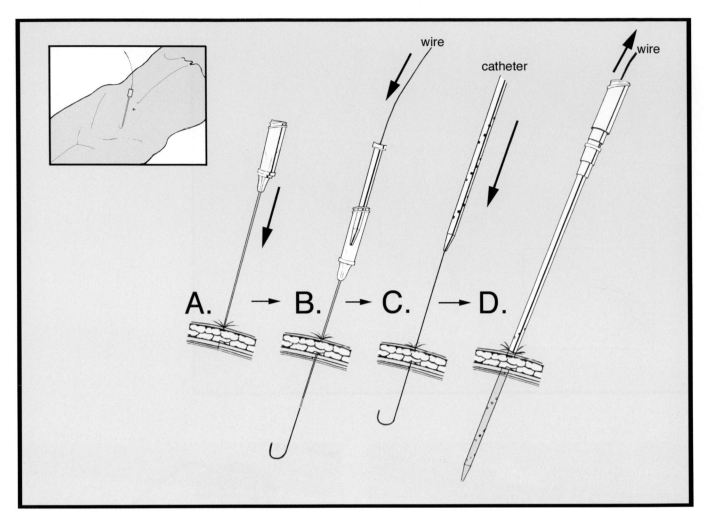

5.3F. Illustration of closed DPL with introduction of the catheter intraperitoneally with the guide-wire technique. The needle is inserted intraperitoneally (A). The guide-wire is introduced into the peritoneal cavity through the needle (B), and the needle is withdrawn. The plastic catheter is inserted over the guide-wire (C), and the wire is removed (D). A syringe is attached on the catheter, and aspiration for free blood is performed. If the aspiration is negative, one liter of warm fluid (or 20 cc/Kg for children) is infused for subsequent analysis of the returned fluid.

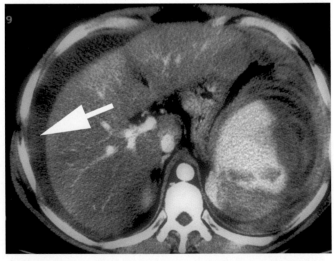

5.3G. CT scan shows free fluid around the liver secondary to a splenic injury.

5.4 Splenic Injuries

Commentary

The clinical presentation of a splenic rupture may vary from mild left hypochondrial pain to severe hypovolemic shock. The diagnosis is suspected from the clinical examination (pain in left upper abdomen often radiating to the left shoulder, signs of hypovolemia) or trauma ultrasound showing free intraperitoneal fluid and confirmed by CT scan or laparotomy.

Most isolated splenic injuries can safely be managed nonoperatively (about 90% in children, 70% in adults). The criteria for nonoperative management are hemodynamic stability and a soft abdomen. The abdominal CT scan may be very helpful in determining the need for surgical intervention: Grades IV or V splenic injuries often fail nonoperative management, and the presence of blushing on CT scan is suggestive of active bleeding or a false aneurysm. In these cases, depending on the clinical condition of the patient, operative intervention or angiographic embolization should be considered. Caution should be exercised in the selection of patients for nonoperative management in the presence of multiple associated severe injuries. Severe splenic injuries treated nonoperatively should be followed up by serial CT scans until there is satisfactory healing or absorption of any large hematomas.

Postsplenectomy complications may be systemic (postsplenectomy sepsis or thrombocytosis) or local (subdiaphragmatic abscess, pancreatic pseudocyst or fistula, gastric dilatation, necrosis of the fundus of the stomach, thrombosis of the splenic vein, left pleural effusion and atelectasis). To avoid postsplenectomy sepsis, pneumococcal vaccine should be administered to all patients. In addition to the vaccine, some authors advocate that in children and immunosuppressed adults, prophylactic penicillin be given. The patient should be advised that medical care should be sought with the first signs or suspicion of any infections.

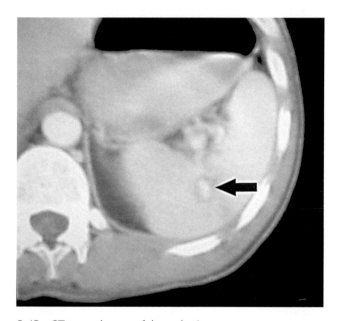

5.4B. CT scan shows a false splenic aneurysm.

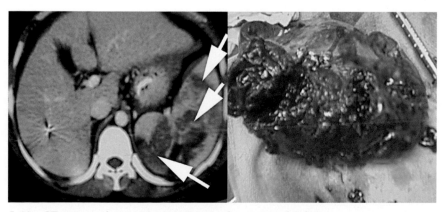

5.4A. CT scan and operative specimen of a ruptured spleen.

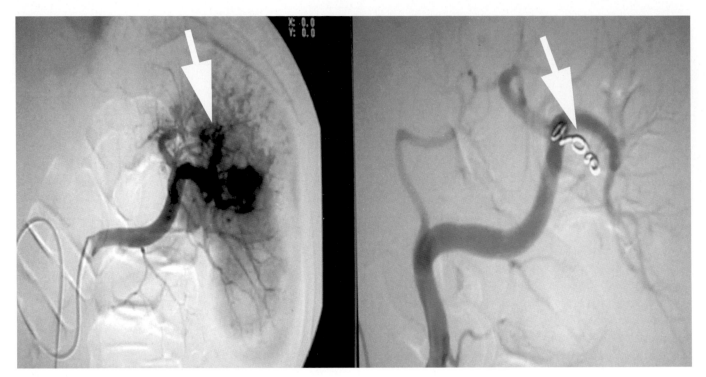

5.4C. Angiograms before (left side) and after (right side) successful embolization of the false splenic aneurysm in the previous case.

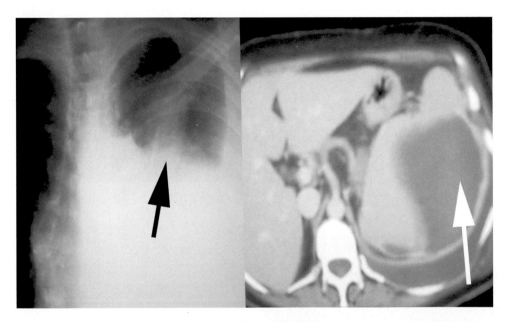

5.4D. Chest x-ray shows an elevated left diaphragm and pleural effusion (left side). CT scan shows large splenic subcapsular hematoma (right side).

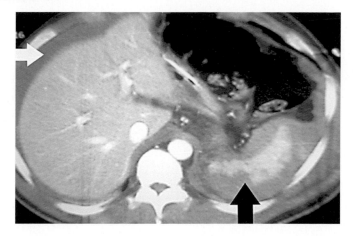

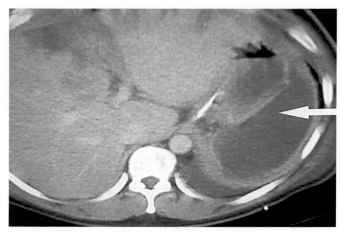

5.4E. CT of a major splenic rupture, which was successfully managed nonoperatively. There is also free blood around the liver.

5.4G. CT with postsplenectomy fluid collection in the splenic bed.

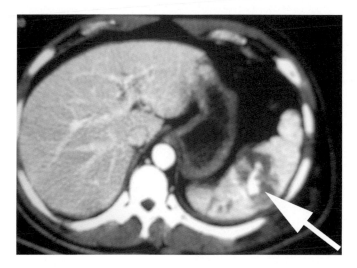

5.4F. Splenic fracture and active bleeding seen by "blushing" on CT.

5.5 Liver Injuries

Commentary

The clinical presentation of a liver injury may vary from minor pain in the right upper abdomen to peritonitis or hypovolemic shock. The diagnosis is suspected from the physical examination and trauma ultrasound and confirmed by CT scan or laparotomy. Most minor and moderate liver injuries (grades I–III) and even some severe injuries (grades IV, V) may be successfully managed nonoperatively, provided the patient is hemodynamically stable and the abdomen is soft. The operative management may vary from simple suturing and draining to liver packing or nonanatomical lobectomy. In addition, angiographic embolization is a very effective adjuvant modality in complex cases.

Post-traumatic liver complications include liver abscess, biloma, false aneurysms, and hemobilia (bleeding into the biliary tree). Most of these complications can be managed with percutaneous drainage or angiographic embolization.

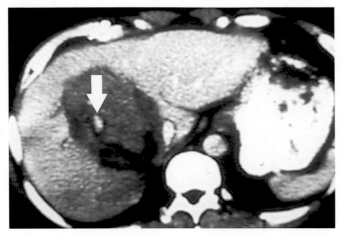

5.5A. Abdominal CT scan shows a false aneurysm in the liver.

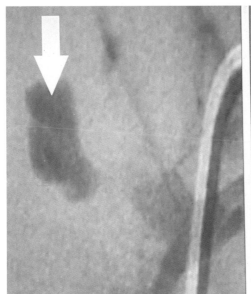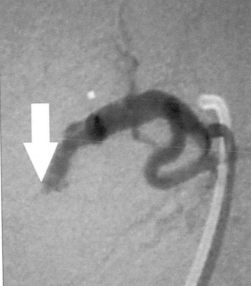

5.5B. Angiography before (left side) and after (right side) embolization of the previous aneurysm.

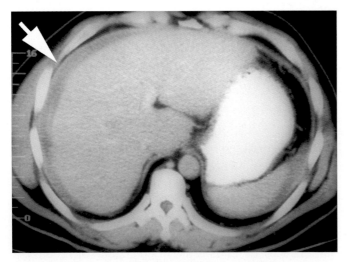

5.5C. CT scan of a subcapsular liver hematoma.

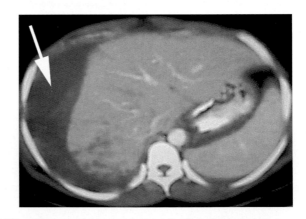

5.5D. CT scan of large subcapsular liver hematoma.

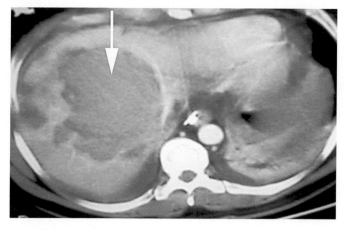

5.5E. CT of large intrahepatic hematoma successfully managed nonoperatively.

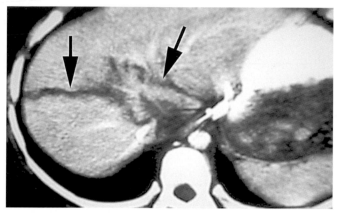

5.5F. CT of grade IV liver injury successfully managed nonoperatively.

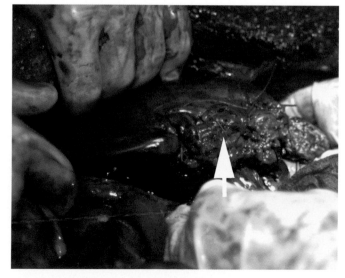

5.5G. Intraoperative photograph of extensive left lobe injury requiring nonanatomic lobe resection.

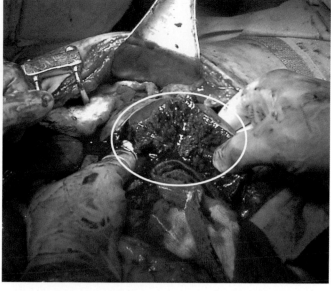

5.5H. Intraoperative photograph of grade III liver injury.

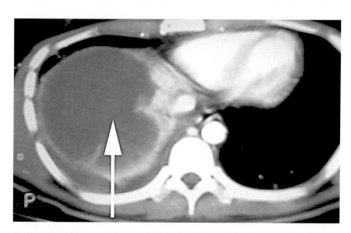

5.5I. CT of large biloma following liver injury.

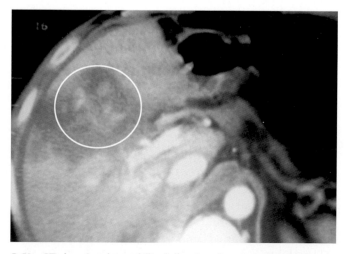

5.5J. CT showing hemobilia following liver trauma. The patient had large amounts of blood in the nasogastric tube.

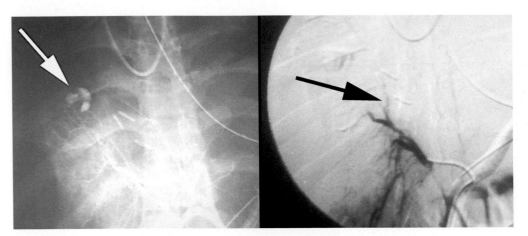

5.5K. Angiographic confirmation of false aneurysm of the previous case of hemobilia (left side) and successful embolization (right side).

5.6 Pancreatic Injuries

Commentary

Most pancreatic injuries due to blunt trauma occur at the neck of the pancreas, caused by crushing of the organ against the spine. The clinical presentation may vary from mild epigastric pain to obvious peritonitis. The diagnosis is suspected from the history of abdominal trauma and confirmed by specific investigations or at operation. The initial serum amylase may be elevated in about 70% of patients, and serial amylase measurements should be performed in suspected cases. The CT scan is usually diagnostic, although the early CT scan may not show the injury. It is essential that in suspected cases a repeat CT scan be performed 6–8 hours after the initial investigation. Endoscopic retrograde cholangiopancreatography (ERCP) or MRCP is useful in determining any damage to the duct. The MRCP does not require endoscopy and is not uncomfortable for the patient. Many superficial pancreatic injuries not involving the duct may be managed successfully without operation. However, in cases with proven ductal injury or clinical signs of peritonitis, an operation should be performed. In the presence of distal ductal injury (to the left of the superior mesenteric vessels), a distal pancreatectomy is the procedure of choice. In severe injuries to the head of the pancreas or severe combined pancreatoduodenal injuries, a Whipple's pancreatoduodenectomy may be necessary. In injuries to the head of the pancreas when the integrity of the duct cannot be determined by inspection or intraoperative pancreatography, simple drainage of the area is safer than major resections.

Local complications directly related to the injury include pancreatic pseudocyst, pancreatitis, abscess, and fistula. Many of these complications can be managed nonoperatively or by percutaneous drainage. It is not common that any of these complications will require an operation.

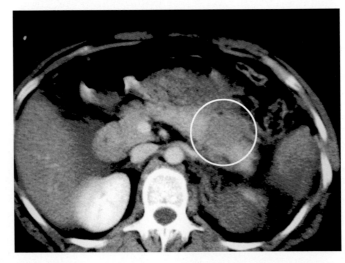

5.6A. CT scan shows distal pancreatic transection. Note the absence of contrast uptake by the transected distal pancreas.

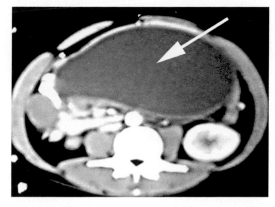

5.6D. CT showing post-traumatic pancreatic pseudocyst.

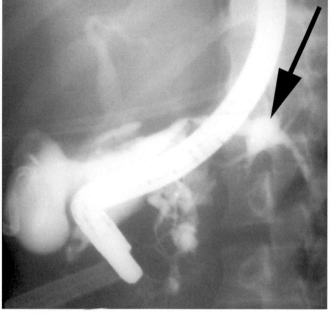

5.6B. ERCP (endoscopic retrograde cholangiopancrea-tography) shows distal pancreatic injury with partial transection and extravasation.

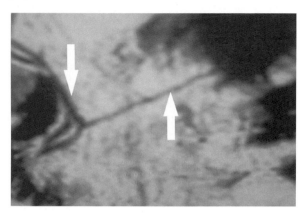

5.6E. Normal MRCP (magnetic resonance cholangio-pancreatography), showing the common bile duct (left arrow) and the pancreatic duct (right arrow).

5.6C. Post-traumatic pancreatic pseudocyst on CT scan (left side) and transection of the duct on ERCP (right side).

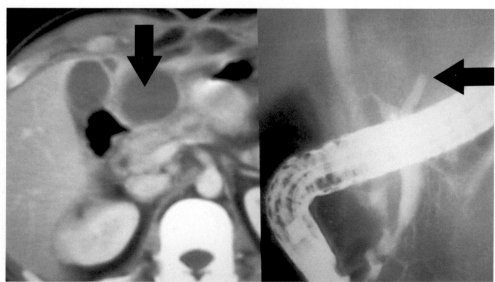

5.7 Renal Injuries

Commentary

A kidney injury may manifest clinically with pain in the loin and gross or microscopic hematuria. Ancillary investigations should be reserved for only hemodynamically stable patients with a soft abdomen. The abdominal CT scan with intravenous contrast is the most useful investigation and has largely replaced the intravenous pyelography (IVP). The CT scan may show parenchymal injuries and evidence of active bleeding or false aneurysm. The IVP is reserved for evaluation of the ureters. Angiographic evaluation is useful in cases with persistent gross hematuria or post-traumatic hypertension.

The vast majority of blunt renal injuries can be safely managed nonoperatively. Any attempts to explore and repair a renal injury may result in loss of the kidney. Exploration of the kidney should be reserved for patients with major gross hematuria or intraoperative expansion of the perirenal hematoma.

Complications related to renal injury include false aneurysm, arteriovenous fistula, urinoma, late hematuria, and late hypertension.

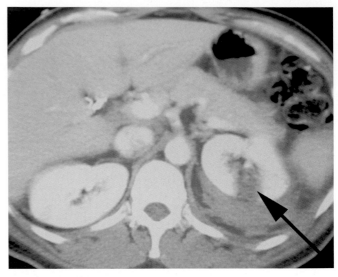

5.7B. CT scan shows hilar injury of the kidney.

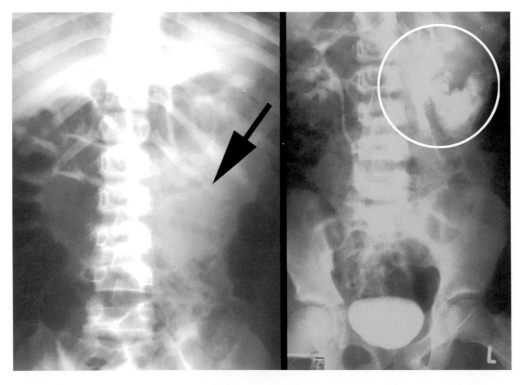

5.7A. Abdominal plain film shows an opacification of the left abdomen due to a renal hematoma (left side). Intravenous pyelogram demonstrates extravasation from the left caliceal system (right side).

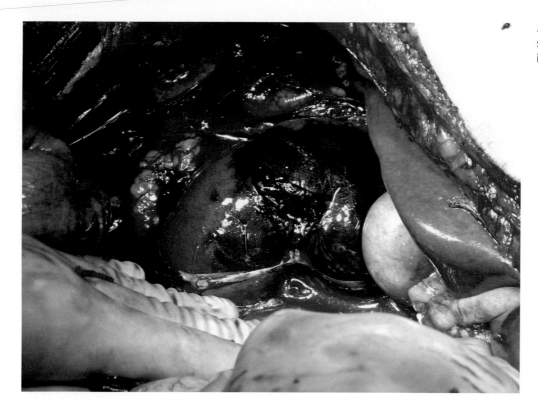

5.7C. Operative view of the same case confirms the hilar injury.

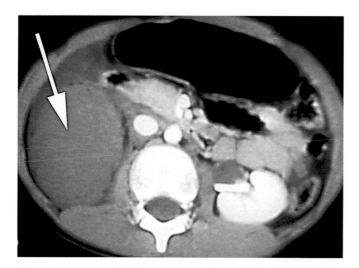

5.7D. CT scan with failure of the right kidney to take up contrast because of disruption of the renal artery. Note the large right kidney hematoma.

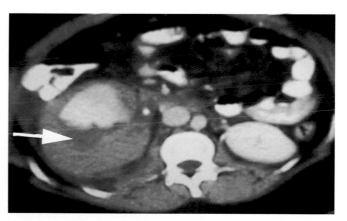

5.7E. CT scan of a patient with gross hematuria showing a large right renal hematoma.

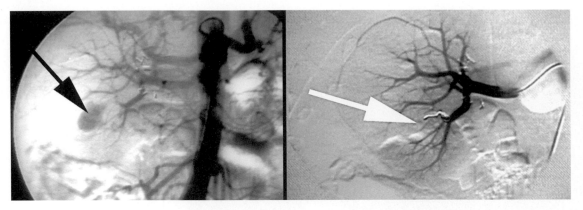

5.7F. Angiogram of the same patient showing a false aneurysm in the kidney (left side), which was successfully embolized (right side).

5.8 Bladder Injuries

Commentary

Bladder injuries are usually due to pelvic fractures or blunt abdominal trauma with a full bladder. The rupture may occur intraperitoneally or extraperitoneally. The patient may present with hematuria or inability to pass urine, and the diagnosis is confirmed by cystogram.

All intraperitoneal ruptures need operation and repair. Most extraperitoneal ruptures can be managed nonoperatively with transurethral catheter drainage for about ten days.

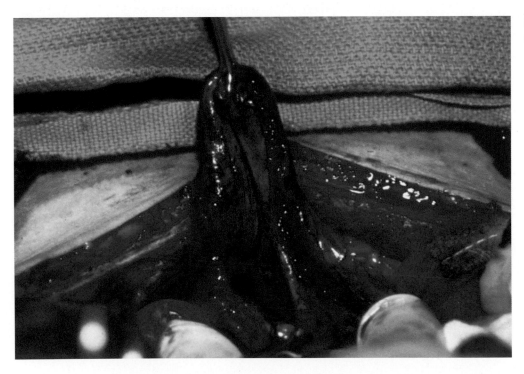

5.8A. Intraperitoneal rupture of the bladder at operation.

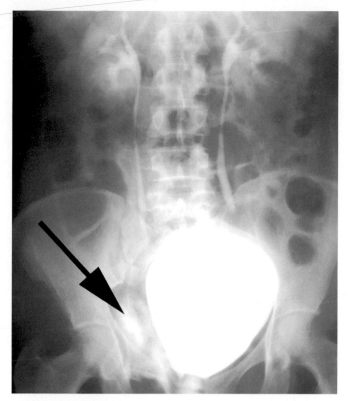

5.8B. Cystogram showing major intraperitoneal bladder rupture.

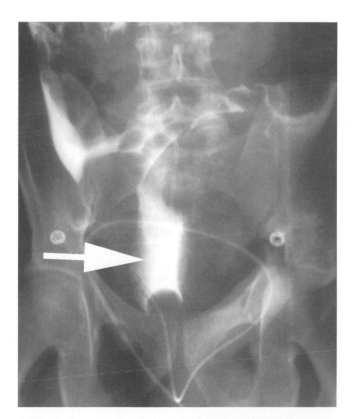

5.8C. Cystogram showing major intraperitoneal bladder rupture.

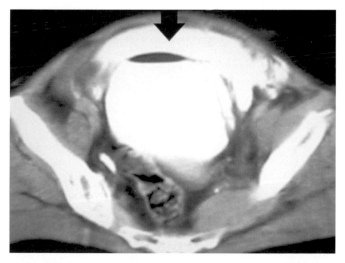

5.8D. CT cystogram of extraperitoneal rupture.

5.9 Urethral Injuries

Commentary

Urethral injuries occur almost exclusively in males, and they are usually associated with anterior pelvic fractures or falls resulting in straddle injuries. The clinical presentation may include blood at the urethral meatus, inability to pass urine, floating prostate on rectal examination, and urine extravasation in the scrotum. The diagnosis is confirmed by urethrogram.

In suspected urethral injuries, avoid transurethral catheterization until a retrograde urethrogram shows integrity of the urethra. The management is nonoperative with a suprapubic bladder catheter for approximately two weeks.

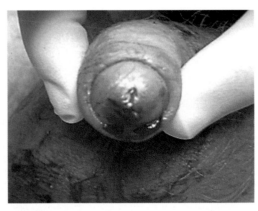

5.9A. Photograph of blood in the urethral meatus in a patient with urethral rupture.

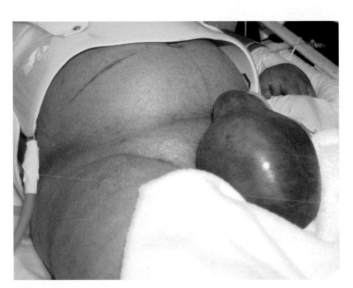

5.9C. Photograph of ruptured urethra due to pelvic fracture and with urine extravasation into the scrotum.

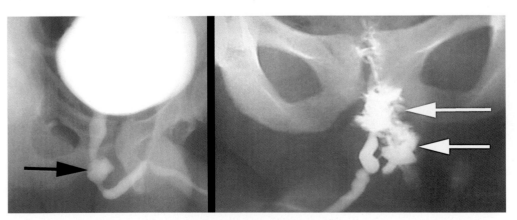

5.9B. Urethral ruptures seen on retrograde urethrograms. Note the dye extravasation.

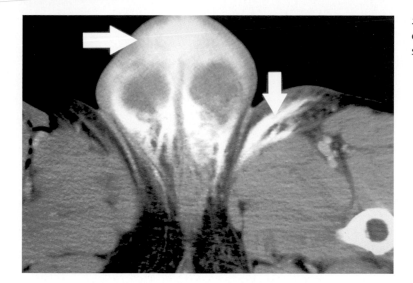

5.9D. CT cystogram with massive extravasation of contrast in the scrotum and extraperitoneal tissues, secondary to posterior urethral rupture.

5.10 Duodenal Injuries

Commentary

Blunt duodenal trauma may occur as a result of direct trauma to the abdomen that compresses the duodenum against the vertebral column or following deceleration injuries. The injury usually involves the retroperitoneal part of the duodenum. The clinical examination may be difficult due to subtle signs and symptoms because of the retroperitoneal location of the rupture. The initial presentation may include minor epigastric tenderness and tachycardia, and signs of peritonitis may appear a few hours later.

Laboratory tests are of little help in the early diagnosis of duodenal rupture. The serum amylase may be elevated and should be monitored at 4- to 6-hour intervals. Plain films may show retroperitoneal air, especially around the upper pole of the right kidney. CT scan with oral contrast or Gastrograffin meal are the definitive studies.

Early diagnosis and surgical repair remain the cornerstones for a good outcome. Common postoperative complications include local infection and fistula formation.

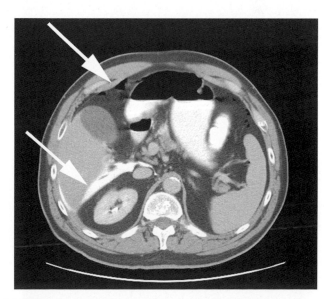

5.10B. CT scan with oral contrast shows contrast extravasation in the mid-abdomen and between kidney and liver (lower arrow). A small amount of free intraperitoneal air is seen in the anterior abdomen (upper arrow).

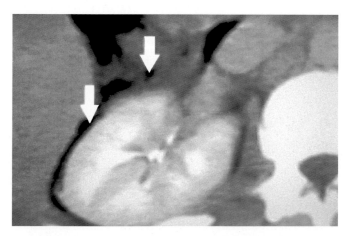

5.10A. CT scan of retroperitoneal duodenal rupture with free air around the kidney.

5.11 Small-Bowel Injuries

Commentary

Small-bowel perforation occurs in about 3% of blunt abdominal traumas. The diagnosis can be very difficult, especially in unevaluable multitrauma patients, and is the one of the most commonly missed injuries. A seat-belt sign is a highly suspicious finding that should alert the physician to the possibility of bowel injury.

The plain abdominal x-ray is usually of little help because in most of the cases it is nondiagnostic and fails to show any free intraperitoneal air. The abdominal CT scan may be diagnostic in about 70% of cases, as it may show small amounts of free air or thickening of the bowel wall or mesentery. The presence of free fluid without evidence of solid organ injury is a highly suspicious finding, and in unevaluable patients it should be an indication for exploratory laparotomy. In suspicious cases, a follow-up CT scan a few hours after the initial one should be considered. Diagnostic peritoneal lavage (DPL) at the early stages is nonspecific and of very little value, though delayed DPL may show an elevated white cell count in the fluid.

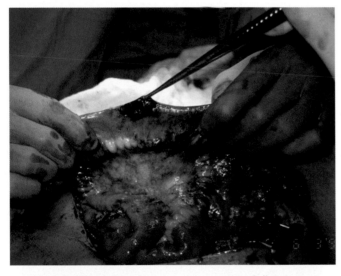

5.11A. Small-bowel perforation at operation following a motor vehicle accident.

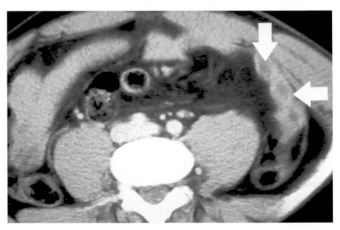

5.11C. CT scan shows a few loops of thickened loops of small bowel secondary to peritonitis due to small-bowel perforation.

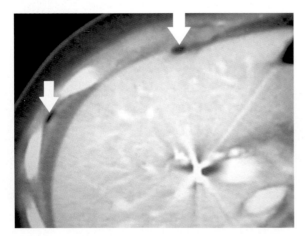

5.11B. CT shows small amounts of free air secondary to small-bowel perforation.

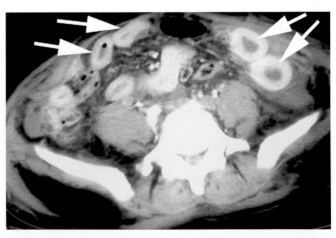

5.11D. CT scan shows multiple thickened loops of small bowel secondary to peritonitis.

5.12 Colorectal Injuries

Commentary

Blunt colorectal trauma may occur in association with pelvic fractures or high-speed deceleration accidents. The diagnosis is usually easy in intraperitoneal injuries because of the presence of peritonitis. However, in extraperitoneal injuries, the physical findings may be unremarkable, and the diagnosis may be delayed. The diagnosis should be suspected in severe pelvic fractures, especially in the presence of blood on rectal examination. A Gastrograffin enema and a careful sigmoidoscopy without excessive insufflation can confirm the injury. Early operation is essential to reduce the possibility of sepsis.

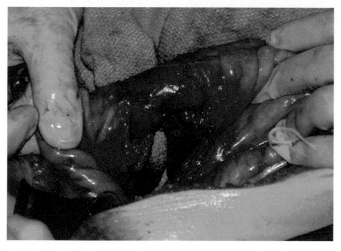 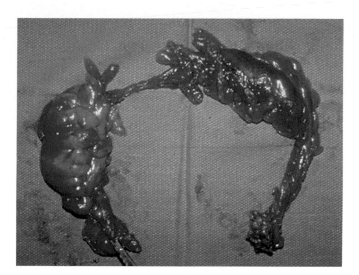

5.12A and B. Photographs of extensive sigmoid colon injuries, including devascularization, secondary to deceleration injuries after high-speed car accidents.

5.13 Mechanism of Injury in Penetrating Abdominal Trauma

Commentary

A distinction should be made between low-velocity and high-velocity penetrating abdominal injuries because the severity of the injury, the treatment, and the prognosis are different. High-velocity injuries cause extensive damage by direct laceration, production of a shock wave, and transient cavitation. Almost all cases require a laparotomy. Low-velocity injuries (knives, most civilian handguns) cause damage only by direct laceration, and often there is no significant intra-abdominal injury requiring surgical repair. Although many centers recommend routine laparotomy, many others practice selective nonoperative management for all low-velocity injuries. Criteria for nonoperative management are hemodynamic stability and a soft abdomen. These patients are closely monitored with frequent hemodynamic and abdominal examinations for 24–48 hours.

Omental or bowel evisceration is associated with significant intra-abdominal injuries requiring operation in about 75% of cases. Some centers practice nonoperative management in carefully selected patients with evisceration who remain hemodynamically stable and whose abdomens are soft after reduction of the protruding viscus.

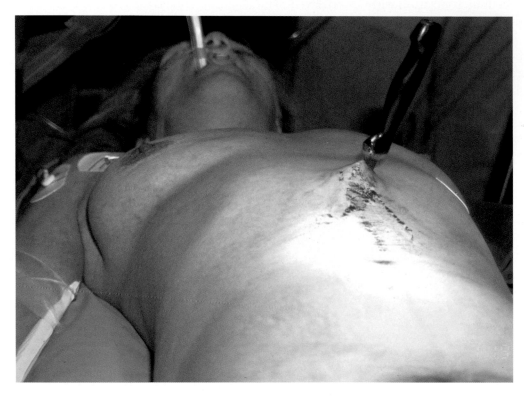

5.13A. Photograph of a stab wound to the abdomen with impaled knife. Such objects should be removed only in the operating room. Fifty percent of stab wound patients do not have significant intra-abdominal injuries.

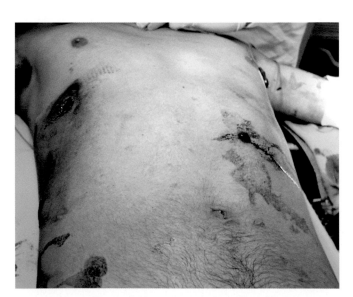

5.13B. Photograph of a low-velocity gunshot wound; about one-quarter of patients do not have significant injury requiring operation.

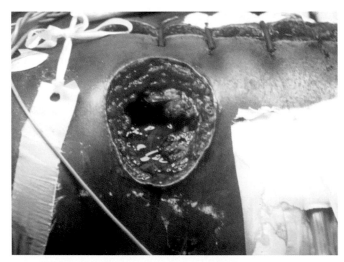

5.13C. Photograph of a shotgun wound to the abdomen. Close-range shotgun injuries are very destructive, with extensive soft tissue loss.

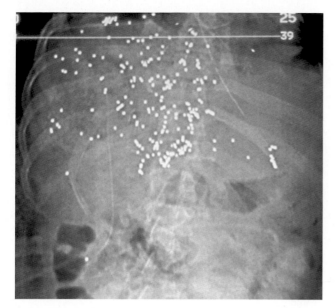

5.13D. Plain radiograph showing multiple intra-abdominal pellets in a shotgun wound victim.

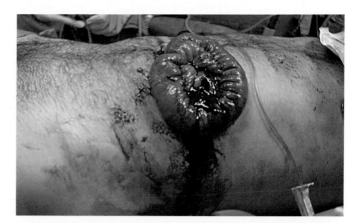

5.13F.

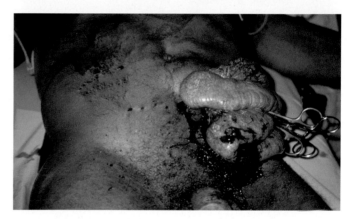

5.13G.

5.13E, F, and G. Photographs of omental and bowel evisceration following stab wounds. In about one-quarter of cases, there is no significant internal injury.

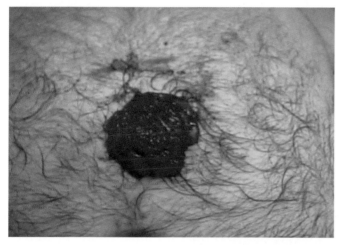

5.13E.

5.14 Investigations in Penetrating Abdominal Injury

Commentary

Investigations should be reserved for only fairly stable patients. Chest and abdominal films are important in gunshot wounds for localization of any missiles or fragments, and they make the operation easier. Also, they may identify any fractures, especially of the spine. Abdominal x-rays are of no value in knife injuries and should not be performed. In selected hemodynami-cally stable patients with minimal or no abdominal signs, abdominal CT scan may be helpful in identifying the bullet track or any solid organ injuries. If the bullet track is extraperitoneal, the patient may avoid an unnecessary operation. For solid organ injuries, the CT scan provides information about the injury grade and the presence of active bleeding or false aneurysm, and it is helpful in planning the optimal treatment.

Laparoscopy is useful in the evaluation of penetrating injuries of the left thoracoabdominal and anterior right thoracoabdominal regions to exclude diaphragmatic injuries. This procedure is discussed extensively in the chest trauma chapter.

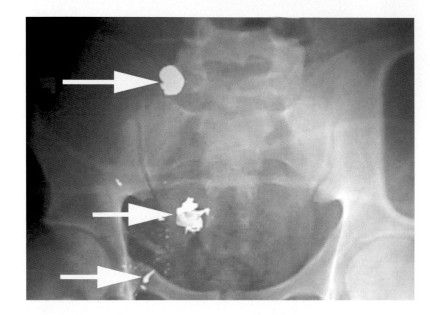

5.14A. Abdominal film showing two missiles and smaller missile fragments.

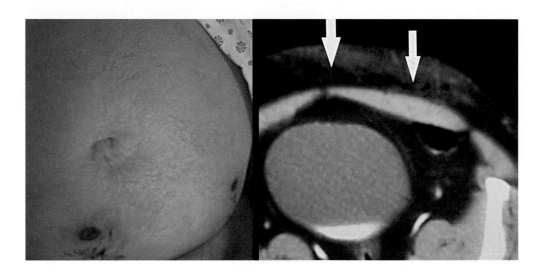

5.14B. Photograph of an abdominal gunshot wound (left side) and the corresponding CT scan (right side), which shows an extraperitoneal bullet track.

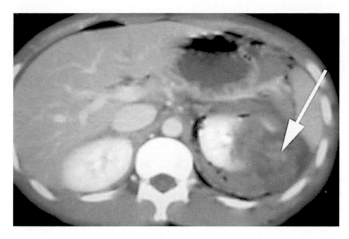

5.14C. CT scan of an abdominal gunshot wound with left kidney injury.

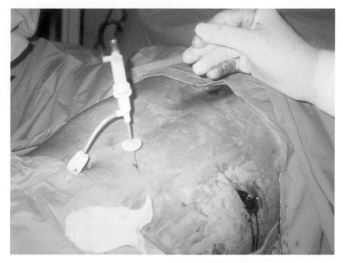

5.14D. Photograph of laparoscopy with a 2-mm laparoscope for a left thoracoabdominal stab wound.

5.15 Transpelvic Gunshot Injuries

Commentary

About half of all transpelvic gunshot injuries are associated with significant injuries requiring surgical repair. The selection of patients for operation or observation should be based on clinical examination and various diagnostic tests. The presence of an acute abdomen, hemodynamic instability, rectal bleeding, or gross hematuria is an absolute indication for an operation.

Injuries to extraperitoneal organs (rectum, urethra) may not give peritoneal signs. Asymptomatic patients should be evaluated by rigid endoscopy and Gastrograffin enema. A CT scan with thin cuts may be useful in delineating the bullet track and identifying patients who may benefit from further investigations.

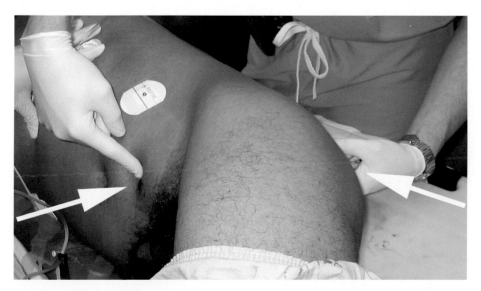

5.15A. Photograph of a transpelvic gunshot wound. Transpelvic injuries are associated with significant injuries in only about half of all patients.

5.16 Penetrating Injuries to the Liver

Commentary

About 30% of all knife wounds to the liver may be managed nonoperatively. Although most trauma centers practice routine laparotomy for all gunshot wounds to the liver, more recent studies have suggested that carefully selected cases (about 10% of all cases or 20% of isolated gunshot wounds to the liver) can be safely managed nonoperatively. The criteria for nonoperative management are hemodynamic stability and a soft abdomen. A CT scan with intravenous contrast should be performed in these cases to assess the extent of the injury and identify any evidence of active bleeding or false aneurysms, which may benefit from angiographic embolization. Hemodynamic instability, the presence of peritonitis, and the need for acute blood transfusions are indications for laparotomy.

Complications of penetrating liver injuries include bleeding, false aneurysm, arteriovenous fistula, hemobilia, biloma, and liver abscess. Most of these complications can be managed successfully with interventional radiology (angiographic embolization or percutaneous drainage).

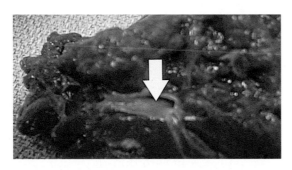

5.16A. Photograph of a stab wound to the liver with transection of a major intrahepatic vessel (arrow).

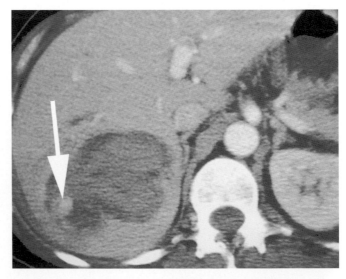

5.16C. CT scan of a gunshot wound to the liver successfully managed nonoperatively.

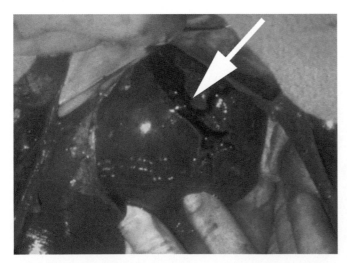

5.16B. Intraoperative photograph of a low-velocity gunshot wound to the liver.

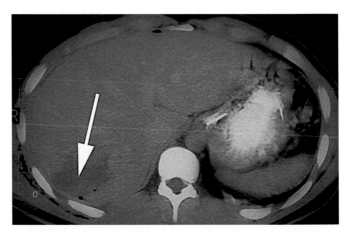

5.16D. Gunshot wound of the liver with a suspicious false aneurysm on the CT scan.

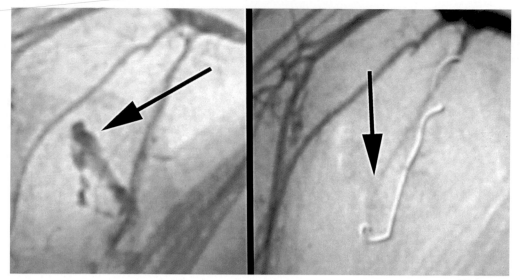

5.16E. Angiographic confirmation (left side) and embolization of the aneurysm (right side) from the same patient. The patient was successfully managed nonoperatively.

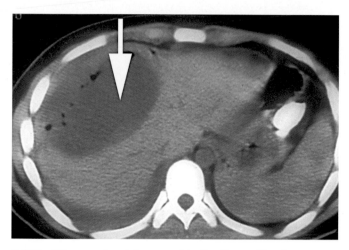

5.16F. CT scan of a stab wound to the liver with a large intrahepatic hematoma. There was successful nonoperative management.

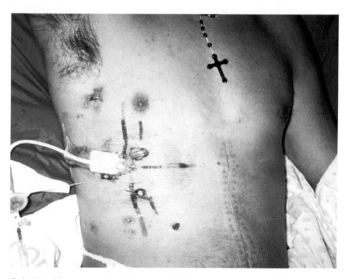

5.16H. Photograph of successful management of the same patient with percutaneous drainage.

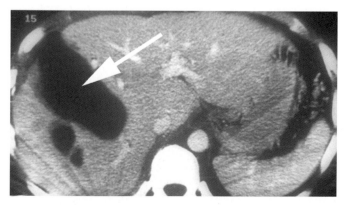

5.16G. Post-traumatic biloma on CT scan.

5.17 Penetrating Splenic Injuries

Commentary

Some penetrating injuries to the spleen can be safely managed nonoperatively, provided the patient is hemodynamically stable and the abdomen is soft. However, in the majority of cases there are associated intra-abdominal injuries or significant bleeding, and the patient needs an emergency laparotomy. Investigations should be reserved for stable patients and should include abdominal CT scanning with intravenous contrast. Laparoscopy should be considered in appropriate cases to exclude diaphragmatic injury.

A

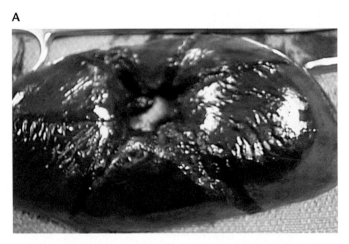

B

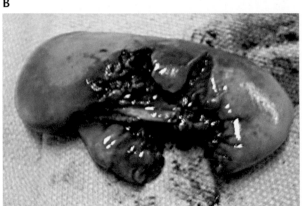

5.17A and B. Photographs of gunshot wounds to the spleen with extensive damage requiring emergency splenectomy.

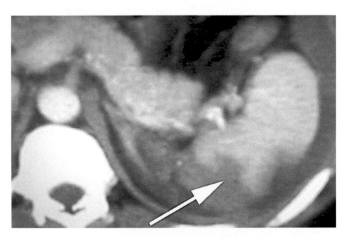

5.17C. CT scan of a gunshot wound to the spleen with successful nonoperative management.

5.18 Penetrating Pancreatic Injuries

Commentary

Almost all penetrating pancreatic injuries require operation because of the severity of the injury and the presence of other associated injuries. The management of the pancreatic injury may vary from simple drainage to distal pancreatectomy or pancreatoduodenectomy.

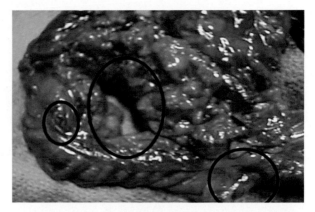

5.18A. Photograph of an operative specimen following pancreatoduodenectomy for extensive injury to the head of the pancreas and the duodenum from a gunshot wound.

5.19 Penetrating Renal Injuries

Commentary

Many isolated penetrating kidney injuries can be managed nonoperatively, provided the patient is hemodynamically stable and has a soft abdomen. A CT scan with intravenous contrast is strongly recommended to assess the extent of parenchymal injury and the presence of pelvicaliceal system leak or vascular lesions such as false aneurysm or arteriovenous fistula. Angiography is recommended in cases with persistent gross hematuria or suspected aneurysm or arteriovenous fistula in which CT findings are not diagnostic.

Post-traumatic complications include urinoma, false aneurysm, arteriovenous fistula, abscess, and hypertension. Most of these complications can be managed with interventional radiology.

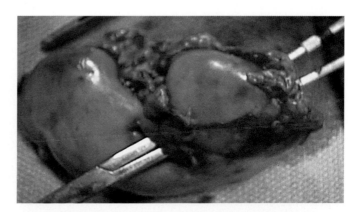

5.19A. Photograph of an operative kidney specimen. Nephrectomy was performed for a through-and-through stab wound to the kidney associated with severe bleeding.

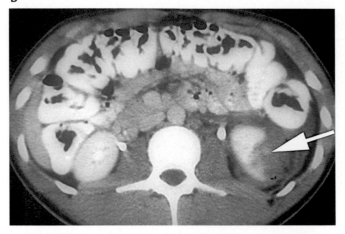

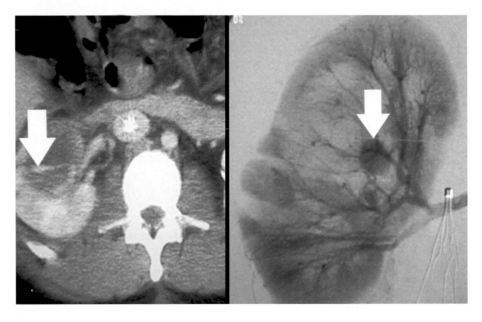

5.19B and C. CT scans of gunshot wounds to the kidney successfully managed nonoperatively.

5.19D. CT scan (left side) and angiography (right side) demonstrate a false aneurysm of the right kidney following a gunshot wound.

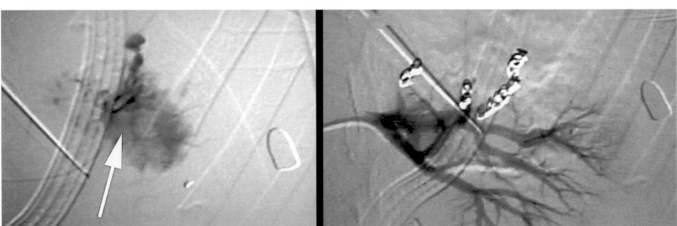

5.19E. Angiography: false aneurysm of the kidney following a gunshot wound (left side) and successful embolization (right side).

5.20 Penetrating Colorectal Injuries

Commentary

Almost all intraperitoneal colorectal injuries give early signs of peritonitis, and they are easy to diagnose. However, small retroperitoneal colonic injuries may not give any early clinical signs. Similarly, extraperitoneal rectal injuries may not give any significant abdominal signs. Rectal examination may show blood in the stool. Abdominal CT scan with a contrast enema may be helpful in diagnosing the injuries. A carefully performed sigmoidoscopy may show blood in the rectum or even the actual perforation.

Early surgical intervention is important to reduce the risk of septic complications. Most colon injuries can be managed safely with primary repair or resection and primary anastomosis. Colostomy is reserved for cases with edematous or ischemic bowel. Small rectal injuries may be managed by primary repair, and large injuries require a proximal colostomy.

The most common complications are abdominal sepsis (intra-abdominal abscess, wound sepsis) and colonic fistula. More than 20% of patients with colonic resection develop severe abdominal septic complications.

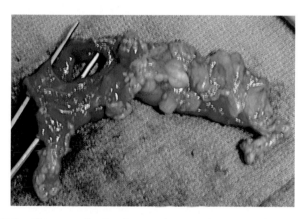

5.20A. Photograph of a destructive gunshot wound to the cecum, requiring right hemicolectomy and ileotransverse anastomosis.

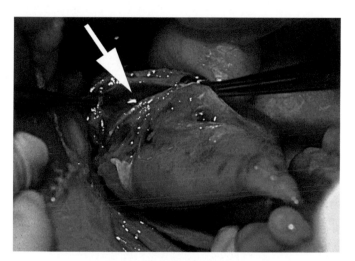

5.20C. Intraoperative photograph of colorectal injury in previous case managed with proximal diverting colostomy.

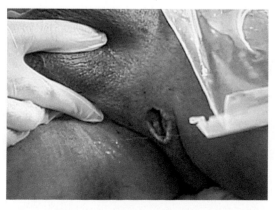

5.20B. Photograph of a gunshot wound to the perineum with rectal injury.

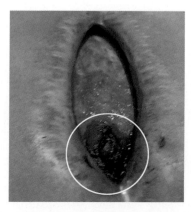

5.20D. Photograph of a colonic fistula. This is a serious complication following colon repair.

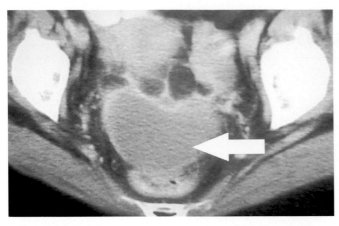

5.20E. CT of pelvic abscess following penetrating rectal injury; percutaneous drainage by interventional radiology is the treatment of choice.

5.21 Abdominal Vascular Injuries

Commentary

Most patients with penetrating abdominal vascular injuries present in shock, although in some cases retroperitoneal containment may prevent rapid exsanguination and early shock. Peritonitis due to associated hollow viscus perforations is a common finding. The diagnosis of vascular injury should be suspected in the presence of severe hemodynamic instability or a rapidly distending abdomen. A trauma ultrasound is often very helpful, although it cannot detect retroperitoneal bleeding.

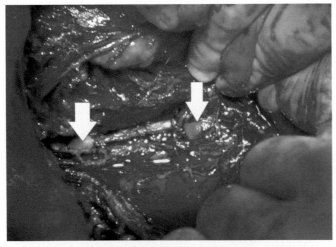

5.21A. Intraoperative photograph of a gunshot wound to the infrarenal inferior vena cava with proximal and distal ligation. Ligation of the inferior vena cava below the kidneys is usually well tolerated.

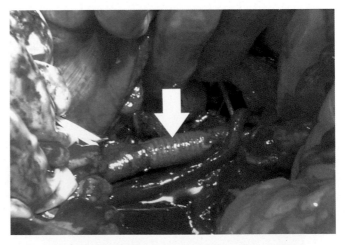

5.21B. Intraoperative photograph of a gunshot wound to the abdominal aorta managed with a prosthetic graft.

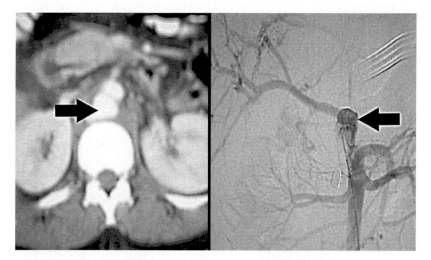

5.21C. Post–gunshot wound false aneurysm of the suprarenal aorta, as seen on the CT scan (left side) and angiogram (right side). The patient required surgical repair with a prosthetic graft. Angiographic stent placement was not an option because of the close proximity of the aneurysm with the superior mesenteric artery.

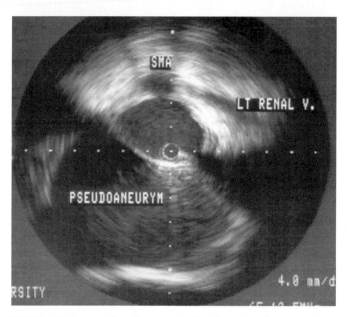

5.21D. Endovascular ultrasound showing pseudoaneurysm in the previous case.

5.22 Retained Bullets

Commentary

Bullets are not sterile, and theoretically retained bullets, especially those that have penetrated the colon, should be associated with a high incidence of local sepsis. However, removal of retained bullets does not reduce the risk of sepsis, and thus bullets should be removed only if they are easily accessible.

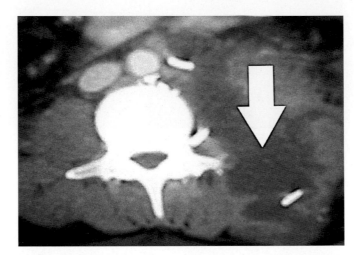

5.22A. CT showing abscess in the bullet track in the psoas muscle, following a gunshot wound in which the bullet traversed the colon and exited from the body.

5.23 Abdominal Trauma in Pregnancy

Commentary

Many physiological changes occur during pregnancy: (a) The blood volume increases by about 50% during the last term, and the trauma victim may lose up to one-third of her volume without any significant hemodynamic changes. (b) The enlarged uterus compresses the inferior vena and impairs venous return. To avoid this problem, the patient should be placed in the left oblique or lateral position, always protecting the spine in appropriate cases. (c) In blunt abdominal trauma, there is a high incidence of placenta abruption. Always look for vaginal bleeding. Ultrasound is very insensitive for abruption, and continuous fetal monitoring is indicated. (d) There is a significant risk of isoimmunization in Rh-negative victims. These patients should receive immunoglobulin. (e) Amniotic fluid embolization may occur and result in severe respiratory failure and disseminated intravascular coagulopathy. (f) Fetal mortality is high, even in moderate severity maternal trauma. In severe trauma, with a nonviable fetus (<24 weeks or weight <500 g) no efforts should be made to stop contractions or deliver the fetus by cesarean section. If the mother needs surgery, it should not be delayed because of the pregnancy. With a viable fetus, a cesarean section should be considered if there is fetal distress and the mother is fairly stable. If the fetus is at term and stable and the mother needs a laparotomy for her injuries, a cesarean section should be performed. A perimortem cesarean section should be performed if the fetus is of a viable gestation (>24 weeks).

In stable patients with advanced pregnancy and blunt abdominal trauma, ultrasound can be used to assess for injury and to evaluate the fetus. These patients should be admitted for continuous fetal monitoring and general examination.

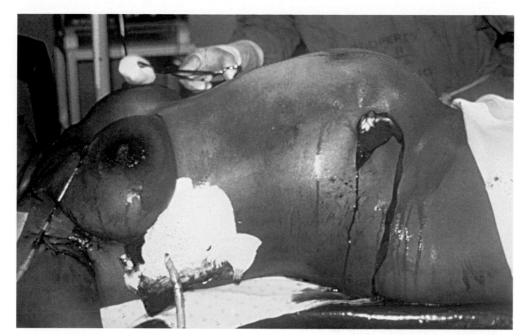

5.23A. Photograph of penetrating abdominal trauma in advanced pregnancy. The patient had signs of peritonitis.

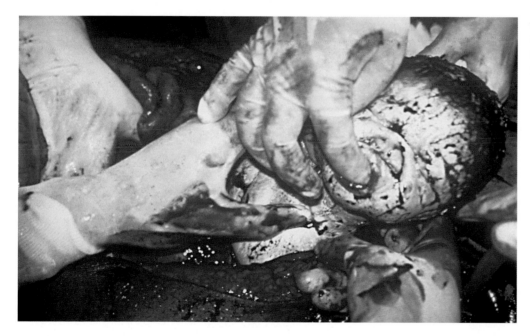

5.23B. Photograph of a cesarean section during exploratory laparotomy for an acute abdomen.

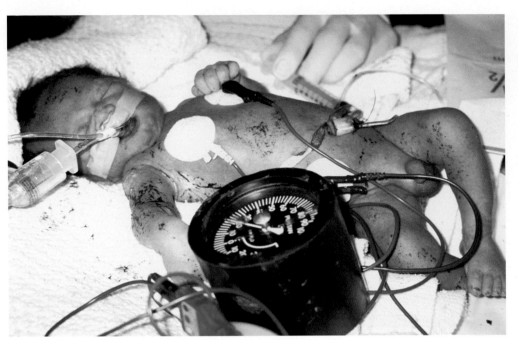

5.23C. Photograph of a baby, delivered by emergency perimortem cesarean section, who survived without any problems.

Musculoskeletal Injury

Introduction

Orthopedic injuries are found in approximately 85% of blunt trauma victims, and thus expert knowledge in their emergency care is necessary. Many injuries are also acutely life-threatening or limb-threatening and thus need to be evaluated and treated in an expedited fashion. Despite the importance of early treatment, the standard primary survey evaluation with the ABCDE approach is necessary to detect other injuries with a greater priority. During the primary survey, the only attention to musculoskeletal injury is acute hemorrhage control with direct pressure.

Clinical Examination

The physical exam is an integral component of detecting acute orthopedic injuries. The overlying skin should be examined for contusions and lacerations. Lacerations need a more detailed evaluation for neurovascular injury, tendon injury, foreign bodies, and proximity to fracture sites. Cool, pale skin may indicate acute vascular insufficiency. Capillary refill and peripheral pulses should be checked and compared with the unaffected limb. In some cases Doppler ultrasound may be required to detect poor pulses. The compartments should be palpated for firmness that may indicate an acute compartment syndrome. General range of motion and areas of tenderness help guide necessary radiographs. Careful peripheral nerve exam is also important, as nerve injury may be part of the injury complex. Some injuries may not present with any fracture, but ligamentous injury is important to detect.

Investigations

1. Plain radiographs are necessary for most orthopedic injuries. Fractures are usually evident on plain radi-

ographs, but occasionally the fracture is occult, requiring further imaging. An AP pelvis film is standard in multisystem blunt trauma, and other radiographs should be guided by the clinical exam. X-rays should view the affected bone in at least two planes and provide a full view of the involved bone, including the joints above and below. Depending on the spectrum of injuries, full radiographic imaging may need to be delayed to stabilize the patient from life-threatening injuries.

2. Computed tomography (CT) scanning is useful in evaluating patients with continued pain and with normal plain radiographs, such as in acute hip injuries. CT scan provides much more detail of an identified injury and allows 3D reformatting.

3. Magnetic resonance imaging (MRI) is rarely needed to acutely evaluate musculoskeletal injury. It is useful in detecting occult fractures, as in hip injuries, and is also useful in delineating ligamentous and cartilaginous injury, such as may be seen with acute knee injury. It has a prominent role in spinal injuries.

4. Bone scanning at 72 hours is occasionally used to follow up patients who may have occult fractures of the scaphoid.

5. Doppler ultrasound and arteriography, in conjunction with the ankle-brachial index, are used to evaluate patients with possible vascular injury.

6. Intracompartment pressures can easily be measured with portable equipment and can help guide the management of patients with possible compartment syndrome.

General Management

Life-threatening injuries receive priority, and thus many orthopedic emergencies may receive more extensive evaluation and treatment in the postoperative phase. Some orthopedic injuries require special mention as they are life-threatening and need similar prioritization. Major pelvic fractures are associated with significant retroperitoneal hemorrhage that is difficult to control. Liberal blood transfusions, external stabilization, and emergency angiography with embolization may be necessary to hemodynamically stabilize the patient. Major arterial injury with exsanguination may occur with penetrating injury or by blunt force with fracture or dislocation-induced vessel laceration. Depending on the involved vessel and the clinical status of the patient, emergency operative therapy may be necessary to control bleeding. Acute crush syndrome causes traumatic rhabdomyolysis that will lead to acute renal failure if not promptly managed with vigorous intravenous hydration, diuretics, and alkalinization.

Open fractures and open joints are limb-threatening and need irrigation, tetanus immunization, and parenteral antibiotics. Formal operative debridement will be necessary on an emergent basis. Traumatic amputations will need to be considered for emergency reimplantation, and the amputated part appropriately cooled and carefully cared for. Compartment syndrome may develop over hours, and thus high-risk injuries need serial physical examinations and compartment pressures evaluated. Dislocations need prompt reduction with deep sedation and neurovascular status checked before and after the reduction. Closed fractures need at least gross alignment with splinting in the emergency department to decrease pain and to avoid further displacement. Definitive closed or open reduction can be completed once the patient has been stabilized from other injuries.

Common Mistakes and Pitfalls

1. Significant occult blood loss can occur with fractures of large bones such as the femur and the pelvis and can often account for acute hemorrhagic shock. Anticipate large blood loss with these injuries while excluding other causes of occult hemorrhage.

2. Compartment syndrome may insidiously develop in the polytrauma patient, and thus repeat clinical examination is paramount for early diagnosis of this condition. Pain out of proportion to the apparent injury is an early symptom and will need to be evaluated by assessing compartment pressures. Segmental fractures in long bones such as the tibia are especially susceptible to compartment syndrome, and thus a high index of suspicion must be maintained.

3. Neurovascular injury complicates many fractures and needs to be carefully sought. Ankle-brachial index, Doppler ultrasound, and/or arteriography may be needed to delineate acute vascular injury.

4. Occult fractures should be suspected in patients with significant pain but with normal radiographs. Further radiographs, CT scanning, MRI, or bone scan may be necessary for fracture identification.

5. Pediatric radiographs are inherently more difficult to interpret because of osseous growth plates. At times, comparison views of the other extremity will be necessary, and occult fractures should be suspected in children with tenderness over the physis.

6.1 Classification of Fractures

Commentary

Correct terminology is necessary and allows clear communication when describing orthopedic injuries. Fractures are first described by anatomic location, and long bones are usually divided in thirds in describing the location of the injury. Open or compound fractures refer to fractures with a break in the overlying skin, in contrast to closed fractures that have normal skin integrity.

The fracture line or pattern is then described and follows the following common convention:

1. Transverse: fracture line perpendicular to the long axis of the bone

2. Oblique: fracture line oblique to the long axis of the bone

3. Spiral: fracture line curved in a spiral fashion

4. Comminuted: fracture with two or more pieces

5. Segmental: fracture at two distinct levels

6. Torus: wrinkling or buckling of bone cortex, seen in pediatrics

7. Greenstick: incomplete fracture, seen in pediatrics

Displacement refers to the degree of offset of the bone ends relative to one another, and thus completely displaced fractures tend to be more unstable injuries. Displacement is described by outlining the position of the distal bone relative to the proximal end. A bayonet deformity refers to injuries with 100% displacement and overriding of the bone ends with shortening of the affected extremity.

Angulation refers to the angle between the longitudinal axes of the main fracture segments. Fractures with significant angulation generally require reduction to maintain good function. Angulation may be described by the relationship of the bone distal to the fracture site with respect to the proximal end or by describing the direction the apex of fracture angle is pointing.

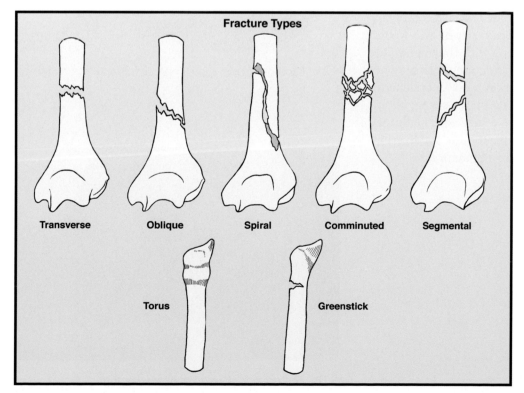

6.1A. Illustration of fracture pattern types.

6.2 Open Fractures

Commentary

Open or compound fractures are true orthopedic emergencies. They are defined as fractures in contact with the outside environment and thus require a break in the skin covering the fracture site. This skin break may be large and obvious or a small puncture wound injury, and thus determination if a fracture is open can sometimes be difficult.

Below is the Gustilo classification that is often used when describing open fractures:

Type I: Puncture wound <1 cm and relatively clean

Type II: Laceration longer than 1 cm but without extensive soft tissue damage, flaps, or avulsion and with a minimal to moderate crushing component

Type IIIA: Adequate soft tissue coverage of the fracture despite extensive soft tissue laceration or flaps, or high-energy trauma irrespective of the size of the wound.

Type IIIB: Extensive soft tissue injury loss with periosteal stripping and bone exposure

Type IIIC: Open fracture associated with arterial injury requiring repair

Staphylococcus aureus commonly causes osteomyelitis, and thus antibiotic therapy is guided against this organism. Emergency therapy includes covering the wound with sterile saline dressings, along with the appropriate tetanus immunization. All open fractures of large bones require early operative irrigation and debridement. Patients needing emergent operation for severe associated injuries can have external fixation performed whereas stable patients are eligible for internal fixation. Mangled extremities may require amputation.

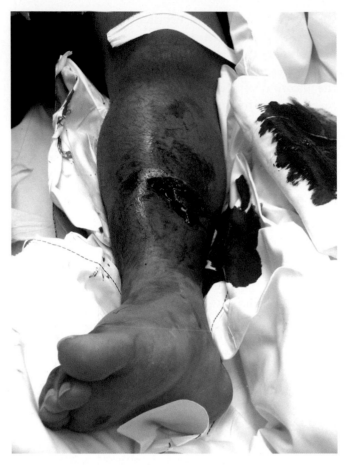

6.2A. Photograph of a type II open fracture of the mid tibia.

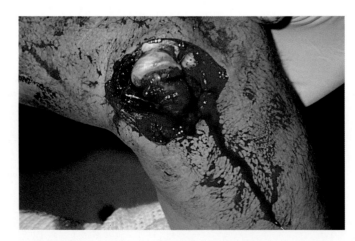

6.2B. Photograph of an open elbow fracture.

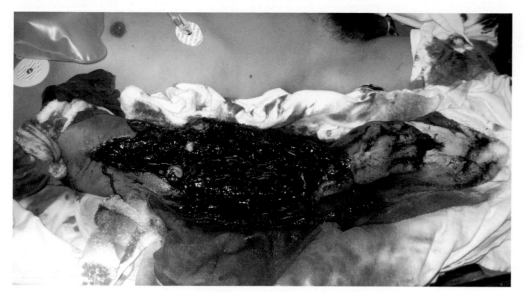

6.2C. Photograph of a mangled right arm with severe crush injury. This patient accidentally placed his arm into an industrial mixer. Amputation was required.

6.3 Open Joint Injury

Commentary

Open joint injuries are serious orthopedic emergencies, with septic arthritis and osteomyelitis being common complications. Detection may be straightforward on physical exam or may be subtle, requiring a high index of suspicion or adjunctive testing. Any deep wound in proximity to a joint should be considered as entering the joint.

Plain x-rays can show an associated fracture, air, or a foreign body within the joint but may be normal. Careful exploration under sterile conditions may reveal a wound track directly penetrating the joint capsule. In questionable cases, a saline or methylene blue arthrogram may provide the answer by revealing dye leakage through the wound site. Emergency therapy includes parenteral antibiotic coverage and tetanus immunization. All major open joints require formal operative exploration and irrigation.

6.3A. Photograph of an open volar dislocation of the metacarpal joint.

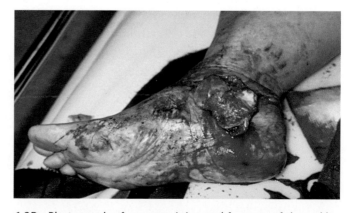

6.3B. Photograph of an open joint and fracture of the ankle.

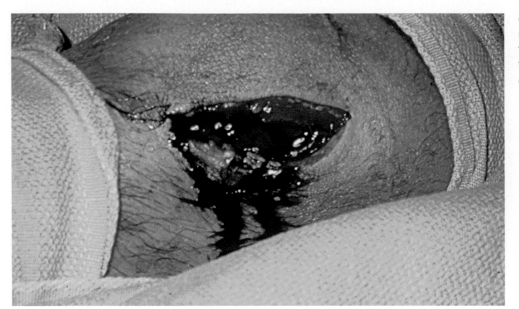

6.3C. Photograph of a methylene blue arthrogram of the knee with leakage through the proximal wound signifying an open joint.

6.4 Salter-Harris Classification

Commentary

In a growing child, the epiphyseal plate is a weak cartilaginous structure and is predisposed to injury. Injuries most often occur in the zone of hypertrophic cartilage cells, and the germinal cells are usually undamaged; thus, fortunately growth is often not affected.

The most commonly used classification of epiphyseal injuries is the Salter-Harris classification. In this classification, prognosis becomes progressively worse with higher numerical order.

Type I: A very common slip through the zone of provisional calcification without fracture. No germinal layer is involved, and the fracture usually heals without consequence. Comparison radiographs are often necessary for diagnosis.

Type II: An epiphyseal plate slip with an associated fracture through the metaphysis, forming a triangular fragment. This is a very common type and forms three-quarters of all epiphyseal injuries. Prognosis is good.

Type III: An epiphyseal plate slip with a fracture through the epiphysis involving the articular surface. This fracture involves the germinal layer, and thus accurate reduction is necessary but does not guarantee avoidance of growth complications.

Type IV: Epiphyseal fracture involving both the plate and metaphysis. These fractures are complicated, and significant growth disturbance can occur unless good anatomic reduction is achieved. Operative intervention is often needed in this type of fracture.

Type V: Impaction injury in which the epiphyseal plate is destroyed. They are rare and difficult to diagnose. Unfortunately, growth arrest is the rule in this injury.

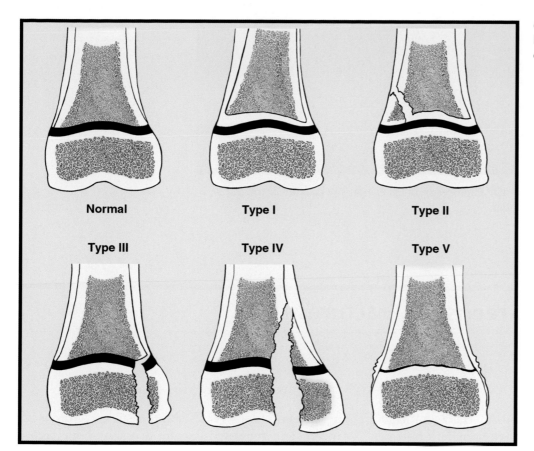

6.4A. Illustration of the Salter-Harris pediatric fracture classification.

Normal **Type I** **Type II**

Type III **Type IV** **Type V**

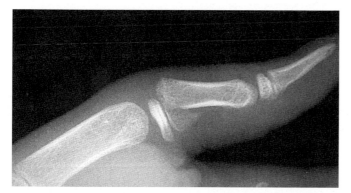

6.4B. Radiograph of Salter-Harris II fracture involving the proximal phalanx of the thumb.

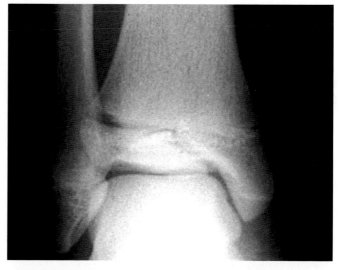

6.4C. Radiograph of Salter-Harris III fracture of the ankle.

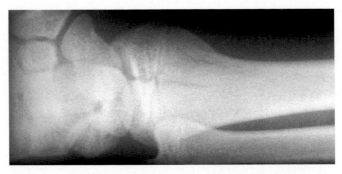

6.4D. Radiograph of Salter-Harris IV fracture of the distal radius.

6.5 Torus and Greenstick Fractures

Commentary

Pediatric bones are much less brittle than adult bones and thus are less likely to have complete fractures through the bone. A torus fracture is an incomplete fracture with a small fold in the cortex. It is often seen at the end of long bones. A greenstick fracture is an incomplete angulated fracture of a long bone recognized by a bowing appearance. These pediatric variants are common and can easily be missed.

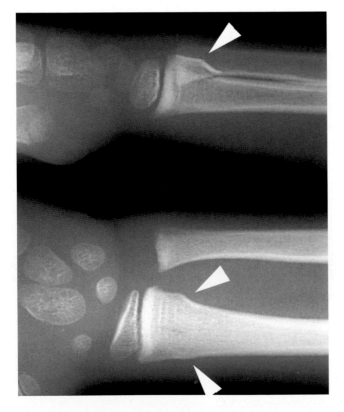

6.5A. Radiograph of a distal radius torus fracture.

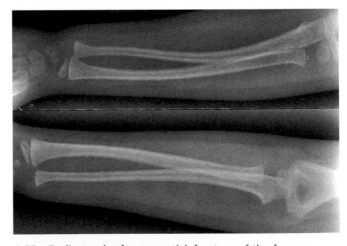

6.5B. Radiograph of a greenstick fracture of the forearm.

6.6 Supracondylar Fracture

Commentary

Distal humeral fractures that are proximal to the epicondyles are termed supracondylar fractures, and most of these fractures occur in children age 5–10 years. In children, the ligaments and joint capsule are stronger than the bone and thus hyperextension injury often causes bone fracture, while adults often suffer a posterior dislocation of the elbow with a similar mechanism.

Supracondylar fractures are of two common types: flexion and extension, with extension fractures the overwhelming majority. These extension injuries are often the result of a fall on an arm with the elbow fully extended. On exam, the elbow will be swollen, often with a joint effusion and with significant pain and tenderness. In addition, the olecranon will be more prominent as it is attached to the posteriorly displaced distal fragment. Careful neurovascular examination of the arm is necessary as many of these fractures are complicated with brachial artery and median, radial, or ulnar nerve injury. In addition, compartment syndrome can be seen with displaced fractures and needs to be considered.

Radiographically, these fractures are often detected on the lateral view of the elbow. Because many of these fractures are transverse they may not be readily visible on the AP view. In addition, up to 25% of these fractures are of the greenstick variety with the posterior cortex remaining intact. The only abnormality seen may be a posterior fat pad sign or an abnormal anterior humeral line. A high degree of suspicion for supracondylar fracture must be maintained for any child with acute elbow trauma, pain, and normal radiography. Most undisplaced fractures are treated nonoperatively with casting, and most displaced fractures will undergo percutaneous pinning.

6.6A. Photograph of a swollen elbow of a child suffering a supracondylar fracture.

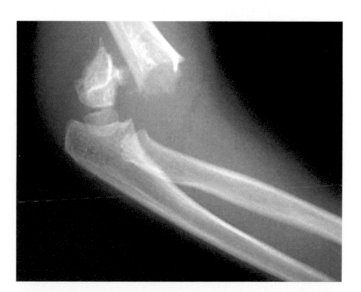

6.6B. Radiograph of a displaced extension supracondylar fracture.

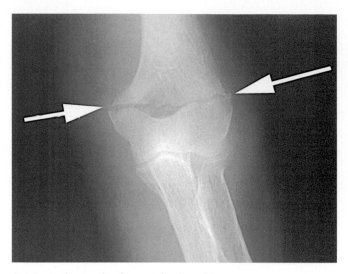

6.6C. Radiograph of an undisplaced transverse supracondylar fracture.

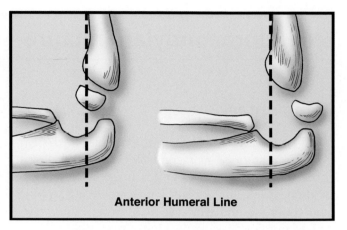

Anterior Humeral Line

6.6D. Illustration of the anterior humeral line. Normally this line will intersect the middle of the capitellum. With an extension fracture, this line will intersect the anterior one-third of the capitellum or pass entirely anteriorly.

6.7 Amputations

Commentary

Amputations are devastating injuries and require expert knowledge in the care of the patient and the amputated part. The area affected is important in the decision to consider reimplantation. Lower extremity reimplantation is rarely indicated, given the frequency of associated crush injury and the efficacy of current prostheses. In contrast, upper extremity amputations, especially involving the thumb, are often reimplanted, given the severe disability that occurs with the loss of that single digit. Time elapsed since the injury is also an important consideration. Reimplantation is less likely to be successful if the warm ischemia (room temperature) time has been >6–8 hours. If the part has been properly cooled and cared for, then this window of time may be successfully extended to 12–24 hours. In addition, clean, sharp amputations are more likely to be successful than crush injuries. In general, all amputated parts should be considered as candidates for reimplantation, and even severely crushed parts can be used for skin coverage.

The amputated part must be cared for properly to maximize the chance of successful reimplantation. The part should be handled minimally with no anti-septics. In addition, no debridement should occur. The part should be irrigated with normal saline and then sterile saline-soaked gauze used to cover the part. It should then be placed in a watertight plastic bag and the bag placed in an ice water mixture.

The patient's stump should also be irrigated with normal saline and direct pressure used to control any bleeding. No antiseptics should be used, but prophylactic antibiotics and tetanus immunization should be administered.

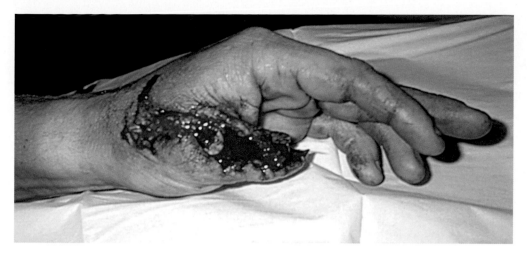

6.7A. Photograph of a hand with thumb amputated secondary to a power saw injury.

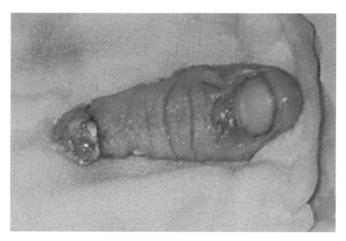

6.7B. Photograph of an amputated thumb.

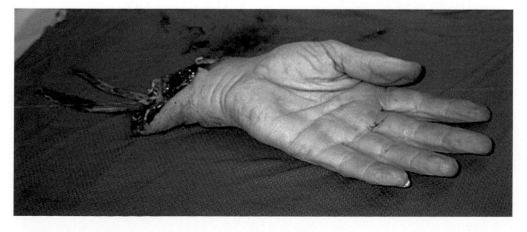

6.7C. Photograph of an amputated hand.

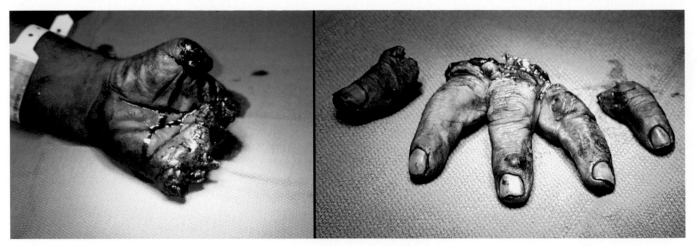

6.7D. Photographs of multiple finger amputations secondary to the hand being caught in a gear mechanism. This patient was a reimplantion candidate.

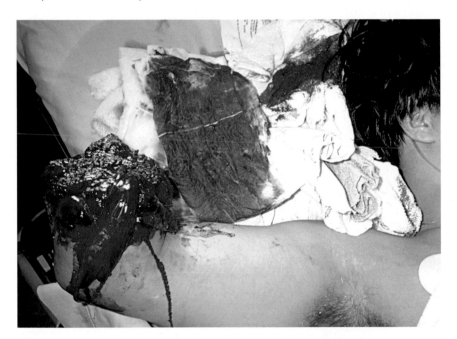

6.7E. Photograph of a proximal forearm amputation secondary to a motor vehicle accident. Direct pressure to the amputated stump is used to control bleeding.

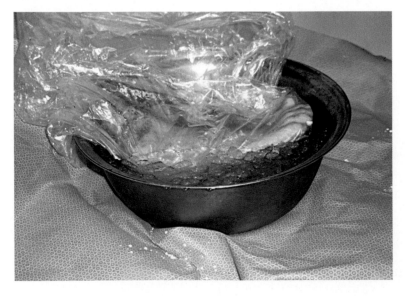

6.7F. Photograph of an amputated foot being cooled in ice water slurry.

6.8 Tendon Injury

Commentary

Tendon lacerations are important injuries to detect, and full examination of the hand will usually detect complete lacerations. Partial injuries are more difficult to diagnosis, as tendon function is usually still intact. A careful examination of the laceration through full range of motion is necessary, as the injured area of tendon may retract out of the field of view.

Flexor tendon repair is difficult and fraught with complications. Flexor tendon repair should be performed by an experienced hand surgeon, often in an operating room setting, although extensor tendon injury over the hand and fingers can be repaired in the emergency department. Prophylactic antibiotic, tetanus immunization, and splinting are essential components of emergency management.

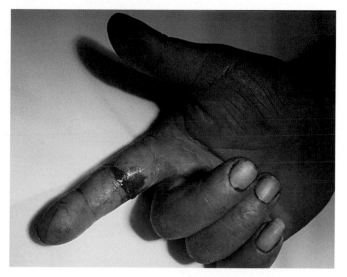

6.8A. This photograph illustrates the classic position of extension in a patient with finger flexor tendon injury.

6.9 Peripheral Vascular Injury

Commentary

Most peripheral vascular injuries occur as a result of acute penetrating trauma, with gunshot wounds being more damaging than stab wounds. Fortunately, blunt trauma rarely causes vascular injury except with markedly displaced fractures and dislocations. Prompt identification and repair is important, given the relatively short "golden period" of about six hours, after which irreversible limb ischemia insult will occur.

A careful physical examination is important for early diagnosis, and most authors divide examination findings into "hard" and "soft" signs. Hard signs of vascular injury include the following: pulsatile bleeding, absent peripheral pulse, an expanding hematoma, palpable thrill, audible bruit, and evidence of regional ischemia such as a pale and cool extremity. In the presence of any of these signs, operative exploration is usually recommended.

Soft signs include moderate hematoma formation, injury in proximity (1–2 cm) to major neurovascular tracts, peripheral nerve injury, and diminished but palpable pulses. To assist the evaluation of diminished pulses, the arterial pressure index (API; Doppler-determined arterial pressure in the affected limb divided by the pressure in an unaffected arm) is often used to screen for injury. An index of >0.9 generally excludes significant injury, and an index <0.9 mandates further investigation. Though there are variations in the stepwise approach, all patients with soft signs should undergo further diagnostic testing such as color flow Doppler ultrasound or arteriography to exclude serious injuries requiring operative attention.

Besides acute limb loss, patients with these injuries are also at risk for acute compartment syndrome. Late complications of missed injuries include pseudoaneurysm formation, delayed thrombosis, arteriovenous fistula, and intermittent claudication.

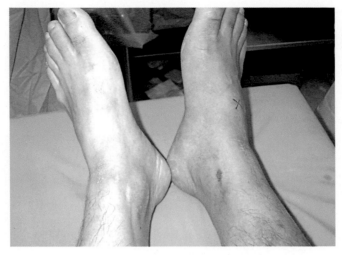

6.9A. Photograph of hard signs of vascular injury: Left foot is cool and pale and has no pulse on examination.

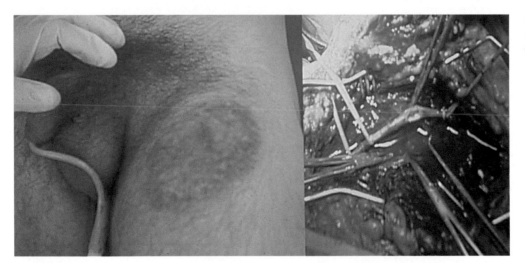

6.9B. Photographs of gunshot wound to the thigh with large groin hematoma (left side) and operative view revealing associated femoral artery injury (right side).

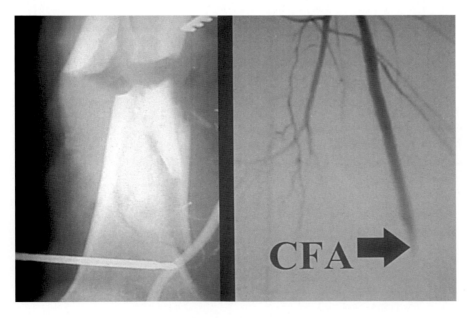

6.9C. Plain x-ray of a displaced fracture of the femur (left side) with angiogram showing acute common femoral artery occlusion (right side).

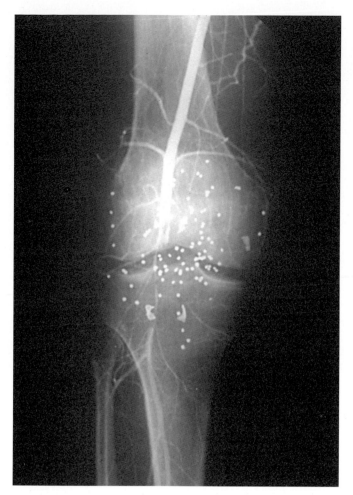

6.9D. Angiogram of shotgun pellet injury to the knee with popliteal artery injury.

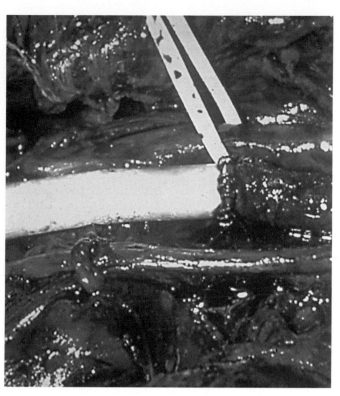

6.9F. Photograph of operative repair of the femoral artery injury in the previous patient.

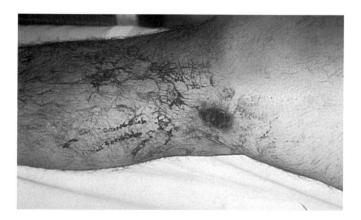

6.9E. Photograph of a gunshot wound to the knee.

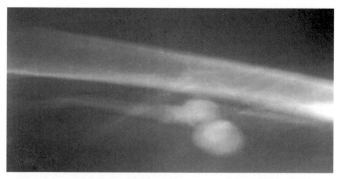

6.9G. Complicating false aneurysm seen on angiogram.

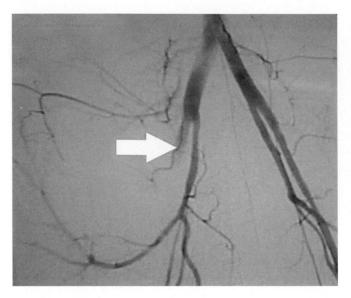

6.9H. Angiography revealing external iliac thrombosis in a blunt trauma patient.

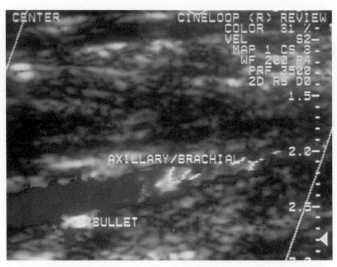

6.9I. Color flow Doppler revealing axillary artery injury.

6.10 Peripheral Nerve Injury

Commentary

Peripheral nerve injuries, though not life-threatening, can cause significant long-term disability. Nerve injuries are generally classified in the following three groups:

1. Neuropraxia: Mild transient nerve dysfunction without gross anatomic disruption to the nerve. Often secondary to contusion, local ischemia, or local pressure.
2. Axonotmesis: More extensive injury with interruption of the axons and myelin sheath but with preservation of the endoneural tube. Complete loss of motor and sensory function is seen distal to the site of injury. Spontaneous recovery is possible and is dependent on the distance between the site of injury and the peripheral muscles to be reinnervated.
3. Neurotmesis: Complete severance of the nerve or damage to the point where spontaneous regeneration is impossible. This injury is often seen follow-

ing direct lacerations, severe contusions, crushing or ischemic compressive injuries, electrical and thermal burns, and chemical injections.

A careful physical examination can exclude peripheral nerve injury. Penetrating injury proximal to a nerve will need careful examination and exploration. In addition, these injuries may have coexistent vascular or tendon injury to be excluded. Certain orthopedic injury complexes are more likely to harbor coexistent nerve injuries and the following tables outline common injury patterns.

Completely severed nerves will need microsurgical repair. In clean, sharp wounds, such as from a knife or glass, ideally this repair can be done early. If the injury is from a missile or crushing injury or if the wound is grossly contaminated, then the nerve should have a delayed exploration and repair.

Upper Extremity Patterns	
Nerve Injury	Upper Extremity Injury
Ulnar	Elbow injury
Distal median	Wrist dislocation
Median, anterior interosseous	Supracondylar fracture
Musculocutaneous	Anterior shoulder dislocation
Radial	Distal humeral shaft fracture, anterior dislocation of shoulder
Axillary	Anterior shoulder dislocation, proximal humeral fracture

Lower Extremity Patterns	
Nerve Injury	Lower Extremity Injury
Femoral	Pubic rami fracture
Obturator	Obturator ring fracture
Posterior tibial	Knee dislocation
Superficial peroneal	Fibular neck fracture, knee dislocation
Deep peroneal	Fibular neck fracture, compartment syndrome
Sciatic	Posterior hip dislocation
Superior and inferior gluteal	Acetabular fracture

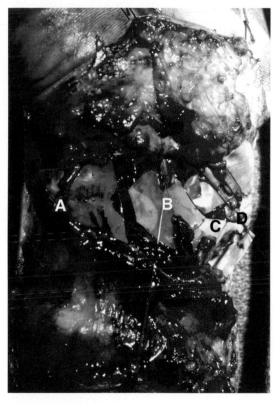

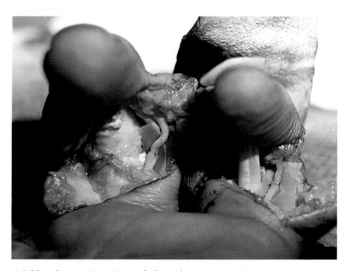

6.10B. Operative view of digital nerve injuries post repair.

6.10A. Operative view of a "spaghetti" wrist with neurovascular injury. A, radial artery; B, median nerve; C, ulnar artery; and D, flexor carpi ulnaris.

6.11 Metacarpal Fractures

Commentary

Metacarpal fractures are commonly seen in the emergency department and are often secondary to direct force, such as a clenched fist injury. Fourth and fifth metacarpal neck fractures of this nature are often referred to as "boxer's fractures." Metacarpal fractures can be classified in four types:

1. Head fractures: Rare injury.
2. Neck fractures: Very common fracture with the apex of the fracture being dorsal. Second and third metacarpal fractures require accurate reduction for good hand function, while the fourth and fifth fractures can heal well with angulation up to 35 and 45 degrees, respectively.
3. Shaft fractures: Can be transverse, oblique, spiral, or comminuted. Rotational deformities can occur, especially with oblique and spiral fractures, and will need identification and correction. This is best evaluated clinically by having the patient flex the fingers into a fist. Rotational deformities will be recognized by an abnormal lie of the affected digit. Normally the fingertips of the flexed hand all point toward the scaphoid at the wrist.
4. Base fractures: Uncommon fractures that are usually stable.

Most metacarpal fractures will have closed reduction, although comminuted, spiral, and oblique fractures may need operative fixation.

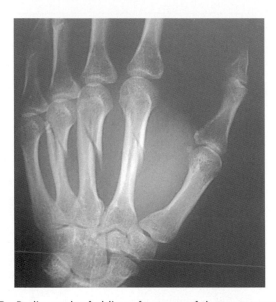

6.11B. Radiograph of oblique fractures of the metacarpal bones.

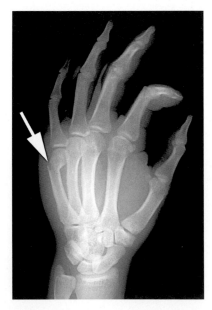

6.11A. Radiograph of a boxer's fracture of the fifth metacarpal bone.

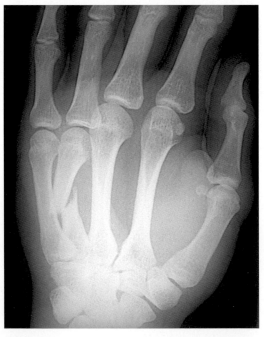

6.11C. Radiograph of a displaced oblique fracture of the fourth metacarpal.

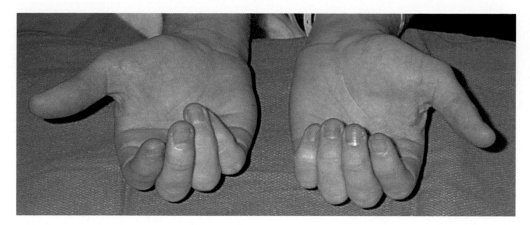

6.11D. Photograph of a rotational injury evident on physical exam. All fingertips should normally point toward the scaphoid. The patient's right fifth digit has a rotational abnormality.

6.12 First Metacarpal Fractures (Bennett's and Rolando's Fractures)

Commentary

First metacarpal fractures are classified as articular or less commonly nonarticular, with the latter being either transverse or oblique. Articular fractures are further described in two common patterns.

Bennett's fracture is an oblique fracture that involves the carpometacarpal joint. It is usually due to direct axial force on a partially flexed thumb, such as in a fistfight. The characteristic finding is a small triangular proximal fragment that remains anatomically correct while the shaft is displaced in a dorsal-radial fashion by the pull of the abductor pollicis longus and the abductor pollicis. Anatomic reduction is important, and these fractures are usually treated with percutaneous pinning or open reduction.

Rolando's fracture is a comminuted fracture at the base of the first metacarpal. It is a relatively rare fracture often caused by a similar mechanism to a Bennett's fracture. The treatment is controversial and may vary from closed to open reduction, depending on the degree of comminution and displacement.

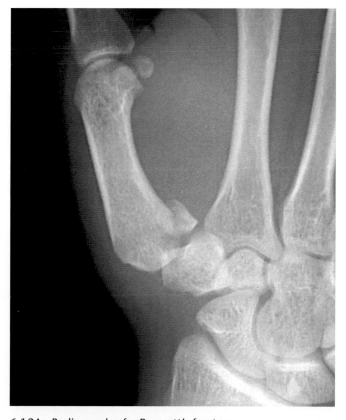

6.12A. Radiograph of a Bennett's fracture.

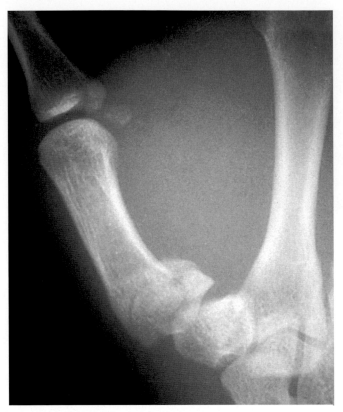

6.12B. Radiograph of a Rolando fracture.

6.13 Scaphoid Fracture

Commentary

Fractures of the scaphoid bone are common and usually occur from a fall on an outstretched hand. Pain as well as tenderness is usually demonstrated in the anatomical snuffbox. Pain with axial force along the metacarpal will also help identify scaphoid injury.

Scaphoid fractures are classified as proximal one-third, middle third, and distal third fractures. The proximal third does not have its own blood supply, and thus these fractures are particularly at high risk for avascular necrosis if treatment is delayed or improper. Plain radiographs are often diagnostic, but up to 20% may present with normal radiographs initially. Patients with scaphoid tenderness and normal radiographs are placed in a thumb spica cast and will need a follow-up exam. A bone scan may be done in three days, or the patient may have repeat radiographs in ten days to detect occult fractures. Nondisplaced scaphoid fractures are treated with thumb spica immobilization, and displaced or unstable fractures often need open reduction.

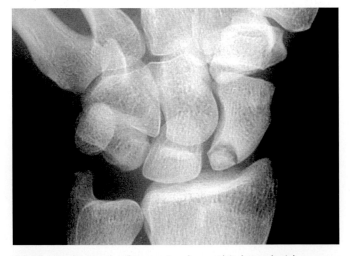

6.13A. Radiograph of a proximal one-third scaphoid fracture.

6.14 Scapholunate Dislocation

Commentary

Scapholunate ligamentous injury is often secondary to forced dorsiflexion of the wrist, as occurs in a fall on an outstretched hand. There is pain and tenderness on the radial aspect of the wrist just distal to Lister's tubercle.

This injury is commonly missed, and radiographs should be carefully examined for an abnormal gap between the scaphoid and lunate on the PA view. This joint space is normally less than 3 mm, and any widening of this space is representative of a scapholunate ligamentous injury. This injury may be treated with closed reduction and percutaneous pinning or may require open reduction. Missed scapholunate injuries often cause chronic arthritis and pain or may cause ischemic necrosis of the lunate (Kienböck's disease).

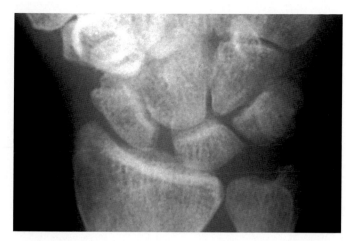

6.14A. Widening of the joint space between the scaphoid and the lunate in a radiograph of a scapholunate dislocation.

6.15 Lunate and Perilunate Dislocation

Commentary

Lunate and perilunate dislocations are relatively uncommon injuries that can easily be missed if the treating physician is not familiar with normal carpal relationships. The injury often involves high energy, such as a fall or motor vehicle accident, that causes extreme hyperextension, ulnar deviation, and midcarpal dorsiflexion.

In the normal wrist, the lateral view reveals that the distal radius, lunate, and capitate align themselves forming three Cs atop each other. This relationship is significantly altered with a lunate or perilunate dislocation, and thus a lateral radiograph usually reveals the injury pattern.

A lunate dislocation will demonstrate the lunate pushed off the distal radius in a "spilled teacup" sign on the lateral view. On the AP view, the lunate will appear as a "piece of pie" sign. A perilunate dislocation demonstrates a capitate that is posterior or anterior to the lunate, while the lunate maintains contact with the distal radius. The AP view is less specific and shows an obliterated joint space between the lunate and the capitate. Treatment involves anatomical alignment with closed reduction, though open reduction may be necessary.

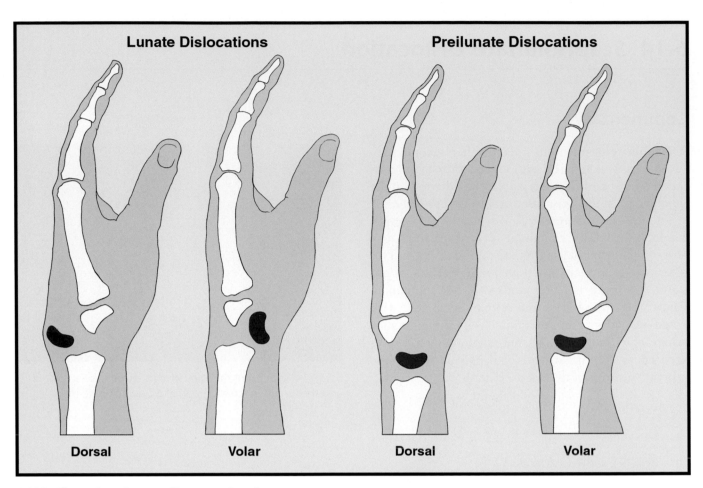

6.15A. Illustration of types of lunate and perilunate dislocations.

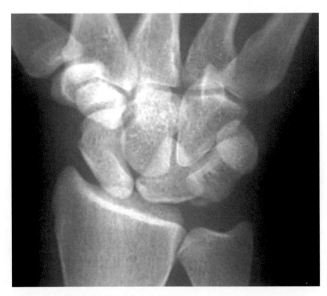

6.15B. AP x-ray of the wrist showing a lunate dislocation with a "piece of pie" lunate bone.

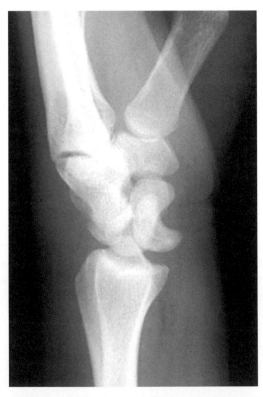

6.15C. Lateral radiograph view of the wrist with a volar lunate dislocation.

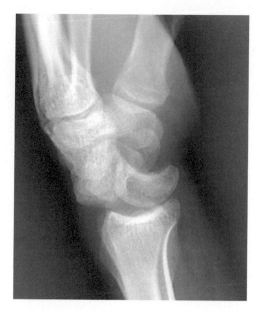

6.15D. Lateral radiograph view of the wrist with a dorsal perilunate dislocation.

6.16 Colles' Fracture

Commentary

A Colles' fracture is the most common fracture of the wrist. It is a transverse fracture of the distal radius metaphysis, which is dorsally displaced and angulated. The fracture may also be intra-articular and can involve the ulnar styloid.

The usual mechanism is a fall on an outstretched hand, and the wrist may demonstrate the classic "dinner fork" deformity on exam. The treatment is usually closed reduction, though more comminuted and displaced fractures will need open reduction and fixation.

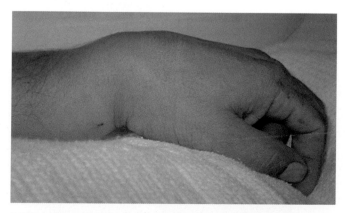

6.16A. Photograph of the classic "dinner fork" deformity seen with dorsal radius fractures.

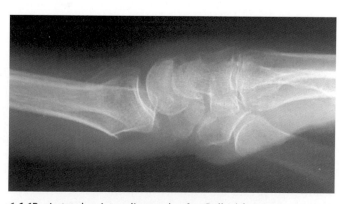

6.16B. Lateral wrist radiograph of a Colles' fracture.

6.17 Forearm Fractures

Commentary

When evaluating forearm fractures, it is important to remember that isolated fractures in this area are rare. Injuries may encompass two fractures at similar or separate sites or may involve a single fracture with ligamentous injury and with or without dislocation. Careful examination of the wrist and elbow joints is imperative, as these are commonly involved sites. Some common patterns are seen in forearm fractures and thus knowledge of these injury patterns is important.

Both bones fractures (involving both the radius and ulnar shafts) are often seen in children secondary to minor falls on an outstretched hand. They are only rarely seen in adults and are then from high-energy mechanisms or severe direct impact. In a child, radiographs can reveal buckle or torus fractures, incomplete fractures, complete fractures, or a combination. Closed reduction is often successful in children because small amounts of residual angulation will resolve with bone remodeling. Complete fractures are more common in adults, and open reduction is often required.

The Monteggia fracture complex, first described in 1814, is a proximal ulnar fracture with an associated radial head dislocation. It is uncommon, about 7% of all forearm fractures. The injury is caused by forced pronation of the forearm during a fall on an outstretched hand. Local pain and tenderness are seen, and the radial nerve should be examined, as it is commonly injured. Radiographs easily reveal the proximal ulnar fracture, and in these cases the radial head should be carefully evaluated. In the normal position, the radial head should align with the capitellum when a line is drawn through the radial shaft. Monteggia fractures are treated with open reduction.

The Galeazzi fracture complex is a distal fracture of the radius with an associated dislocation or subluxation of the distal radial-ulnar joint. The injury occurs with a fall on an outstretched hand with the wrist in extension and the forearm forcibly pronated, or with a direct blow to the dorsoradial aspect of the wrist. This injury is relatively rare and accounts for only 7% of all forearm fractures. The AP radiograph reveals a fracture of the radius at the junction of the middle and distal thirds, and an increase in joint space between the distal radius and ulna may be seen. The lateral view will demonstrate dorsal angulation of the radial fracture, and the head of the ulna will be displaced dorsally. Galeazzi fractures are unstable and require operative fixation.

Isolated ulnar shaft fractures or nightstick fractures are relatively common. They occur as a result of a direct force to the ulna, often happening when raising one's arm in natural defense to a blow from an object such as a stick. In proximal ulnar fractures, the radial head should be carefully examined to exclude the presence of a Monteggia fracture. Associated injuries are rare but include compartment syndrome and vascular injury. Most undisplaced fractures are treated with plaster immobilization, while displaced fractures (>50% of width of ulna) may need open reduction.

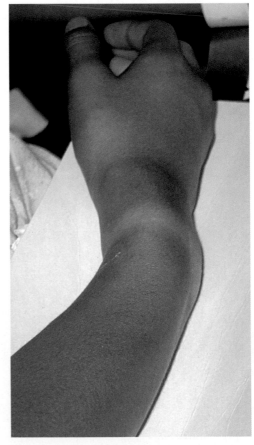

6.17A. Photograph of a child with a "both bones" fracture.

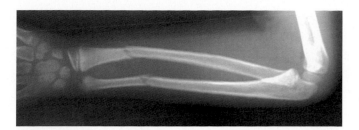

6.17B. Radiograph of a both bones fracture.

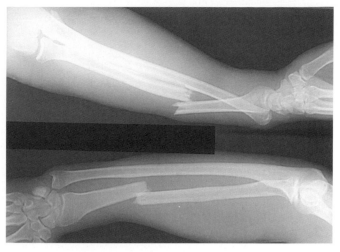

6.17D. AP and lateral radiographs of a Galeazzi fracture.

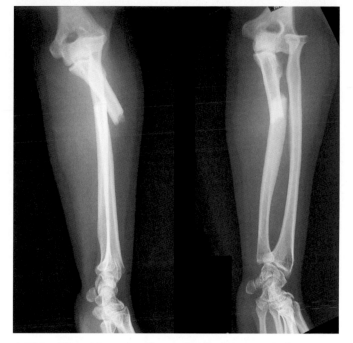

6.17C. AP and lateral radiographs of a Monteggia fracture.

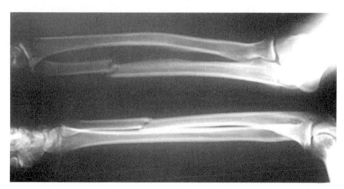

6.17E. AP and lateral radiographs of a nightstick fracture.

6.18 Elbow Dislocation

Commentary

Elbow dislocations account for about 20% of all dislocations and are the next most common dislocation after the shoulder and fingers. They are usually the result of a fall on an outstretched hand with the arm extended and abducted. Most elbow dislocations (>90%) are posterior, and the patient will present with the elbow in 45 degrees of flexion, with a prominence of the olecranon process posteriorly. The collateral ligaments are torn, and careful neurovascular assessment is important as brachial artery and median nerve injuries can complicate this injury.

Radiographs will reveal a dislocation. Most often the coronoid process will slip posteriorly, but occasionally a fracture of the process will be noted. Reduction is performed by countertraction with flexion of the elbow.

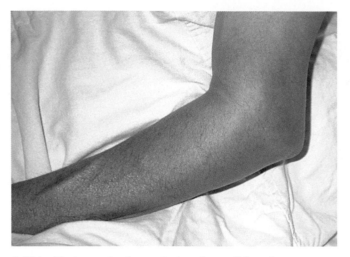

6.18A. Photograph of a posterior elbow dislocation

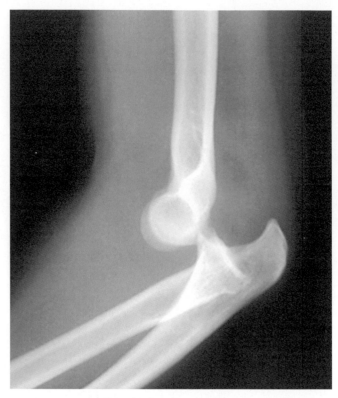

6.18B. Posterior elbow dislocation on x-ray.

6.19 Radial Head Fracture

Commentary

Radial head fractures are common injuries of the elbow that usually occur with a fall on an outstretched hand or by direct trauma. The injury can result in damage to the articular surface, depression of the radial head, or an angulated fracture of the radial head and neck. Often a fracture is seen on radiographs, but they may reveal only a fat pad sign indicative of an effusion and an occult fracture. Nondisplaced or minimally displaced fractures are treated with a sling or posterior splint. Fractures that are displaced more than 3 mm or involve more than one-third of the joint surface are usually treated operatively with the insertion of small screws. Comminuted fractures are treated conservatively, though the treatment of severely comminuted and displaced fractures is controversial and includes excision of fragments and/or the radial head with or without the insertion of Silastic implants.

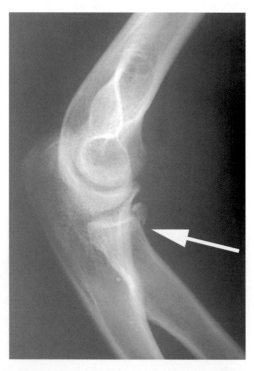

6.19A. Radiograph of a radial head fracture involving the articular surface.

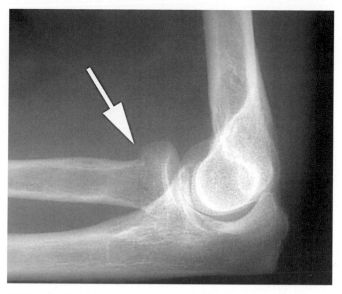

6.19B. Radiograph of an impacted radial head fracture.

6.20 Humeral Fracture

Commentary

Humeral shaft fractures are often the result of direct blows to the arm, motor vehicle accidents, or minor falls in the elderly. Physical exam reveals severe tenderness localized to the fracture area. Radial nerve injuries complicate up to 20% of humerus fractures, though median and ulnar nerve injuries are rarely seen.

Plain radiographs are most often diagnostic, and conservative treatment is used for the majority of closed injuries. The sugar tong splint and hanging cast are good techniques for immobilization. Open fractures, severely comminuted fractures, and fractures that are not adequately aligned by closed reduction are treated with open reduction.

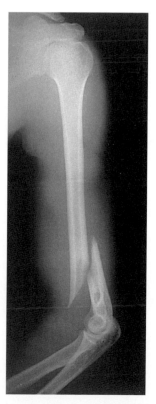

6.20A. Radiograph of an oblique distal one-third humeral fracture.

6.21 Shoulder Dislocations

Commentary

The shoulder is the most commonly dislocated joint. Shoulder dislocations can be classified as anterior, posterior, or inferior (luxatio erecta).

Anterior dislocations are ~90% of all shoulder dislocations. They are usually the result of a fall on an outstretched hand with the arm abducted, extended, and externally rotated. On examination, the arm is held in slight abduction and external rotation. The humeral head is palpable anteriorly, and a slight hollow is noticed in the shoulder laterally. Axillary nerve injury complicates shoulder dislocations in up to 10% of cases.

Standard radiography includes AP and lateral views and either a transscapular **Y** view or an axillary view. Radiographs may reveal a compression fracture in the humeral head termed a Hill-Sachs deformity. In addition, a small anteroinferior glenoid rim fracture called a Bankart lesion may be seen.

Multiple techniques that use traction, leverage, or a combination can be used to reduce this injury, including traction-countertraction, external rotation, Stimson technique, scapular rotation, and the hippocratic technique. Closed reduction is successful in the majority of cases, though operative reduction is used in irreducible cases, unstable joints, large glenoid rim fractures, >5–10 mm of displacement of avulsed greater or lesser tuberosity fractures, intrathoracic dislocations, and many posterior dislocations.

Posterior dislocations are rare injuries, about 5% of all dislocations. They can be difficult to diagnose, and up to 50% of cases are thought to be initially misdiagnosed. The injury occurs with an axial load on an adducted internally rotated and forward flexed arm, direct blow to the shoulder, or severe muscular contraction as from a seizure or electrical injury. The arm is usually internally rotated on exam, and the patient is unable to elevate the arm above 90 degrees. The AP radiograph may look nearly normal, and thus the transscapular **Y** view or axillary view is necessary to exclude the diagnosis. Reduction is accomplished by slow in-line traction, usually with general anesthesia.

Inferior dislocation, also known as luxatio erecta, is a very rare dislocation forming ~1% of all shoulder dislocations. The injury occurs with forced abduction of the arm, and the patient presents with a fully abducted arm and the elbow flexed with the forearm on or behind the head. Neurovascular compromise is common because these structures are inferior to the joint. Plain radiographs easily demonstrate the dislocation, and closed reduction is usually successful with in-line traction.

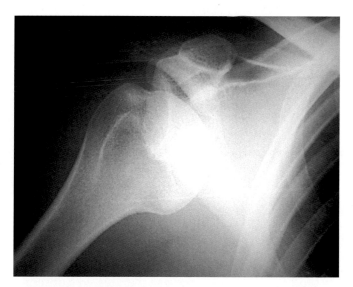

6.21A. Illustration of types of shoulder dislocations.

Anterior Dislocation

Luxatio Erecta Dislocation

Posterior Dislocation

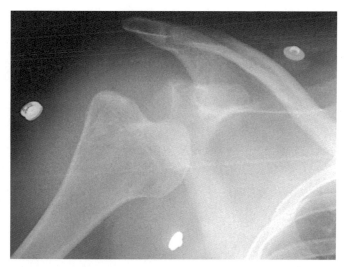

6.21B. AP radiograph of an anterior shoulder dislocation.

6.21C. AP radiograph of an anterior shoulder dislocation with a large Hill-Sachs deformity.

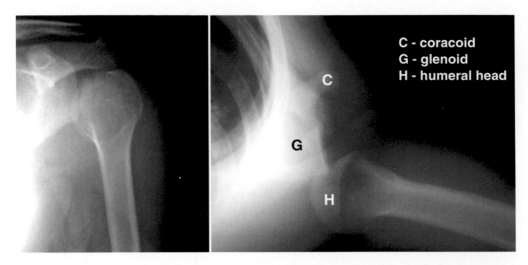

6.21D. AP view of a posterior dislocation (left side) and axillary view of same patient (right side).

C - coracoid
G - glenoid
H - humeral head

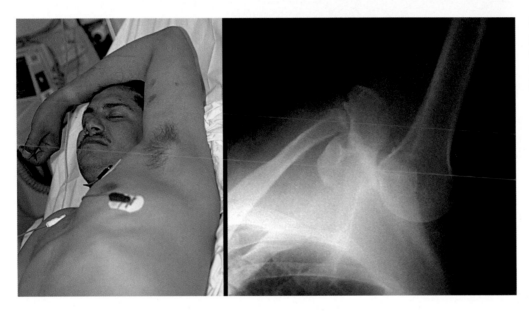

6.21E. Photograph of a patient with a luxatio erecta dislocation (left side) and corresponding radiograph (right side).

6.22 Clavicle Fracture

Commentary

Clavicle fractures are common and can occur from a direct blow to the clavicle or from a fall on an outstretched hand. Localized tenderness is found on examination, and radiography easily delineates the fracture. Complications are unusual but can include a host of serious injuries, including pneumothorax, subclavian vessel injury, tracheal injury, pacemaker malfunction, and thoracic outlet syndrome with brachial plexus injury.

Most clavicle fractures can be treated conservatively with a sling or a figure-of-eight bandage. Open reduction is usually not necessary and is reserved for patients with open fractures, irreducible fractures with soft tissue interposition, unstable fractures, associated acromioclavicular dislocation, associated brachial plexus injury, or nonunion.

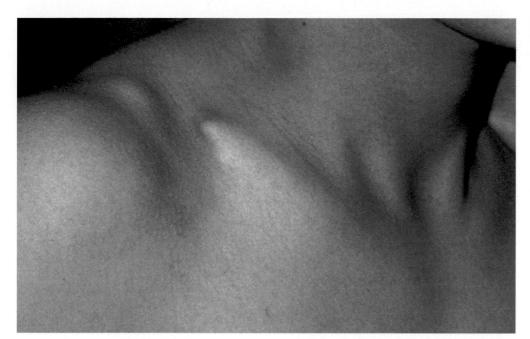

6.22A. Photograph of skin tenting seen with a displaced clavicle fracture.

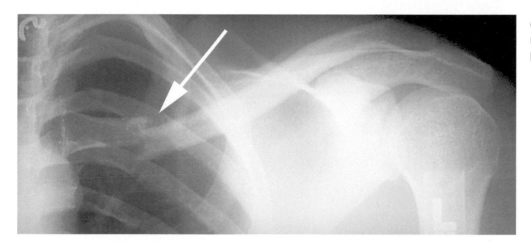

6.22B. A slightly displaced medial clavicle fracture on plain radiography.

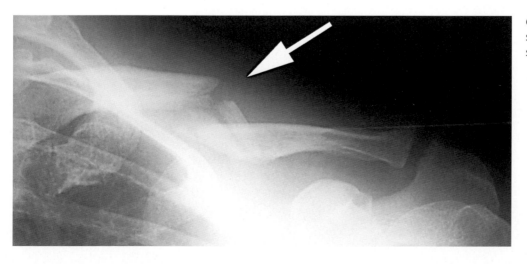

6.22C. Plain radiograph showing a comminuted mid-shaft clavicle fracture.

6.23 Sternoclavicular Dislocation

Commentary

The sternoclavicular joint is the articulation of the medial aspect of the clavicle and the manubrium portion of the sternum. It is a "ball and socket" joint, and thus dislocations may occur in any direction. The injury is rare, accounting for 1.5% of all dislocations, and usually caused by high-energy mechanisms such as motor vehicle accidents or contact sports.

These injuries are classified as:

- First degree: incomplete injury/stretching

- Second degree: mild subluxation

- Third degree: complete dislocation

The majority of these dislocations are anterior (~90%). The less commonly seen posterior dislocation is associated with life-threatening vascular injury, tracheal injury, and brachial plexus injury. First- and second-degree injuries are treated conservatively, but third-degree injuries require reduction. Reduction is accomplished by having the patient lie supine with the arm abducted while traction is placed to the arm by an assistant.

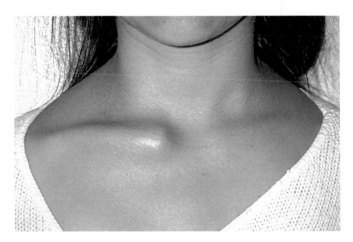

6.23A. Photograph of a woman with a right-sided anterior sternoclavicular dislocation.

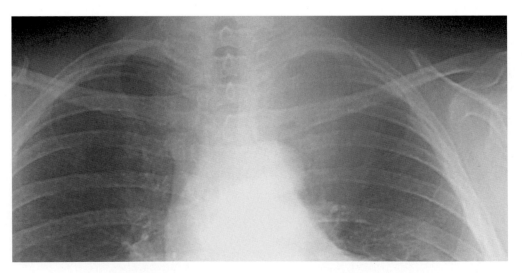

6.23B. Chest radiograph showing asymmetry of the clavicles with respect to the sternum in an anterior right sternoclavicular dislocation.

6.24 Scapula Fracture

Commentary

The scapula is integral to the normal function of the shoulder, and it is rarely injured, given its protection by thick surrounding musculature. Scapula fractures can be classified as the following:

- body fracture
- acromion fracture
- scapula neck fracture
- glenoid fracture
- coracoid fracture

Body fractures are the most serious of these types and form ~1% of all fractures. Mechanisms of injury include direct trauma, motor vehicle accidents, sports injuries, falls, and crush injuries. Examination reveals tenderness over the body of the scapula. Associated injuries are common, given the high energy required to fracture the scapula, and thus they need to be excluded. These injuries can include rib fractures, pneumothorax, hemothorax, pulmonary contusion, clavicle fracture, subclavian vessel injury, spine fracture, and skull fracture.

AP and transcapular radiographic views are usually sufficient to delineate the injury. In general, these fractures are managed conservatively with sling and swathe, though some authors prefer operative therapy.

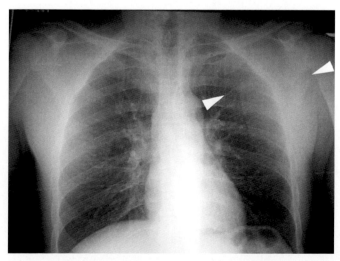

6.24A. Chest radiography demonstrating a mid-body scapula fracture.

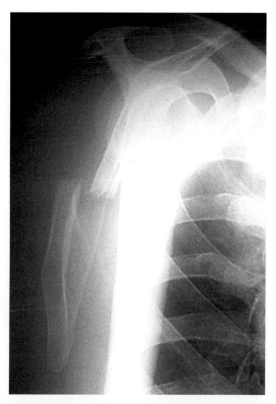

6.24B. Scapular view radiograph illustrating a mid-body fracture.

6.25 Pelvic Fractures

Commentary

Pelvic fractures account for significant morbidity and mortality, and their emergency management is challenging. Though minor pubic rami fractures are often seen in the elderly with ground-level falls, major pelvic fractures usually require significant force, and thus motor vehicle accidents, falls, and auto-versus-pedestrian accidents are the leading causes. Overall mortality is 5–15%, and other extrapelvic injuries are commonly seen.

The pelvic bones form a sturdy ring, but when a break in this ring occurs, especially if at two places, complications can be significant, with the most serious being acute hemorrhage within the retroperitoneal space. In the male, a urethral transection is identified clinically by the presence of blood at the urethral meatus, a scrotal hematoma, or a high-riding prostate. The presence of any of these signs mandates a retrograde urethrogram to exclude urethral injury before placement of a Foley catheter. In addition, the bladder, rectum, vagina, uterus, and sacral nerve roots are all at high risk of injury from pelvic bone fractures.

Persistent retroperitoneal bleeding can be extremely difficult to manage, accounting for 65% of deaths from pelvic fractures, and therefore prompt identification of the bleeding source in the pelvic fracture victim in shock is critical. These seriously injured patients are also at high risk for intraperitoneal, intrathoracic, and long bone fractures that could account for extensive blood loss. Bedside ultrasound, computed tomography, and diagnostic peritoneal lavage are all useful adjuncts in the proper identification of the bleeding source. Proper disposition is imperative, as laparotomy has a limited role in hemorrhage control in the modern management of pelvic fractures and associated retroperitoneal bleeding and may worsen mortality. In addition to aggressive blood resuscitation, tightly wrapped sheets, special pelvic binders, or a MAST suit can be helpful in stabilizing the pelvis. Emergency external fixation is most helpful in stabilizing anterior arch fractures but less helpful for bleeding associated with posterior pelvic injuries. Serious retroperitoneal bleeding is best treated by angiography; selective embolization of small pelvic arteries may be lifesaving in the critical patient.

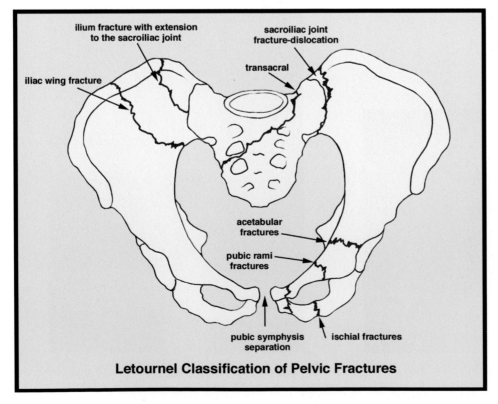

6.25A. Illustration of Letournel's anatomic classification of pelvic fractures.

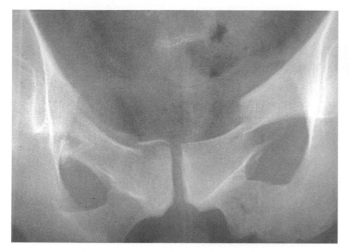

6.25B. Pelvic x-ray showing bilateral pubic rami fractures.

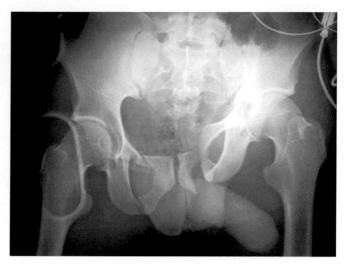

6.25D. Pelvic x-ray showing unstable Malgaigne fracture with bilateral pubic rami fractures and left sacroiliac joint disruption.

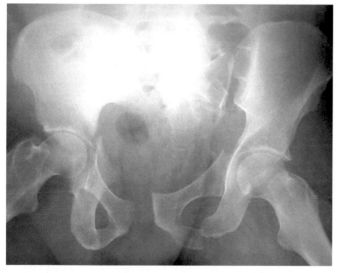

6.25C. Pelvic x-ray showing unstable Malgaigne fracture with widening of symphysis pubis, right acetabular fracture, left rami fracture, and left sacroiliac joint disruption.

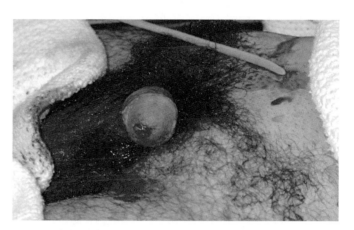

6.25E. Photograph of blood at urethral meatus with suprapubic cystostomy.

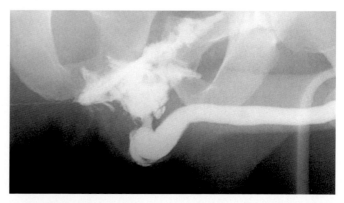

6.25F. Retrograde urethrogram with gross dye extravasation indicating urethral injury.

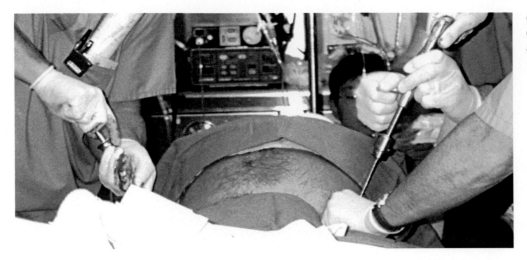

6.25G. Photograph of external fixation in progress in an unstable pelvic fracture.

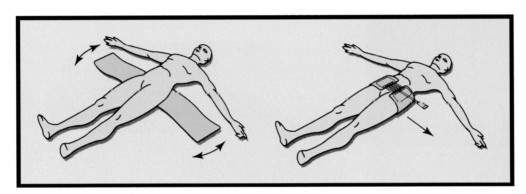

6.25H. Illustration of external pelvic binder device being placed (courtesy of Biocybernetics Inc.).

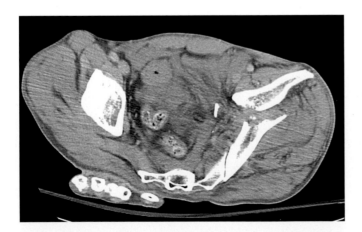

6.25I. CT scan showing a large pelvic hematoma with pelvic fracture.

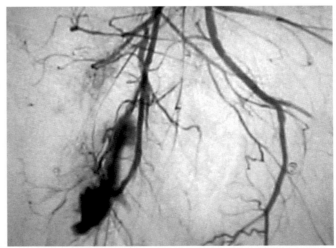

6.25J. Angiogram showing acute bleeding from the internal pudendal artery.

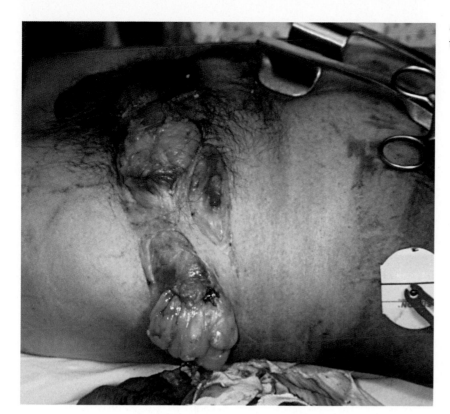

6.25K. Photograph of an open pelvic fracture from a motor vehicle accident.

6.26 Hip Dislocation

Commentary

Hip dislocations occur from high-energy trauma such as motor vehicle accidents and are true orthopedic emergencies because of the risk of ischemic necrosis to the femoral head. Because many patients present with severe associated trauma, other injuries may take priority, but the hip dislocation should be addressed before other orthopedic concerns. Ninety percent of all hip dislocations are posterior, with only about 10% being anterior dislocations. Rarely seen are central dislocations in which there is a concomitant fracture in the floor of the acetabulum. Given the energy involved, a femoral head fracture may also be present, and radiographs should provide good views of the femoral head and neck. In addition, the sciatic nerve is at risk with posterior dislocations, whereas the femoral nerve and vessels may be damaged with anterior dislocations, and thus the affected lower extremity requires a careful neurovascular examination.

Early closed reduction is paramount, as the femoral head has a limited blood supply. The average rate of avascular necrosis is 20%, and the risk rises to 50% in reductions performed twelve hours or more after the injury. Reduction can usually be accomplished using the Allis or Stimson techniques (see 6.26D and E) with appropriate deep sedation, though some patients will require operative reduction.

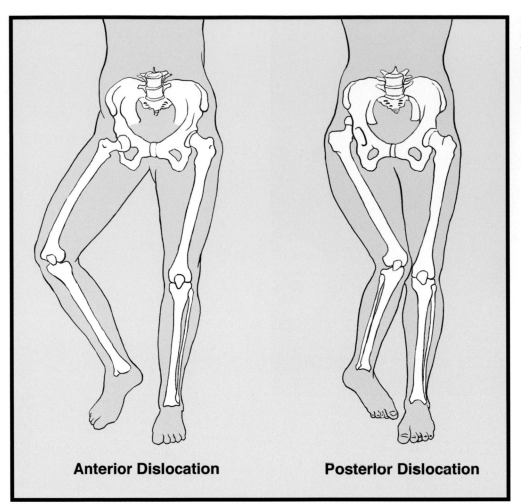

6.26A. Illustration of the classic position of adduction, flexion, and internal rotation seen in a posterior hip dislocation, and extension and external rotation seen in anterior hip dislocation.

Anterior Dislocation

Posterior Dislocation

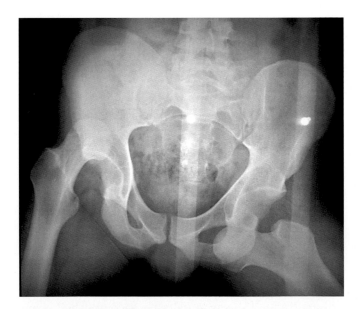

6.26B. AP pelvis radiograph reveals both a posterior (right hip) and an anterior hip dislocation (left hip) occurring simultaneously in a patient involved in a motor vehicle accident.

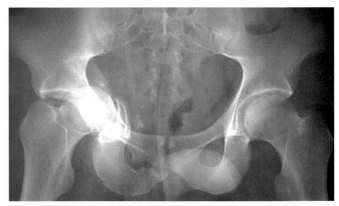

6.26C. AP pelvis radiograph showing a right central hip dislocation with acetabular fracture.

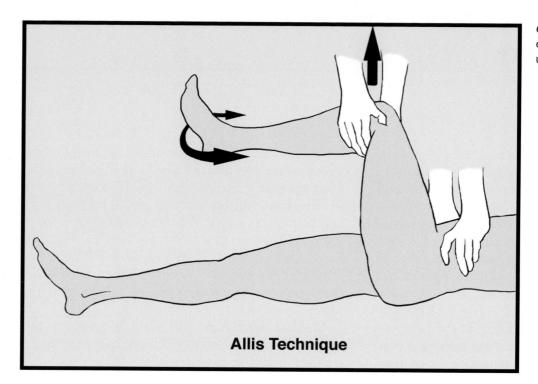

6.26D. Illustration of Allis closed reduction technique used for posterior dislocations.

Allis Technique

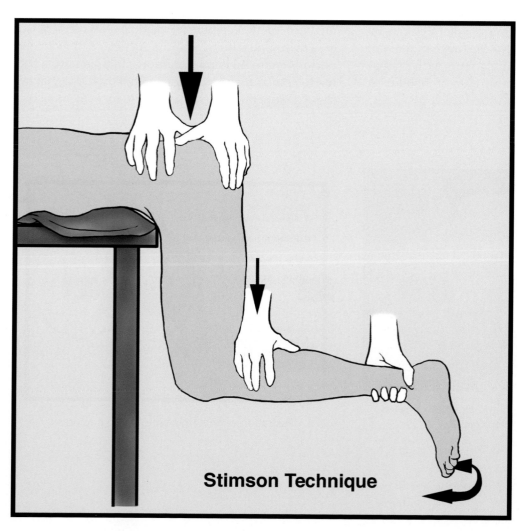

6.26E. Illustration of Stimson closed reduction technique used for posterior dislocations.

Stimson Technique

6.27 Hip Fracture

Commentary

Hip fractures are commonly seen in the elderly, who are prone to osteoporosis and minor falls. Fractures in patients younger than fifty often require high-energy mechanisms or a pathological process affecting the hip. Most patients complain of pain in the medial thigh or groin, and there is significant discomfort with internal or external rotation. In addition, the affected leg is often shortened and externally rotated, though neurovascular status is usually intact.

Hip fractures can be classified as femoral head fractures, neck fractures, intertrochanteric fractures, and subtrochanteric fractures. Standard radiographic evaluation includes an AP pelvis, along with coned views of the hip and a lateral view of the hip. On the AP pelvis view, it is important to examine the trabeculae carefully and to look for a disruption of Shenton's line (Figure 6.27C). Detection of minor fractures can be difficult, and plain radiographs can appear normal; thus, CT or MRI is indicated in patients with normal plain radiographs but persistent hip pain or inability to bear weight on the affected leg.

Femoral head and neck fractures are intracapsular fractures and have limited blood supply, making avascular necrosis a serious concern. In contrast, both intertrochanteric and subtrochanteric fractures have excellent blood supply. Prosthetic hip replacement or internal fixation is used to manage most hip fractures. Early mobilization of elderly patients avoids numerous complications associated with prolonged immobilization, such as pulmonary embolus, pneumonia, and sepsis.

Children differ from older adults in respect to this injury. Children's bones and periosteum are much stronger, and thus more severe trauma is required to produce hip fractures in this population. Comminution is not seen as often, and the periosteum often remains intact, thus limiting displacement of the injury. The presence of the epiphyseal plate predisposes to late growth complications, and the incidence of avascular necrosis is also higher. In addition, children have a better tolerance to bedrest and immobilization, making these treatment options a possibility for some injuries.

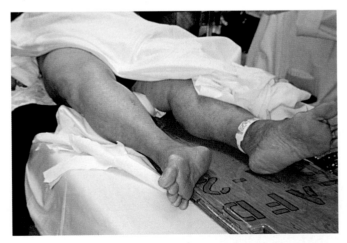

6.27A. Photograph of a shortened and externally rotated leg, the classic leg position after a hip fracture.

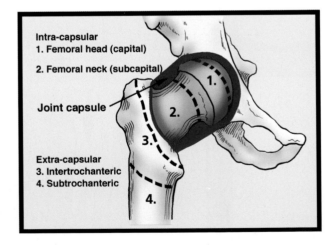

6.27B. Illustration of anatomic types of hip fractures.

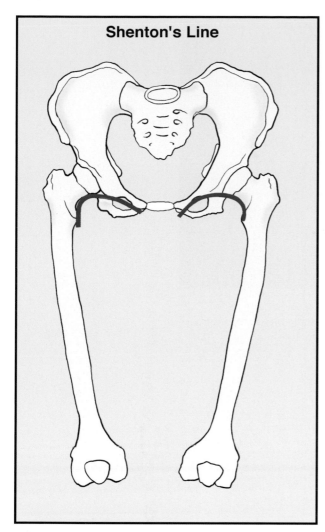

6.27C. Illustration of Shenton's line.

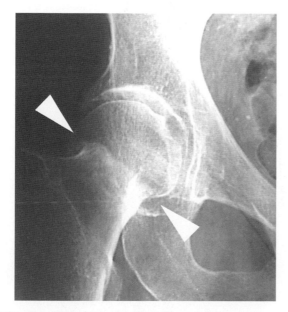

6.27D. Hip radiograph of a femoral neck fracture.

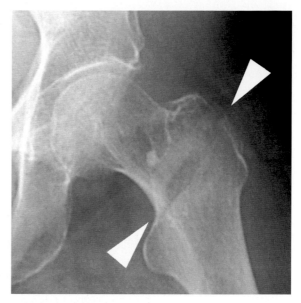

6.27E. Hip radiograph of a intertrochanteric hip fracture.

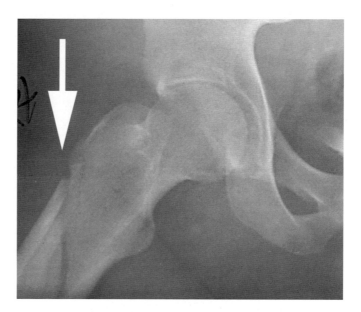

6.27F. Hip radiograph of a subtrochanteric hip fracture.

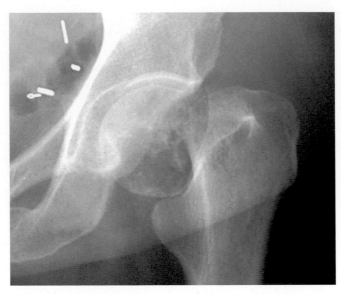

6.27G. Hip radiograph of a pathological femoral neck fracture in a young adult with metastatic breast carcinoma. Note the poor bone density at the fracture site.

6.28 Femoral Shaft Fracture

Commentary

The femur is the longest and strongest bone in the body, and thus fractures often require high-energy mechanisms such as major falls, motor vehicle accidents, or gunshot wounds. Physical examination reveals gross laxity of the femur, thigh swelling, and severe pain.

Significant blood loss can occur, and each fractured femur can easily lose three units of blood. Consequently, femur fractures are an important cause of hemorrhagic shock in the trauma victim. Gentle traction will reduce displaced fractures, and the limb should be splinted to maintain anatomic positioning to minimize soft tissue injury and blood loss. A careful physical examination is necessary to exclude neurovascular injury or compartment syndrome that may be present. Plain radiographs usually reveal the fracture clearly but should not delay the resuscitation of a critical patient, as they rarely will alter acute management. Emergency department treatment includes appropriate analgesia with limb traction. Orthopedic consultation is necessary, and most mid-shaft fractures will be operatively treated with an intramedullary rod.

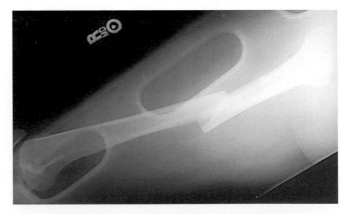

6.28A. Plain radiograph of a displaced femoral shaft fracture.

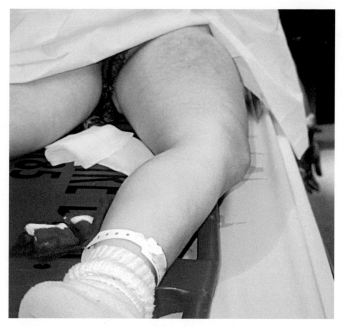

6.28B. Photograph of a swollen thigh in a patient with a femoral shaft fracture.

6.29 Patellar Fracture

Commentary

Patellar fractures account for approximately 1% of skeletal fractures, and most are associated with direct trauma to the knee. On examination, there is often point tenderness over the patella, with significant swelling and ecchymosis. A large hemarthrosis may occur with patellar fractures, and joint aspiration may be necessary for pain relief. The quadriceps extensor mechanism may be affected and thus should be tested for integrity by asking the patient to extend the knee against gravity. Radiographic assessment should include AP, lateral, and skyline views, though small undisplaced fractures can still be difficult to detect, and a bipartite patella can be a confusing normal variant. Three types of fractures are commonly seen: transverse, longitudinal, and stellate.

Most patellar fractures can be successfully treated by conservative therapy with cylindrical casting or a bulky Jones dressing for smaller fractures. Operative repair is done for open fractures, widely displaced fractures, severe articular disruptions, osteochondral fractures, and longitudinal fractures.

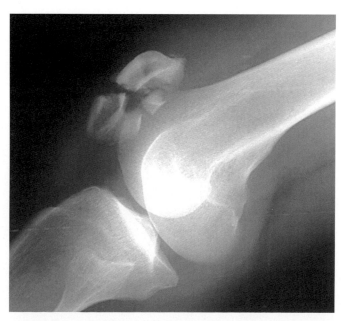

6.29A. Radiograph shows an obvious transverse fracture through the mid-body of the patella.

6.30 Tibial Plateau Fracture

Commentary

Tibial plateau fractures are often the result of direct shear forces. With most car bumpers being twenty inches high, the tibial plateau is at high risk in auto-versus-pedestrian accidents. Swelling, hemarthrosis, point tenderness, and pain with any motion of the knee make weight bearing impossible. Ligamentous injury may coexist and thus should be sought out on the clinical examination. Standard AP and lateral radiographs with oblique views will make the diagnosis in most cases, but occasionally CT scanning may be needed to further define the injury. The medial plateau is stronger, and thus fractures usually involve the lateral plateau. Generally the fractures are of two varieties: split and/or depressed. Split fractures tend to occur in younger patients with stronger bone, and depressed fractures more often occur in the elderly patient with osteoporosis.

As tibial plateau fractures involve the articular surface of a major joint, they are at high risk for persistent pain and arthritis and thus should be managed by an orthopedic surgeon. In the past, these fractures have generally been casted, but because of the residual stiffness often associated with casting, surgical intervention and early mobilization are increasingly being used.

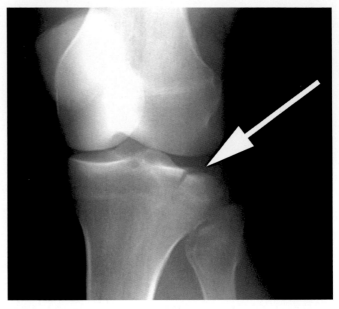

6.30B. This AP view of the knee reveals a lateral split plateau fracture.

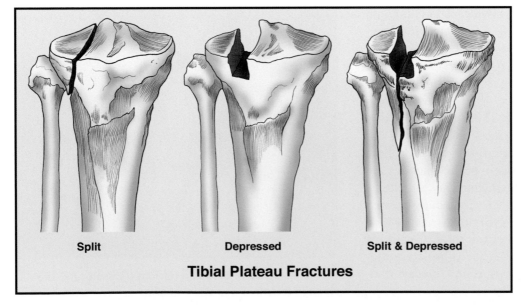

Split   **Depressed**   **Split & Depressed**

Tibial Plateau Fractures

6.30A. Illustration of types of plateau fractures.

6.31 Knee Dislocation

Commentary

Knee dislocation is rare but extremely important to recognize, as missed coexistent popliteal artery injury can lead to limb loss. This injury requires a high-energy mechanism and is often seen in the context of multiple trauma. Knee dislocation is classified according to the position of the tibia relative to the femur. There are five major types of dislocation:

- Anterior: Anterior dislocation is often caused by severe knee hyperextension.

- Posterior: Posterior dislocation occurs with anterior to posterior force to the proximal tibia, such as a dashboard type of injury or a high-energy fall on a flexed knee.

- Medial, lateral, or rotatory: Medial, lateral, and rotatory dislocations require varus, valgus, or rotatory components of applied force.

More than half of all dislocations are anterior or posterior, and both of these have a high incidence of popliteal artery injury. Physical exam of the affected limb will often show gross deformity around the knee, with swelling and immobility. The finding of varus or valgus instability in full extension of the knee is suggestive of a complete ligamentous disruption and a spontaneously reduced knee dislocation.

A careful vascular examination is essential, as popliteal artery injury occurs in 35–45% of all knee dislocations, and the presence of normal pulses does not rule out a significant vascular injury. All patients should be initially evaluated using the ankle-brachial index and color flow Doppler ultrasound. Patients with abnormal findings on these studies will need formal angiography. In addition, coexistent peroneal nerve injury occurs in 25–35% of cases and manifests with decreased sensation at the first webspace with impaired dorsiflexion of the foot.

Emergency treatment consists of prompt reduction with gentle in-line traction. Definitive treatment includes identification of vascular injury and operative repair of the ligamentous injury. Limb loss occurs in about a third of all cases.

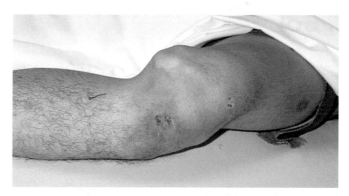

6.31B. Photograph of a lateral knee dislocation.

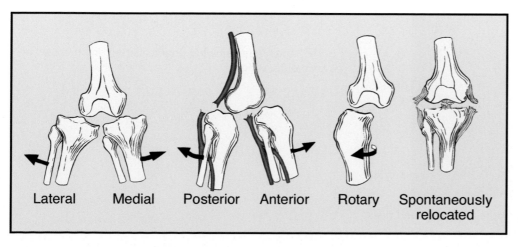

Lateral   Medial   Posterior   Anterior   Rotary   Spontaneously relocated

6.31A. Illustration of types of knee dislocation.

6.31 Knee Dislocation   211

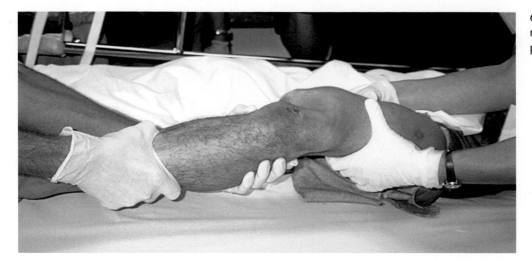

6.31C. Photograph of knee reduction in progress of the previous case.

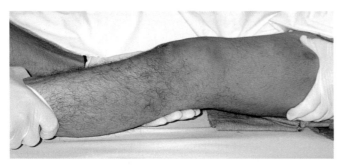

6.31D. Post-reduction photograph showing knee in good position in previous case.

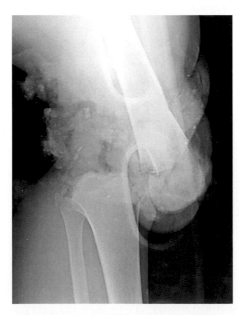

6.31E. Radiograph of a posterior knee dislocation and distal femur fracture.

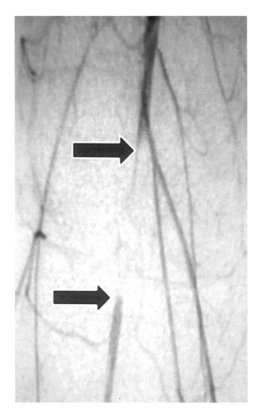

6.31F. Angiogram showing popliteal artery injury following a knee dislocation.

6.32 Maisonneuve Fracture Complex

Commentary

The Maisonneuve fracture complex represents 5–7% of all ankle fractures and can easily be missed if the treating physician is not familiar with this injury pattern. The mechanism typically involves external rotation of the inverted or adducted foot. The complex includes a combination of a proximal oblique fibular fracture, disruption of the tibiofibular ligament distally, and a medial malleolar fracture or deltoid ligament tear. In addition, the interosseous membrane may be torn.

Typically the patient has severe ankle pain but with pain also throughout the entire lower leg. Careful examination reveals medial malleolar tenderness, and this fracture complex underscores the importance of noting coexistent tenderness at the proximal fibula. Plain radiographs reveal a medial malleolar fracture and/or widening of the medial mortise with an oblique proximal fibula fracture. Treatment is directed toward restoring integrity of the ankle mortise. Although some patients are treated conservatively with casting, most patients need operative repair.

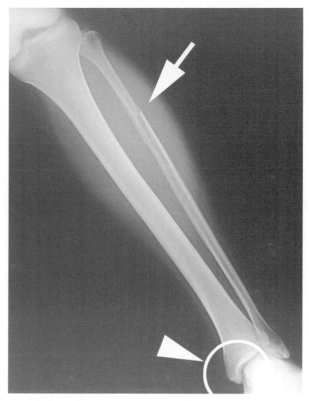

6.32A. Plain radiograph showing widening of the medial ankle joint and a proximal fibular fracture.

6.33 Ankle Dislocation

Commentary

Ankle joint dislocations are often secondary to sudden rotational forces, such as from sports injuries, falls, and motor vehicle accidents. Dislocations of the ankle are described according to the direction of displacement of the talus and foot in relation to the tibia and are most commonly lateral, although medial, posterior, and anterior dislocations are also seen. Dislocation without fracture is rare.

Neurovascular status should be checked, although most often this remains intact. Reduction is relatively straightforward and accomplished by flexing the knee to 90 degrees, stabilizing the lower leg, plantar flexing the foot, and pulling forward and reversing the direction of the dislocation. Gross ligamentous disruption with or without fracture is consistently present, and thus surgical stabilization is necessary in this injury.

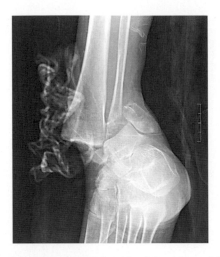

6.33A. Radiograph of lateral ankle dislocation with bimalleolar fracture.

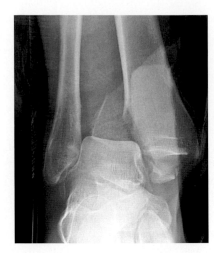

6.33B. Radiograph of a medial ankle dislocation with distal tibia fracture.

6.33C. Photograph of a medial ankle dislocation in a patient injured in a motor vehicle accident.

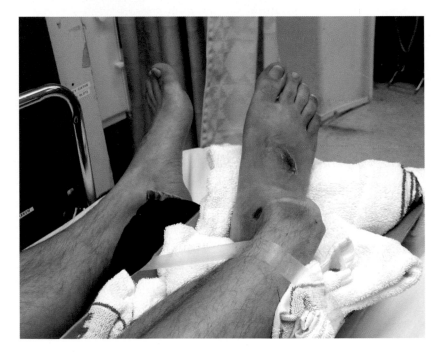

6.34 Subtalar Dislocation

Commentary

Subtalar or peritalar dislocation requires the disruption of both the talocalcaneal and talonavicular joints without affecting the tibiotalar joint. This uncommon injury is usually the result of severe torsional forces, such as in falls or motor vehicle accidents. Dislocations can be anterior or posterior, although medial and lateral are the most common. Obvious deformity is present, and an AP radiograph can be used to confirm the diagnosis.

Reduction should not be delayed and can usually be accomplished by in-line traction and reversal of the deformity. Most cases are managed conservatively, with a below-knee cast, with good results although chronic limitation of motion at the subtalar joint may affect the gait.

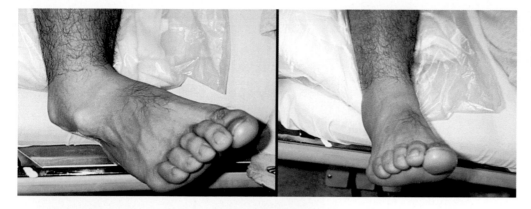

6.34A. Photograph of a medial subtalar dislocation (left side) and post reduction (right side).

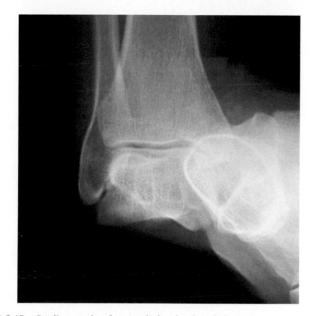

6.34B. Radiograph of a medial subtalar dislocation.

6.35 Lisfranc Fracture/Dislocation

Commentary

The tarsometatarsal joints are commonly called the Lisfranc joints, and dislocation or fracture/dislocation injury to this area is termed a Lisfranc injury. The joint consists of articulations between the bases of the first three metatarsals with their respective cuneiforms and the fourth and fifth metatarsal with the cuboid. These joints are normally held in place by strong ligaments, and thus this injury is most commonly seen with high-energy mechanisms such as motor vehicle accidents.

Because of the strong ligamentous attachments, associated fractures of the metatarsals are often seen. Usually the injury to the foot is clinically evident, with significant swelling and tenderness of the forefoot. Occasional vascular injury may occur in a branch of the dorsalis pedis artery, which forms the plantar arch. Radiographically, the fracture dislocation may be grossly evident or quite subtle. The first four metatarsals should align with their respective tarsal articulations along their medial edges. Disruption in this area or widening around the bases of the first three metatarsals is suggestive of an injury. Therapy of Lisfranc fractures usually involves closed reduction with internal fixation using percutaneous Kirschner wires.

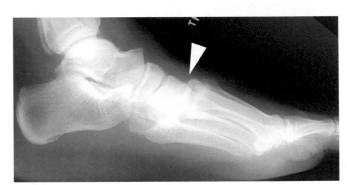

6.35A. Illustration of types of tarsometatarsal dislocations.

Homolateral   **Divergent**

Lisfranc Fracture/Dislocations

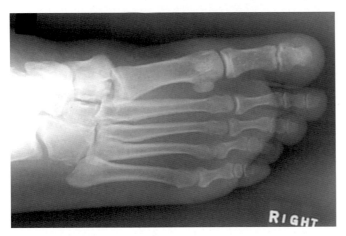

6.35B. Homolateral tarsometatarsal dislocation seen on the AP foot x-ray.

6.35C. Lateral foot radiograph of previous patient.

6.36 Metatarsal Base Fractures

Commentary

When assessing fractures of the base of the fifth metatarsal, it is important to distinguish isolated tuberosity fractures from diaphyseal fractures as the treatment and incidence of complications varies significantly. Avulsion fractures usually occur with sud-den inversion of the plantar flexed foot. The insertion of the peroneus brevis has been implicated in these fractures by causing avulsion of the styloid process. Fortunately, these fractures usually heal well without complication. Treatment of these isolated tuberosity fractures ("dancer's fractures") will be determined by the degree of pain and discomfort present, as these fractures may be treated with a compressive dressing, stiff shoe, or a short walking cast.

Diaphyseal fractures usually occur with running or jumping injuries, and transverse fractures within 15 mm of the proximal bone are often termed Jones frac-tures. Undisplaced fractures of this type are usually treated with non-weight-bearing casting for six to eight weeks but may require longer immobilization or surgery. Displaced fractures are usually treated opera-tively. Complications of this diaphyseal fracture are common and include delayed union, nonunion, and recurrent fracture.

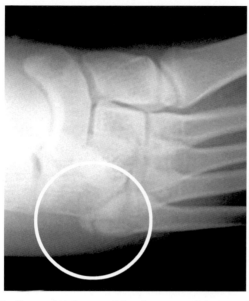

6.36A. Radiograph of an avulsion fracture of the proximal fifth metatarsal.

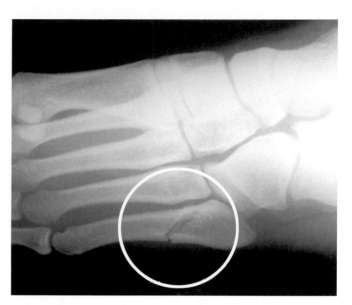

6.36B. Radiograph of a diaphyseal fracture of the proximal fifth metatarsal.

6.37 Calcaneal Fracture

Comentary

The calcaneus is the largest bone within the foot and requires high energy such as a major fall for fracture to occur; thus associated injuries are also common and are important to detect. These include bilateral cal-caneal injuries, lower leg injury, and vertebral injury. Typically, significant pain and deformity around the heel is noted, and weight bearing is impossible. Com-partment syndrome can complicate this injury and must be considered.

Standard radiograph views include a lateral AP view shooting down the foot and an axial calcaneal view shooting down the posterior half of the calca-neus (Harris view). Comminution is commonly seen, as the bone is cancellous in nature. For examining the radiographs, Bohler's angle can assist in determining if compression has also occurred. This angle is normally 20–40 degrees, and loss of this angle suggests compres-sion of the calcaneus. In addition, subtalar joint involvement is important to recognize, as many of these patients are treated operatively. In contrast, nondisplaced extra-articular fractures will often be treated with casting for six to eight weeks. Despite optimal therapy, chronic pain and joint dysfunction is seen in 50% of patients.

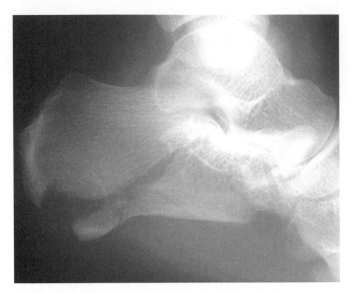

6.37A. X-ray of a mid-body fracture of the calcaneus involving the subtalar joint.

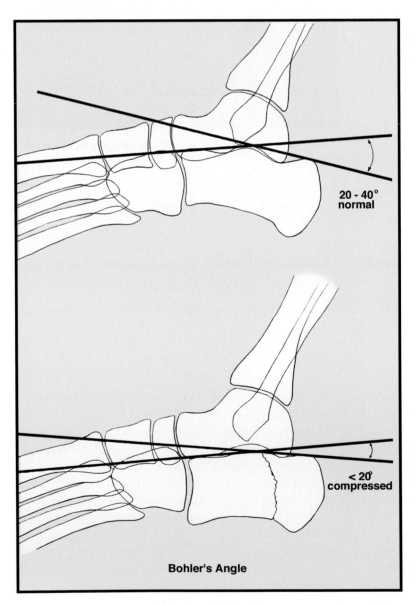

6.37B. Illustration of Bohler's angle. This angle is seen on the lateral view and is the angle between lines connecting the three highest points of the calcaneus.

20 - 40°
normal

< 20°
compressed

Bohler's Angle

7

Spinal Injury

Introduction

One of the most devastating consequences of trauma is spinal cord injury. In the United States, approximately 10,000 spinal cord injuries yearly result in permanent disability. Although spinal fractures can occur in any age group, the peak incidence is in males from ages 18 to 25. Certain conditions predispose to spinal fracture or dislocation: old age, rheumatoid arthritis, osteoporosis, Down's syndrome, and spinal stenosis. Even relatively minor mechanisms can result in spinal fracture in these groups. Forces that injure the spinal column include flexion, extension, axial loading, shear force, and rotational acceleration.

Clinical Examination

All multiple trauma victims must undergo evaluation for possible spinal column fracture, dislocation, or spinal cord injury. Blunt trauma patients should have the spine immobilized at first medical contact and remain in spinal immobilization until the integrity of the cord and spinal column can be verified. In patients with multiple severe injuries, this verification can be deferred until more critical injuries have been addressed, provided that immobilization of the spine is maintained.

Patients with spinal fractures experience pain, and examination will reveal tenderness. However, patients who are unable to report pain because of concomitant head injury or intoxication may harbor occult spinal injuries and should remain immobilized until they can be accurately evaluated. Patients with spinal cord injury manifest symptoms according to the spinal cord level affected. With complete cord transection, all motor and sensory function below the level of the lesion is lost. The highest intact sensory level should be marked on the patient to determine whether the cord lesion is progressing proximally on subsequent examinations. A careful motor examination should corroborate the level

of the cord lesion. Assessment of rectal tone and perianal sensation is important in detecting any sparing of lower cord segments that significantly improves the prognosis. Spinal shock is common in the immediate period after injury and consists of loss of all spinal reflexes and flaccid paralysis below the level of the lesion. During this phase the bulbocavernosus reflex (anal sphincter contraction with stimulation of the glans or urethra) is absent. No prognostication regarding the presence or level of the spinal cord lesion can be made while spinal shock is present. Once the bulbocavernosus reflex returns, spinal shock is resolved, reflexes become spastic, and the lesion is complete. Priapism is common in males after complete cord transection but resolves quickly in most cases.

Neurogenic shock is the hemodynamic effect of sympathetic denervation that results in vasodilation and hypotension. Because the sympathetic innervation to the heart is similarly disrupted by high cord injuries, reflex tachycardia does not occur in response to hypotension, and the patient is usually hypotensive and bradycardic. Regardless of the presence of neurogenic shock, hypotension must be assumed to be due to hemorrhage, and a diligent search for sources of blood loss must be made.

Partial cord syndromes may present with a confusing pattern of neurologic deficits. In central cord syndrome, the hands and arms sustain a much denser bilateral paralysis than the lower extremities. In Brown-Séquard syndrome, pain and temperature sensory loss occurs contralaterally, whereas motor loss and all other sensory loss is ipsilateral. With anterior spinal cord syndrome, there is preservation of posterior column function (position and vibration sense) bilaterally, but all other functions are lost. The syndrome of spinal cord injury without radiographic abnormality (SCIWORA) can occur in any age group but is particularly common in children. Neurologic deficits may be delayed many hours, and by definition, radiographs are normal. Consequently, it is difficult to make this diagnosis on initial evaluation. Patients who report persistent paresthesias should undergo CT scan of the spine if the initial radiographs are normal.

Investigations

A standard series of radiographs in a multiple trauma patient includes a cervical spine series, chest x-ray, and AP pelvis views. Additional spinal x-rays are indicated, depending on the detection of spinal tenderness, step-off, or neurologic lesions that suggest thoracic or lumbar spinal injuries. The lateral view of the cervical spine reveals almost 90% of fractures. The addition of open mouth and AP views increases the sensitivity somewhat, but some fractures elude detection on plain films. In some centers, oblique views are included in the standard cervical spine series, but in the absence of radicular symptoms these views usually add little information. Patients showing only abnormal soft tissue swelling on plain films should be evaluated by flexion/extension views of the spine to determine stability of the spinal ligaments, provided they are able to cooperate. A recent large series confirmed the safety of traditional practice that patients who are alert (not intoxicated or head-injured), without neck pain or midline tenderness, with a normal neurologic examination, and without distracting injuries do not need to undergo cervical spinal radiographs and can be cleared clinically. Conversely, normal spinal radiographs in a patient with persistent neck pain, unexplained neurologic deficits, or persistent paresthesias require further investigation. CT scan is sensitive in detecting many of these occult injuries and provides excellent information regarding the spinal cord itself. MRI provides ideal visualization of the spinal cord and soft tissues supporting the spinal column but is often impractical to obtain during the initial stabilization of the patient. Once the patient is stable, MRI can provide accurate visualization of the cord lesion.

General Management

As with severe head injury, prevention of secondary injuries is the highest priority. Although cord lesions may progress in spite of proper medical care, avoidance of hypotension, hypoxia, seizure, hypoglycemia, and mishandling of the patient are essential to avoid unnecessary deterioration.

Airway assessment occurs simultaneously with spinal immobilization. Patients with complete spinal cord injury above the level of C-4 will be apneic, as movement of the diaphragm and all other respiratory muscles is lost. Immediate assisted ventilation is required for the patient to survive, and the best means of accomplishing this is by endotracheal intubation and mechanical ventilation. In the past, concerns were expressed regarding the use of orotracheal intubation for fear that manipulation of the airway with a laryngoscope would cause movement of unstable spinal fractures and result in spinal cord injury. With the use of manual in-line stabilization by an assistant, orotracheal "rapid sequence intubation" using paralytic drugs has been shown to be safe. Alternatively, the nasotracheal method can be used, but this technique cannot be used in apneic patients and is only 70% successful overall.

Once spinal cord injury is identified, administration of high-dose methylprednisolone is recommended, based on the National Acute Spinal Cord Injury Study (NASCIS) that demonstrated improved recovery in patients receiving steroids within eight hours of injury. Methylprednisolone intravenously with a 30 mg/kg initial bolus followed by 5.4 mg/kg/hour for 24–48 hours is the recommended regimen. Steroids have not been studied in children or in penetrating injuries, and no recommendations regarding high-dose steroids can be made in these cases. Administration of steroids beginning more than eight hours after injury results in worse outcome and is not recommended.

Unstable spinal column fractures and dislocations require operative fixation and sufficient immobilization to restore bony stability. Contaminated penetrating injuries should undergo debridement, but relatively uncontaminated wounds are usually managed conservatively. Neurogenic shock usually responds to fluid administration, but pressor agents may be required to avoid hypotension and resultant hypoperfusion of the injured spinal cord. Patients with high spinal cord injury act as poikilotherms, and attention must be paid to their temperature to avoid hypothermia. Placement of a Foley catheter is recommended in the initial phase of treatment, although intermittent catheterization is the standard for long-term management. Nasogastric decompression is indicated if ileus develops. Early care to avoid decubitus ulcers and early institution of a rehabilitation program are beneficial.

Common Mistakes and Pitfalls

1. Failure to assess the spine clinically or radiographically in high-risk patients who present with even relatively minor mechanisms of injury. Elderly patients who present with low-speed vehicular acci-

dents or ground-level falls can have fractured their brittle or osteoporotic spines. A low threshold for obtaining radiographs should be maintained in trauma involving high-risk patients.

2. Failure to recognize partial cord syndromes. In some series, the vast majority of patients with central cord syndrome were initially misdiagnosed because they were intoxicated or because they were thought to be malingering or have conversion disorder. Paralysis of both upper extremities without simultaneous paralysis of the lower extremities was thought by these clinicians to be anatomically impossible because they were unaware of the presentation of the central cord syndrome.

3. Mishandling of the patient with spinal fracture. One older study found that almost half of patients who developed neurologic deficits did so after contact with medical personnel. Although some of these deficits would occur due to progressive edema or ischemia, others were certainly caused by inadequate care in maintaining spinal immobilization during transfer of the patient from stretcher to x-ray table or CT scanner.

4. Intoxicated or head-injured patients should have spinal precautions maintained until they can reliably report pain or neurologic deficits. Patients who report such symptoms require further investigation even if plain radiographs are normal.

5. There is often confusion between *spinal shock* (loss of reflexes and motor/sensory function for up to 24 hours after injury) and *neurogenic shock* (hemodynamic effects of sympathectomy due to high spinal cord lesions manifesting as bradycardia and hypotension). These terms are not interchangeable and should be used correctly to avoid miscommunication.

6. Chance fracture of the lumbar spine is frequently associated with a small-intestinal injury that may be initially occult.

7. Patients who present with calcaneal fracture(s) after jumping from a height should be screened for coexistent lumbar compression fractures because these fractures are commonly associated.

8. Approximately 10% of spinal fractures are associated with another non-contiguous spine fracture, thus the finding of any spinal fracture should initiate a search for other fractures elsewhere in the spine.

7.1 Central Cord Syndrome

Commentary

Central cord syndrome represents 3% of all cervical spine injuries and occurs mainly in older patients with osteoarthritic changes of the cervical vertebrae. It typically results from hyperextension of the neck with resultant inward buckling of the ligamentum flavum. This produces compression of the central portion of the cord, with subsequent edema and variable amounts of hemorrhage. Because of the stereotopic organization of the lateral corticospinal tract, the hands (lying closest to the center of the cord) are more affected than the arms, which in turn are more affected than the lower extremities. Clinically the syndrome consists of motor weakness that is most profound in the hands and arms, patchy sensory deficits, and variable dysfunction of bowel and bladder. Plain radiographs of the cervical spine are often normal because the condition may occur without a fracture or dislocation. CT scan may reveal central cord edema, but MRI is the most sensitive imaging modality in diagnosing this condition.

Because of the apparent incongruity of the clinical presentation, the condition is often misdiagnosed initially in the ED, especially if the patient is concurrently intoxicated. Misdiagnosis of the condition as "malingering" or "conversion disorder" is common.

Treatment is immobilization of the neck and administration of high-dose corticosteroids. Recovery of bowel and bladder function and ambulation is the rule, although recovery of full manual dexterity is rare.

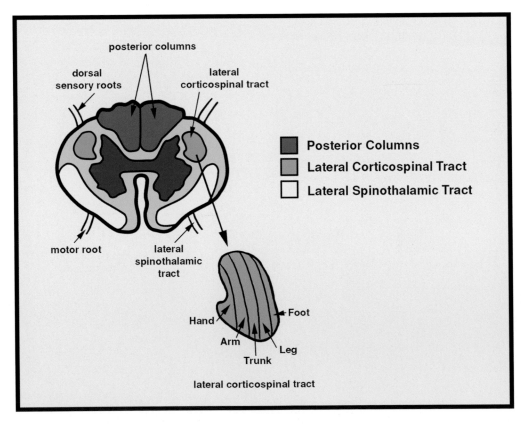

7.1A. Illustration of the cross-section of cervical spinal cord showing ascending sensory and descending motor tracts and stereotopic organization of the lateral corticospinal tract.

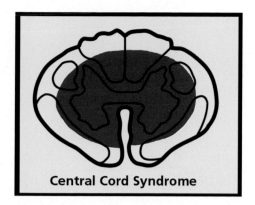

Central Cord Syndrome

7.1B. Illustration of cross-section of cervical spinal cord. The red area shows section of the spinal cord affected in central cord syndrome.

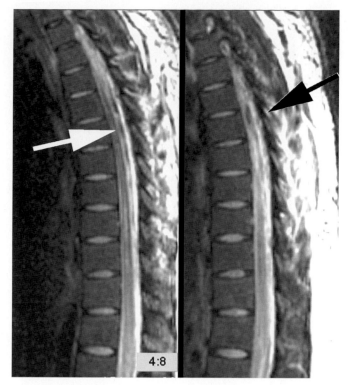

4:8

7.1C. T2 weighted cervicothoracic MRI showing hemorrhagic contusion of the central cervical cord (black arrow) and edema of the adjacent spinal cord (white arrow).

7.2 Brown-Séquard Syndrome

Commentary

Brown-Séquard syndrome is due to an incomplete transection or hemisection of the spinal cord, usually caused by penetrating trauma. It consists of a characteristic constellation of findings with loss of pain and temperature contralateral to the side of the injury and loss of motor function (corticospinal tract), light touch (spinothalamic tract), position, and vibration sensation (posterior columns) ipsilateral to the injury. Although true Brown-Séquard injury is due to an exact hemisection of the spinal cord, the clinical findings may vary if more or less of the cord is transected.

As with other penetrating injuries, the use of high doses of corticosteroids has not been found to be beneficial in prospective series, although it is still sometimes used in individual cases. Broad-spectrum antibiotic coverage is indicated, and surgical debridement may be required. Impaled objects should always be removed in the operating room. Functional recovery is often surprisingly good in spite of the permanent cord lesions.

Neurologic Deficits Distal to Site of Hemisection of Spinal cord in Brown-Séquard Syndrome	
Light touch	Ipsilateral
Position/vibration	Ipsilateral
Motor function	Ipsilateral
Pain sensation	Contralateral
Temperature sensation	Contralateral

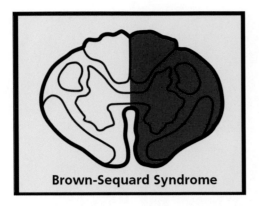

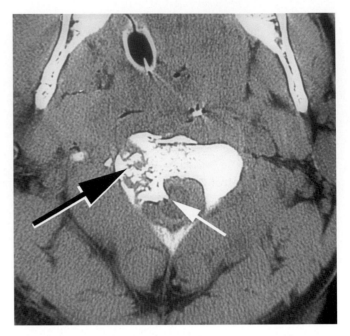

7.2A. Illustration showing spinal cord tracts affected in Brown-Séquard syndrome (red area).

7.2C. CT scan of the cervical spine showing a gunshot wound (black arrow) with bone fragments impinging on the lateral spinal cord (white arrow), resulting in a Brown-Séquard type lesion.

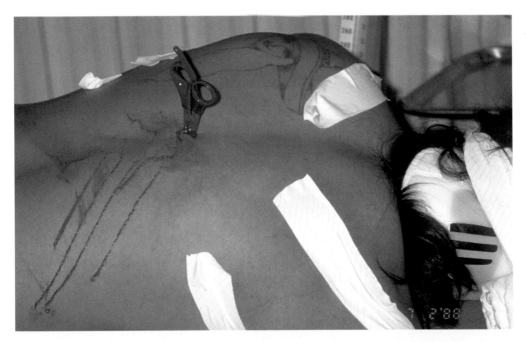

7.2B. Photograph of a patient with scissors embedded in the mid-thoracic spine who manifested classic Brown-Séquard syndrome.

7.3 Anterior Cord Syndrome

Commentary

Anterior cord syndrome results from damage to the anterior spinal artery, producing infarction of the anterior spinal tracts, or by direct laceration of the anterior part of the cord by retropulsed bony fragments. Posterior column function (position and vibration sense) is preserved. Clinically, there is bilateral loss of motor function, light touch, pain, and temperature sensation below the level of the injury.

Anterior cord syndrome is usually seen in elderly patients in conjunction with medical conditions, particularly arterial embolization from the heart. However, it may also result from prolonged cross clamping of the aorta, prolonged hypotension, or direct injury from bone fragments or foreign bodies.

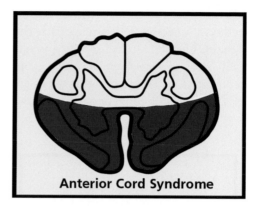

7.3A. Schematic drawing of spinal cord tracts affected in anterior cord syndrome.

7.4 Complete Spinal Cord Transection

Commentary

Complete transection of the spinal cord is a devastating injury. Transection above the level of C-4 results in respiratory failure as the nerve supply to both the diaphragm (C-3–5) and intercostal muscles (T1–12) is lost. Such patients frequently expire in the field unless immediate ventilation is provided.

At more distal levels, acute spinal cord transection results in complete flaccid motor paralysis and anesthesia below the level of the injury. Deep tendon reflexes are absent distal to the lesion. Examination will reveal urinary retention and diminished or absent rectal sphincter tone. In males, transient priapism is very common and indicates complete cord transection, although it often resolves by the time the patient arrives in the ED.

Loss of sympathetic innervation results in loss of vasomotor tone and hypotension. In cervical cord injuries, loss of sympathetic innervation to the heart prevents the normal response of reflex tachycardia.

Consequently, the hemodynamic picture of hypotension, inappropriate bradycardia, and warm, flushed skin constitutes the classic syndrome of neurogenic shock. Inability to vasoconstrict also prevents the normal response to cold stress, and these patients are at risk for hypothermia. Treatment is initially directed at restoring intravascular volume and ensuring that hypotension is not due to occult blood loss. If volume infusion does not restore adequate blood pressure, pressor agents such as dopamine are indicated to improve perfusion and consequently the survival of the spinal cord proximal to the transection.

During the acute phase of spinal cord injury, all distal reflexes are absent, and the patient is said to be in "spinal shock" (not to be confused with neurogenic shock with its hemodynamic manifestations). To confirm that all reflexes are absent, the most distal reflex arc or bulbocavernosus reflex is examined. Stimulation of the glans or clitoris or tugging on a Foley catheter normally produces a reflex anal sphincter contraction. During spinal shock, no response will occur. During this phase, it is possible that spinal cord dysfunction is due to concussion or contusion of the cord, and dramatic recovery of function can occur. Over the ensuing 24–48 hours, spastic reflexes that are typical of an established spinal cord injury begin to appear. The first such reflex to return is the bulbocavernosus reflex. Once this reflex reappears, the period of spinal shock has ended, and significant recovery is unlikely. Sparing of sensation in the perianal area should be elicited, as this represents a positive prognostic sign of potential recovery of spinal function.

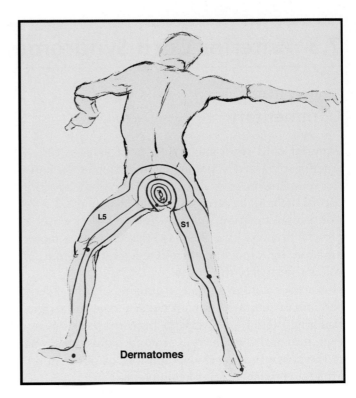

7.4B. Illustration showing posterior dermatomes.

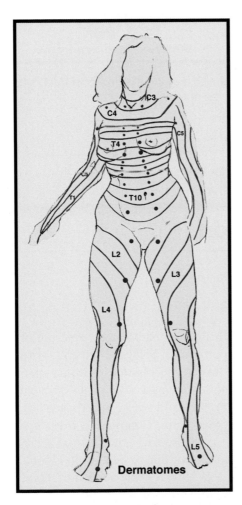

7.4A. Illustration showing anterior dermatomes.

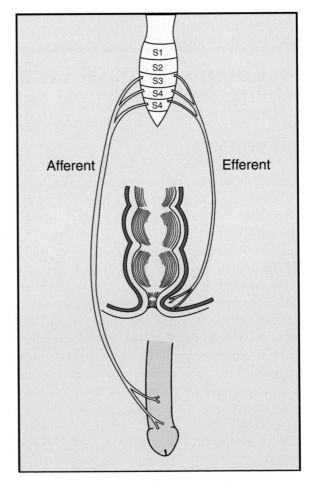

7.4C. Illustration of the bulbocavernosus reflex arc.

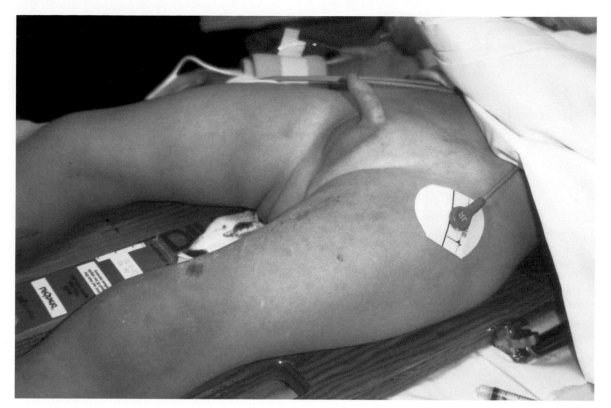

7.4D. Photograph showing priapism in a child with complete transection of the spinal cord.

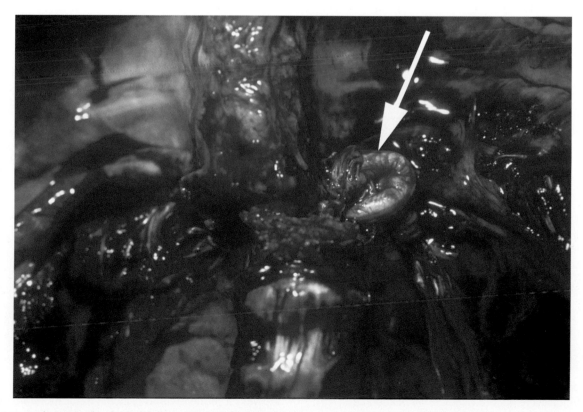

7.4E. Autopsy photograph of severe distraction of the spinal column and extrusion of the spinal cord.

7.5 Atlanto-Occipital Dislocation

Commentary

There are multiple strong ligamentous attachments from the cervical spine to the base of the skull. These include the anterior and posterior longitudinal ligaments, the anterior and posterior atlanto-occipital membranes, the apical ligament from the odontoid, and the capsular ligaments of the atlanto-occipital joint.

Atlanto-occipital dislocation occurs from the application of massive shearing force to the head in an anteroposterior direction as seen in high-speed motor vehicle crashes. The injury is primarily ligamentous, although associated fractures of the face and skull are common.

Separation of the cervical spine from the base of the skull is almost invariably fatal at the scene of the trauma. Fatalities occur from disruption of the spinal cord above the level of C-4 that results in complete paralysis of respiratory effort and asphyxial death or from injury to the brainstem or vertebral arteries. In patients who survive to reach a hospital, mortality is high due to brainstem injury, associated head and systemic trauma, and prolonged coma with its attendant complications. Nevertheless, survivors have been reported, and a full resuscitative effort should be made.

There are several radiologic methods of detecting subluxation or dislocation of the atlanto-occipital joint, although the ratio of Powers is the most commonly used and is described as follows:

The length of the line BC is compared to the length of line OA (see Fig. 7.5C):

Normal:	BC/OA = 0.77
Upper limit of normal:	BC/OA = 1.0
Abnormal:	BC/OA >1.0

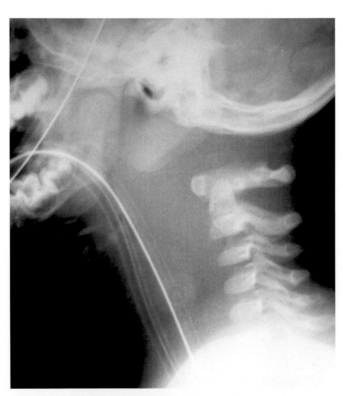

7.5A. Lateral radiograph of the cervical spine in a young child showing severe atlanto-occipital dislocation and massive soft tissue swelling anterior to the spinal column.

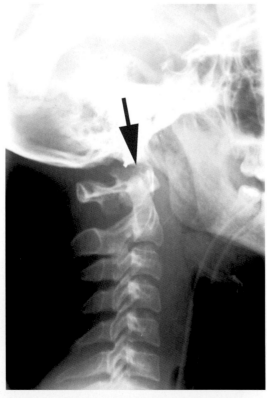

7.5B. Lateral radiograph of the cervical spine in an adult showing a subtler atlanto-occipital dislocation (arrow) with significant soft tissue swelling anterior to the spinal column.

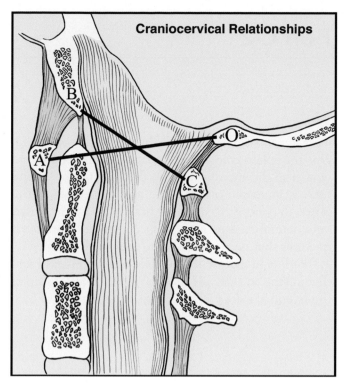

7.5C. Schematic drawing illustrating the measurements used in calculating the "ratio of Powers" to detect atlanto-occipital dislocation.

7.6 Atlantoaxial Dislocation

Commentary

Atlantoaxial dislocation is a rare injury of unclear mechanism. There is disruption of the transverse and alar ligaments that connect the odontoid process to the ring of C-1, which displaces superiorly (see Fig. 7.9A). Neurologic deficits are uncommon with superior dislocation (as shown) or when associated with fracture of the odontoid, although the condition is unstable due to disruption of the ligaments. Anterior dislocation is usually fatal as the spinal cord is compressed against the intact odontoid.

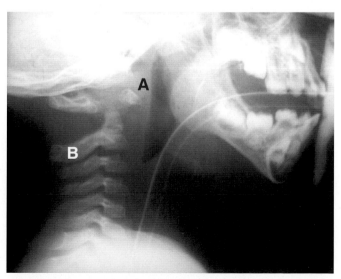

7.6A. Lateral radiograph of the cervical spine in a child showing atlantoaxial dislocation. The ring of C-1 (A) is seen lying completely above the tip of the odontoid process (B).

7.7 Rotatory Subluxation of C-1 on C-2

Commentary

Another form of ligamentous injury in this area is rotatory subluxation of C-1 on C-2 that results from torsional forces applied to the head and neck. Neurologic deficits are rare because the space for the spinal cord is not encroached upon.

The plain radiographic appearance of this injury is subtle and may be confused with a burst fracture of C-1. In the case of rotatory subluxation, one lateral mass rotates anteriorly and the other posteriorly. The anteriorly subluxed lateral mass appears larger and closer to the odontoid process, whereas the other lateral mass appears smaller and farther from the odontoid. On the plain radiographic open-mouth odontoid view, the distance from the odontoid to the lateral mass is increased on one side and decreased on the other, in contrast to a burst fracture of C-1, in which both lateral masses are displaced laterally. In burst fractures that occur on only one side of the ring of C-1, that lateral mass will be displaced laterally, whereas the unaffected side will show a normal relationship of the lateral mass of C-1 to the articular plate of C-2.

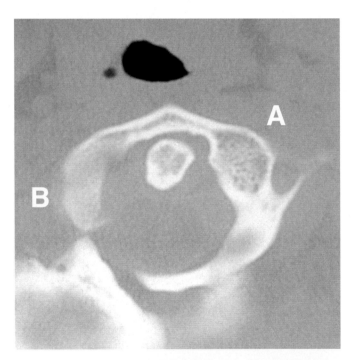

7.7A. CT scan of C-1 and C-2 showing the left lateral mass of C-1 (A) rotated anteriorly and the right lateral mass (B) rotated posteriorly. On a plain radiograph AP view, the left lateral mass will appear larger (because it is farther from the x-ray film) and closer to the odontoid because of the rotation. Conversely, the right lateral mass will appear smaller and farther from the odontoid process.

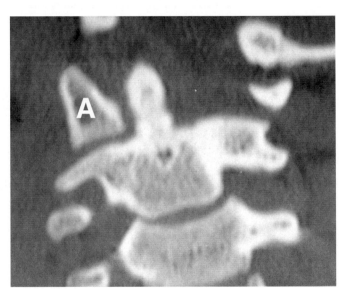

7.7B. CT scan of C-1 and C-2 in the AP orientation. The right lateral mass is seen clearly but the left lateral mass of C-1 has rotated posteriorly out of view.

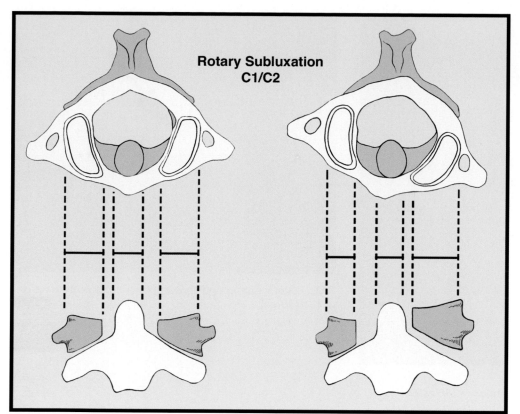

7.7C. Schematic drawing of rotatory subluxation of C-1 on C-2 with the corresponding appearance on the open-mouth plain radiographic view.

Rotary Subluxation C1/C2

7.8 C-1 Burst Fracture (Jefferson Fracture)

Commentary

C-1 or the "atlas" is a ring-shaped vertebra that articulates with the base of the skull superiorly and with C-2 inferiorly. Fractures usually result from axial compression of the head and spinal column (e.g., from diving into a shallow pool or when a passenger's head strikes the inside of the roof of a car in a motor vehicle accident). Because of the angles at which C-1 articulates with the occiput and C-2, the axial force is translated into a lateral force at C-1, causing the fragments to burst outward. Consequently, neurologic deficits are relatively uncommon with C-1 fracture because the space for the spinal cord within the spinal canal is actually increased. A Jefferson fracture is unstable, however, and must be adequately immobilized. An associated fracture of the odontoid process may occur.

On plain films, the open-mouth view is essential to diagnose C-1 fracture. Although some studies question the utility of including an open-mouth view in the standard initial series of x-rays in trauma patients, it is difficult to reliably diagnose a Jefferson fracture on a single lateral view.

CT scan is very accurate in detecting C-1 fractures and is indicated for any suspicious abnormalities or for inadequate visualization on plain radiographs.

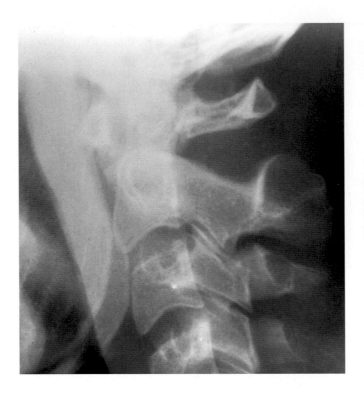

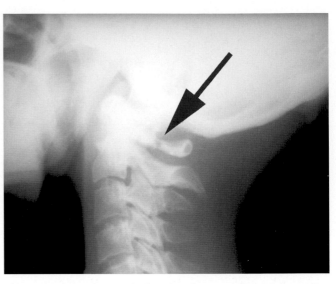

7.8C. Lateral radiograph showing fracture of posterior arch of C-1 (arrow).

7.8A. Lateral C-spine radiograph showing increased preodontoid space and prevertebral soft tissue swelling suggestive of a C-1 fracture. Normal measurements of the preodontoid space are 3 mm in adults and 5 mm in children. A greater space is allowed in children because the odontoid process is incompletely calcified until adolescence. Normal measurements for the prevertebral space anterior to C-3 are 5 mm in adults and 7 mm in children, due to a higher position of the esophagus in children that increases the prevertebral space.

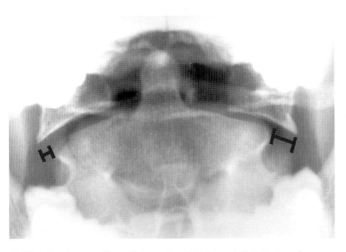

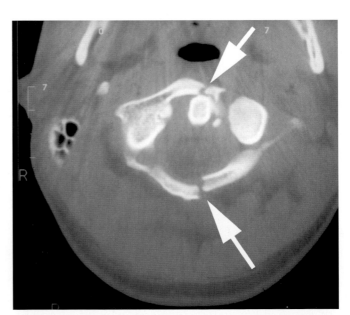

7.8B. Open-mouth radiograph of C-1 and C-2. Lateral displacement of the articular portion of the ring of C1 is the typical finding, as the ring of C-1 generally bursts outward. The distance between the ring and the odontoid process is increased. Displacement of the lateral masses of C-1 on C-2 may be unilateral or bilateral as shown here.

7.8D. CT scan of C-1 showing outwardly displaced fracture fragments. Because C-1 is a ring-shaped structure, at least two fracture sites inevitably exist (arrows). CT scan is particularly useful in a child, whose small mouth and inability to cooperate make the open-mouth view difficult to obtain.

7.9 Odontoid (Dens) Fractures (C-2)

Commentary

There are three types of odontoid fracture. Type I odontoid fracture occurs at the tip of the odontoid process, above the level of the alar ligaments. This is a rare fracture, caused by avulsion of the tip of the odontoid by apical ligaments attached to the base of the skull. It is a stable fracture because the alignment of C-1 on C-2 is maintained by the alar and transverse ligaments (see 7.9A). Neurologic deficit is uncommon.

Type II odontoid fracture occurs at the "neck" of the odontoid process, below the level of the transverse ligaments. It usually results from shear forces that cause anterior-to-posterior displacement of the entire C-1–C-2 complex from the body of C-2. It is a highly unstable fracture, more frequently associated with neurologic deficits, and often complicated by nonunion.

Type III odontoid fracture runs through the vertebral body of C-2. It may be comminuted and unstable. There is usually no associated spinal cord injury unless the fracture is significantly displaced or fragments of C-2 are retropulsed into the canal.

Treatment of odontoid fractures begins with immobilization in a halo vest if there is no evidence of neurologic deficit. Operative reduction may be required for fractures with impingement on the spinal cord or for persistent instability due to nonunion of the fracture fragments.

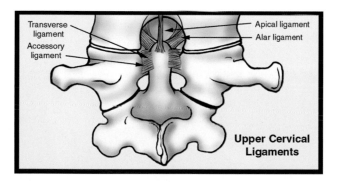

7.9A. Schematic showing the ligamentous attachments of C-1 and C-2.

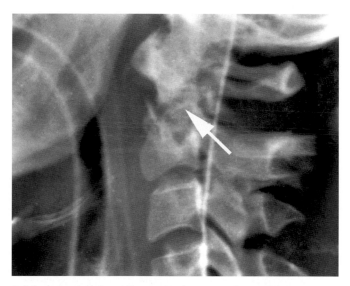

7.9C. Lateral plain radiograph of type II odontoid fracture. Arrow shows fracture line at the base of the odontoid process.

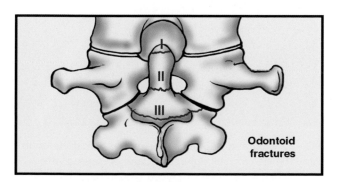

7.9B. Schematic showing the three types of odontoid fracture.

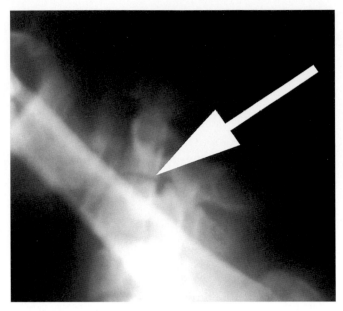

7.9D. Swimmer's view of the cervical spine showing type II odontoid fracture.

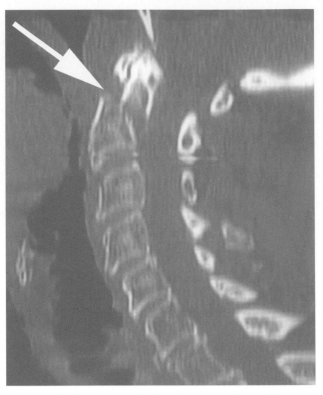

7.9F. Lateral CT showing displaced type II odontoid fracture (arrow).

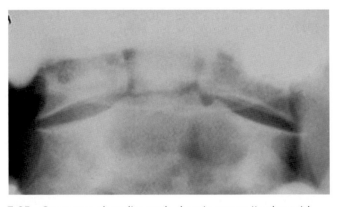

7.9E. Open-mouth radiograph showing type II odontoid fracture.

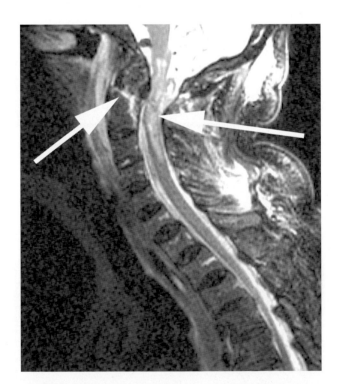

7.9G. T2 weighted MRI of the cervicothoracic spine of an elderly female who fell down stairs and presented with quadriplegia. MRI shows displaced type II fracture of the odontoid (short arrow) with injury to the spinal cord from C-1 to C-3 (long arrow).

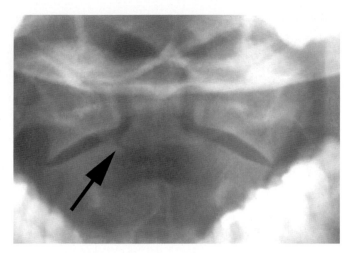

7.9H. Plain radiograph of type III odontoid fracture. Dark arrow shows fracture line through the body of C-2.

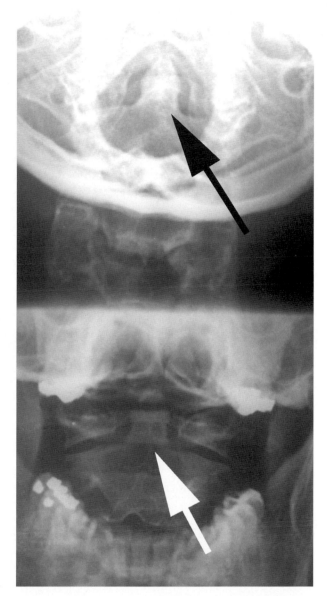

7.9I. Pseudofracture of the odontoid. The lower image appears to show a type II odontoid fracture (white arrow), whereas the upper image (modified open-mouth view) shows a normal odontoid (black arrow). The pseudofracture is due to a "Mach effect," which is a lucency created by the overlap of two bones.

7.10 Hangman's Fracture (C-2)

Commentary

Hangman's fracture is traumatic spondylolisthesis of the pars interarticularis of C-2. In common usage, however, the term is applied to bilateral pedicle fractures of C-2 as well. The fracture results from hyperextension of the neck with compression of the posterior elements of C-2 by the hyperextending occiput. This is the type of injury produced by a judicial hanging, hence the name. Displaced hangman's fractures are commonly associated with severe neurologic deficits. Cord lesions at this level result in paralysis of respiratory muscles and therefore apnea, as well as complete paralysis and sensory loss distal to the lesion.

Nevertheless, patients may sustain this injury without any injury to the spinal cord. These patients should be immobilized in a halo vest and often require operative fixation.

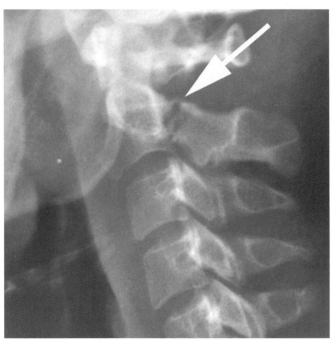

7.10A. Lateral C-spine radiograph showing bilateral pedicle fracture (hangman's fracture) of C-2. Undisplaced hangman's fracture.

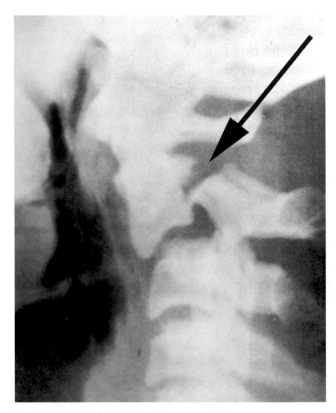

7.10B. Moderately displaced hangman's fracture.

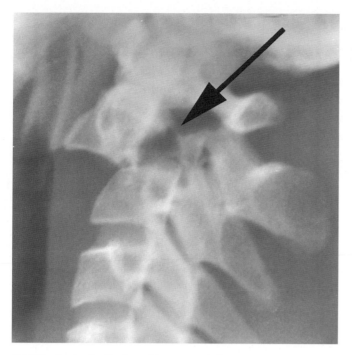

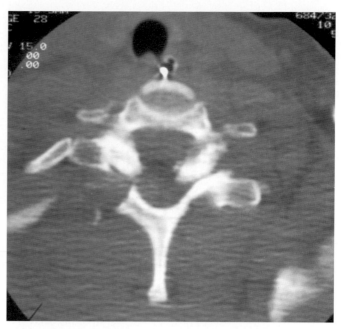

7.10C. Severely displaced hangman's fracture.

7.10D. CT scan of a hangman's type of fracture, extending through the lamina rather than the pedicles of C-2.

7.11 C-3–C-7 Fracture Types

Commentary

Classification of Vertebral Body Fractures

Type I: Anterior inferior fragment (flexion or extension "teardrop" fracture)
Type II: Anterior wedge compression fracture
Type III: Fracture of the anterior half of the vertebral body with minimal or no displacement of the fragments posteriorly
Type IV: Comminuted "burst" fracture of the vertebral body with retroplusion of the fragments into the spinal canal

Vertebral body fractures are common and usually occur as a result of hyperflexion. The severity of the fracture ranges from minor to critical, depending on the degree of comminution and displacement of fragments posteriorly into the spinal canal. Unstable fractures require operative fixation and ultimately spinal fusion.

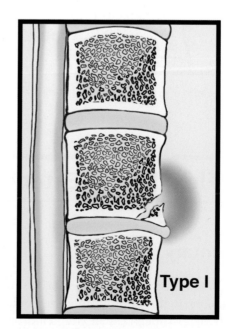

7.11A. Schematic of type I fracture of vertebral body.

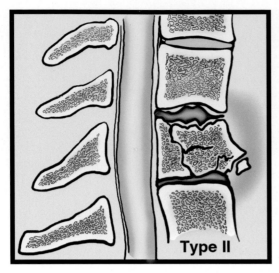

7.11B. Schematic of type II fracture of vertebral body.

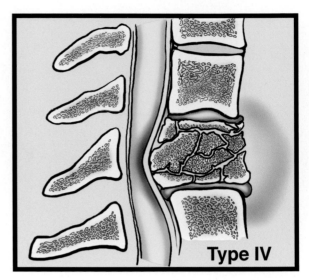

7.11D. Schematic of type IV fracture of vertebral body.

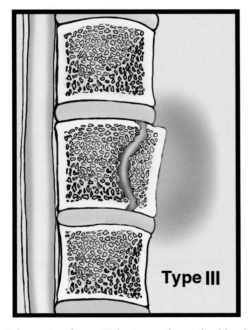

7.11C. Schematic of type III fracture of vertebral body.

7.12 Flexion and Extension Teardrop Fracture

Commentary

The flexion teardrop fracture is seen as a small triangular fragment at the anterior-inferior border of the vertebral body. Although the flexion teardrop fracture appears radiographically innocuous, it is a highly unstable fracture that is associated with spinal cord injury in up to 50% of cases. The injury is caused by hyperflexion of the neck, resulting in disruption of the posterior ligaments. As the flexion continues, the anterior inferior fragment of a vertebral body is fractured off by contact with the subjacent vertebral body. This disrupts the anterior longitudinal spinal ligament, rendering the cervical spine unstable as both anterior and posterior ligamentous support is disrupted. This fracture occurs most commonly at the C-5 level. Often there is associated slight posterior subluxation of the affected vertebral body or of the vertebral column above it.

The extension teardrop fracture appears radiographically similar to the flexion teardrop in that a small anterior fragment is avulsed from either the inferior or superior aspect of the vertebral body. The anterior longitudinal ligament is stretched during hyperextension of the neck and eventually tears, avulsing a small fragment of bone from the anterior aspect of the vertebral body. Because the posterior ligaments remain intact, the fracture is stable with the neck flexed. It may be necessary to perform flexion-extension radiographic views to demonstrate this fracture and determine its stability.

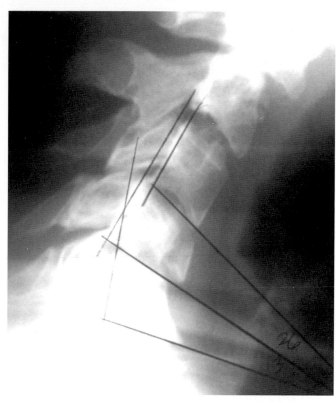

7.12B. Lateral radiograph of the cervical spine showing a flexion teardrop fracture of C-4 with lines showing the posterior displacement and angulation of C-4 on C-5.

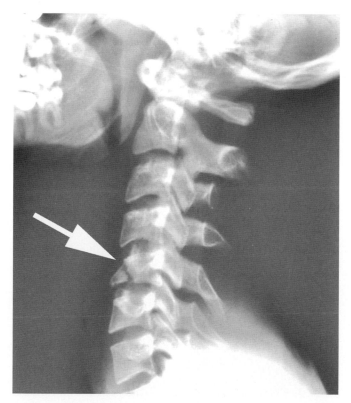

7.12A. Lateral radiograph of a flexion "teardrop" fracture at the base of C-5. Arrow indicates the typical triangular anterior-inferior fragment.

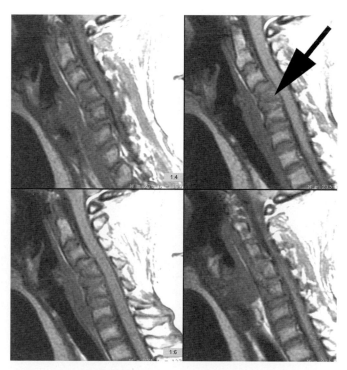

7.12C. T1 weighted MRI of flexion teardrop fracture of C-4 and C-5, with retropulsion of the vertebral bodies into the spinal canal producing slight spinal cord compression.

7.13 Compression or Burst Fracture of the Vertebral Body

Commentary

Axial compression or hyperflexion can produce variable degrees of injury to the vertebral body, ranging from a minor anterior compression "wedge" fracture to complete bursting of the vertebral body with retropulsion of fragments into the spinal canal, causing spinal cord injury.

Anterior compression is apparent on AP radiographs of the spine as loss of height of the anterior vertebral body compared with its posterior height or compared with the adjacent vertebrae. In comparing the normally parallel vertebral endplates, angulation of greater than 11 degrees suggests either ligamentous disruption, facet dislocation, or anterior compression fracture. On the AP radiograph, compression fracture is seen as a loss of height of the vertebral body compared with the adjacent ones, loss of space between adjacent spinous processes, or loss of distance between the pedicles above and below the fracture. Separation of the pedicles laterally compared with those above or below suggests a burst fracture of the vertebral body.

Higher-grade fractures involve comminuted fragments displaced centrifugally. Consequently, plain radiographs reveal loss of vertebral height, increased AP and lateral diameters, and loss of the normal lordotic lines of alignment. A step-off of more than 3.5 mm in the anterior or posterior vertebral lines suggests ligamentous disruption with subluxation, facet dislocation, or burst fracture of the vertebral body. The presence of both anterior and posterior step-offs is diagnostic for burst fracture.

CT scan often reveals more severe comminution of fractures that appear as simple anterior wedge compressions on plain radiographs, and it should be performed when compression fractures are detected on plain films.

All suspicious findings on the initial three-view C-spine series must be delineated further. Use of flexion-extension views for questions of alignment or ligamentous injury can reveal instability that was unsuspected on the initial lateral radiograph. CT scan of the cervical spine can examine regions of the spine that were poorly visualized on plain radiographs and delineate not only the exact extent of the fracture but also its effect on the spinal cord. However, CT scan is not reliable in looking for misalignment and purely ligamentous injuries. MRI is more valuable in visualizing soft tissue disruption in these situations.

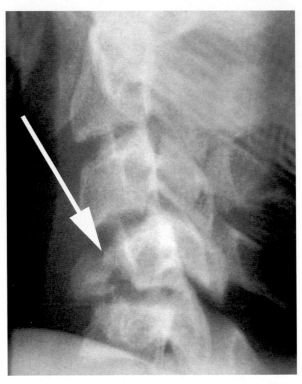

7.13A. Plain radiograph of a flexion-burst fracture (type IV) of C-4 with a large displaced anterior fragment (arrow), slight posterior displacement of the remainder of C-4, and severe angulation at the C-4/C-5 level.

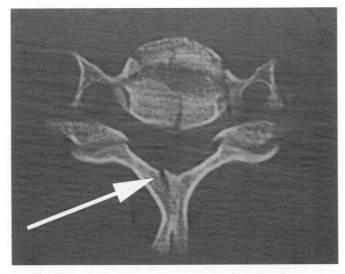

7.13B. CT scan showing a comminuted fracture of the vertebral body with an undisplaced posterior arch fracture (arrow).

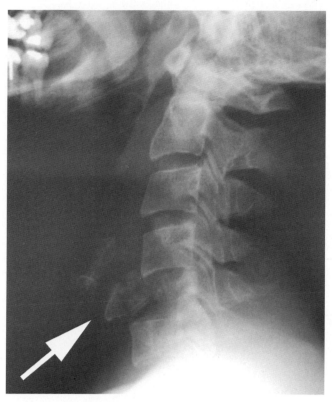

7.13C. Lateral radiograph of a comminuted type III fracture of C-5 (arrow).

7.14 Clay Shoveler's Fracture

Commentary

Clay shoveler's fracture is a painful but stable fracture of the spinous process of C-7. It is caused by forced flexion of the neck against resistance. The spinous process is avulsed by the pull of the posterior ligaments. Treatment is immobilization of the neck for comfort with either a soft or hard cervical collar, as well as appropriate analgesia. Admission is not required unless indicated for other injuries.

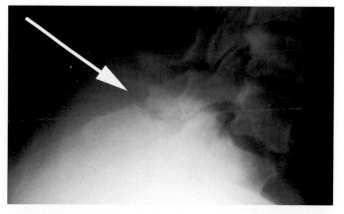

7.14A. Lateral radiograph showing a displaced fracture of the spinous process of C-7, also known as a clay shoveler's fracture.

7.15 Fractures of the Pedicles, Laminae, and Lateral Masses

Commentary

The pedicles and lamina form a diamond-shaped bony encasement of the spinal cord. Isolated fractures of a single pedicle or lamina are usually due to penetrating injury, most commonly a gunshot wound. With blunt trauma, any combination of pedicle and laminar fractures can occur, depending on the angular or rotational forces applied in addition to hyperextension or, less commonly, hyperflexion. Displacement of pedicle or laminar fragments medially can result in direct spinal cord injury. Bilateral pedicle or laminar fractures render the spinal column unstable.

The lateral masses represent the lateral articulations of the spinal column and contain the facet joints. They also form the bony margins of the neural foramina through which nerve roots enter and exit the spinal cord. Consequently, fractures of the lateral masses are often associated with nerve root injury.

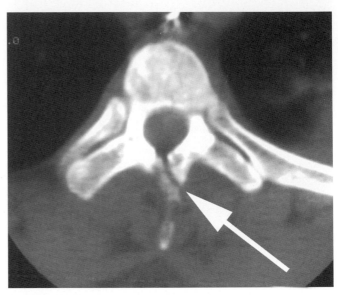

7.15B. CT scan showing fracture of the left lamina of T-1 (arrow).

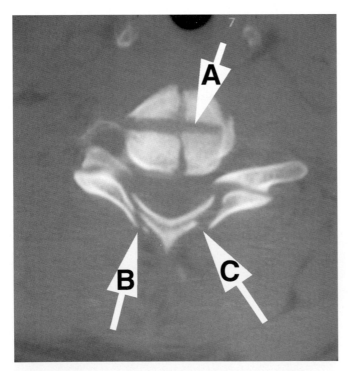

7.15A. CT scan showing a comminuted fracture of the vertebral body (arrow A) with fractures of both laminae (arrows B and C) in a patient who sustained an injury after diving into a swimming pool.

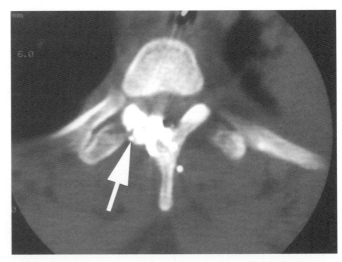

7.15C. CT scan of a patient with a gunshot wound showing fracture and bullet fragments at the right lamina of T-1 (arrow).

7.16 Facet Dislocation

Commentary

Unilateral facet dislocation results from forced flexion of the neck with a rotational component to one side or the other. If sufficient flexion or rotation occurs, one superior facet will become locked anterior to the inferior facet on that side. The opposite side will show normal alignment of the facets. Oblique radiographs of the spine will often more clearly demonstrate the dislocation. Subluxation of the vertebral bodies is less than 50%, and approximately 25% will have associated spinal cord injury. Reduction is accomplished by sedation and simple traction in most cases.

Bilateral facet dislocation results from forced flexion of the neck, causing the superior facets to glide anteriorly on their inferior counterparts. Once the facet joints reach the peak of the inferior facet, they are said to be "perched" atop the inferior facet. If the superior facet continues anteriorly, it becomes locked in the dislocated position. Bilateral facet dislocation results in greater than 50% subluxation of the superior vertebral body on the inferior one and almost inevitably results in complete spinal cord injury.

Plain radiographs are usually sufficient to demonstrate facet dislocation, but CT scan will also demonstrate this injury and may reveal unsuspected fractures of the facets, lateral masses, pedicles, or laminae.

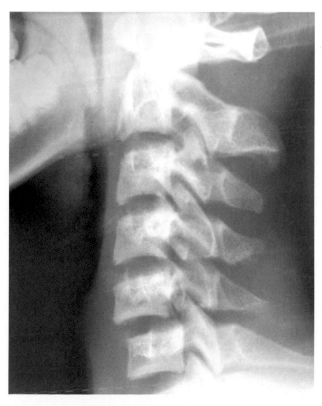

7.16A. Lateral radiograph of the C-spine showing subluxation of C-5 on C-6 due to unilateral facet dislocation of C-5.

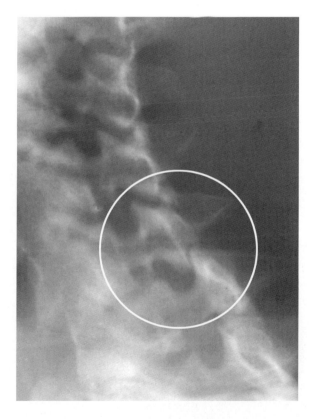

7.16B. Oblique view of unilateral facet dislocation.

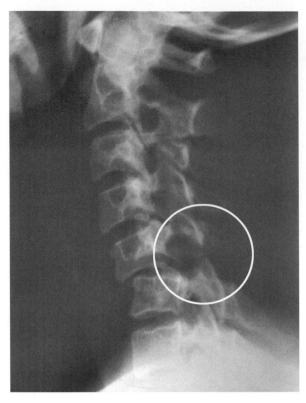

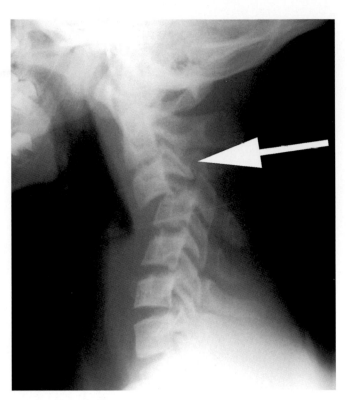

7.16C. Lateral radiograph of the C-spine showing subluxation and angulation of C-5 on C-6. Both superior facets (C-5) are seen resting atop the lower facets (C-6), a condition known as perched facets.

7.16E. Lateral radiograph of a fifteen-year-old girl, injured while jumping on a trampoline, who arrived with quadriplegia. X-ray shows complete bilateral facet dislocation of C-3 on C-4 with significant anterior subluxation and angulation of C-3. (Superior facets are lying anterior to the lower facets; see arrow.)

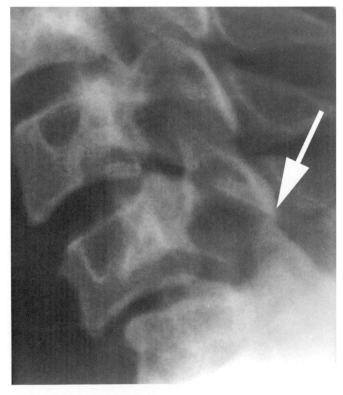

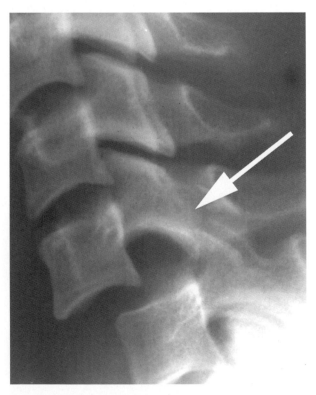

7.16D. Close-up view of perched facets (arrow).

7.16F. Close-up view of bilateral facet dislocation (arrow).

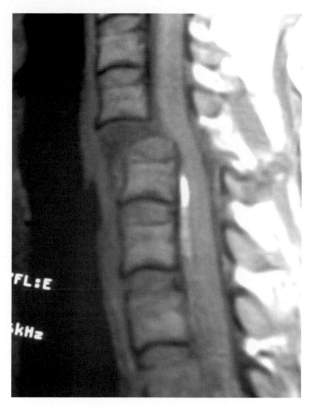

7.16G. T1 weighted MRI of C-5 on C-6 bilateral facet dislocation.

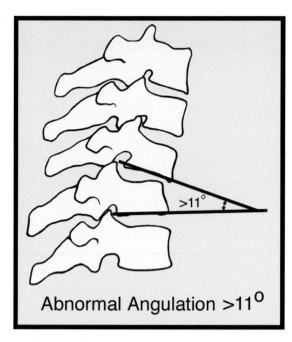

Abnormal Angulation >11°

7.16I. Schematic illustrating abnormal angulation measurements with perched facets.

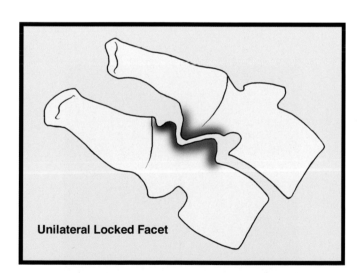

Unilateral Locked Facet

7.16H. Schematic illustrating unilateral facet dislocation.

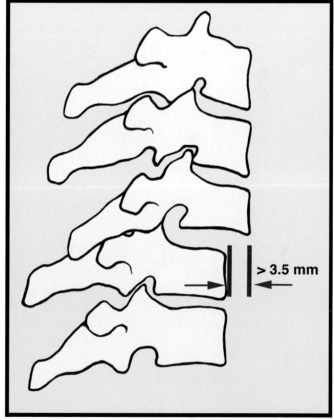

> 3.5 mm

7.16J. Schematic illustrating anterior subluxation with perched facets.

7.17 Cervicothoracic Spinal Injury

Commentary

The junction of C-7 and T-1 is a relatively common location for spinal injury, up to 20% of spinal fractures in some series. Consequently, it is essential to visualize this area with plain radiographs on the initial examination prior to clearing the cervical spine. Visualization of this area is difficult to accomplish in children, patients with large, muscular shoulders, and those with upper extremity injuries that make it difficult to pull on the arms for a lateral x-ray. Unless the lateral x-ray extends to the top of T-1, a swimmer's view is often required to verify alignment in this area. Detection of fractures with the swimmer's view is difficult because of superimposed bones and soft tissues, and CT scan should be used when visualization of the cervicothoracic junction is not possible with conventional radiography or when suspicious areas are identified on the swimmer's view.

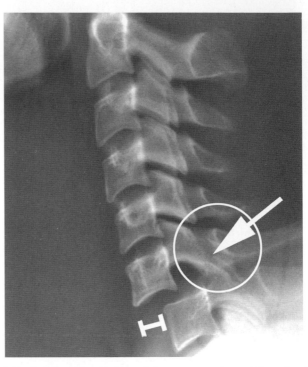

7.17B. Repeat lateral view of the same patient with a clearly apparent bilateral facet dislocation of C-6 on C-7 (arrow) and significant subluxation of C-6 on C-7.

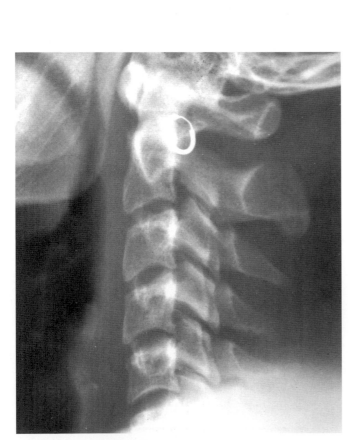

7.17A. Lateral cervical spine radiograph appearing normal to the top of C-6 level.

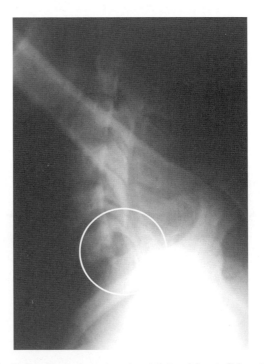

7.17C. Swimmer's view showing bilateral facet dislocation at the cervicothoracic junction.

7.18 Thoracic Spine Injuries

Commentary

Fracture of the thoracic spine is relatively rare because of the stabilizing influence of the ribs and their ligamentous attachments and protection by the large paraspinous musculature posteriorly and by the thorax itself anteriorly. In addition, the anatomy of the thoracic vertebrae inherently limits lateral movement and extension. However, fractures in this segment of the spine are commonly associated with spinal cord injury because of the limited amount of space for the cord within the spinal canal in this area. The most common mechanism is hyperflexion from decelera-

tion injuries or falls. Penetrating injury in this area is another relatively common etiology for thoracic cord injury. Associated thoracoabdominal injuries may take precedence for stabilization, so it is important not to overlook the possibility of concurrent spinal injury.

Visualization of the thoracic spine by plain radiographs is difficult on account of numerous overlying structures. Consequently, CT scan is often necessary to clearly delineate the nature and extent of the injury, as well as the impact on the spinal cord.

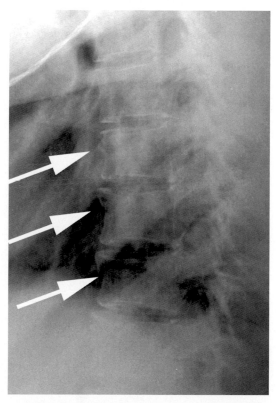

7.18A. Lateral radiograph of the thoracic spine showing three contiguous vertebral compression fractures (arrows) in a young woman who was in a motor vehicle accident.

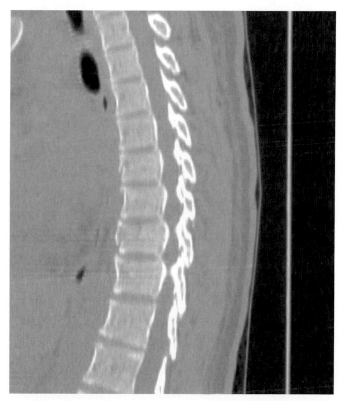

7.18B. Lateral CT scan of the thoracic spine showing anterior compression fractures in the previous patient.

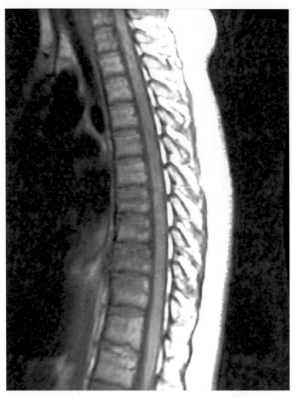

7.18C. T1 weighted MRI of the spine showing the same compression fractures without damage to the spinal cord.

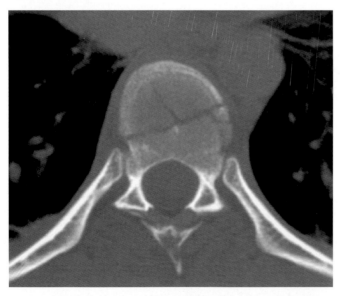

7.18D. CT scan showing a comminuted thoracic vertebral body fracture.

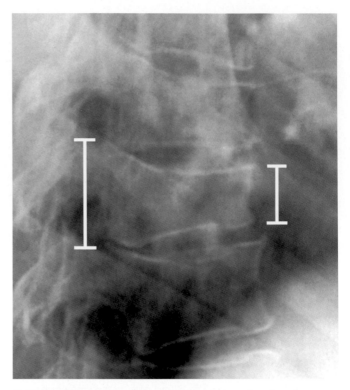

7.18E. Lateral radiograph of the thoracic spine showing anterior wedge compression fracture of T- 6.

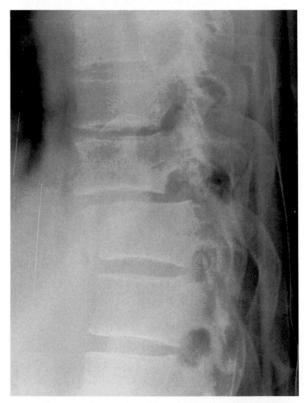

7.18F. Series of spine images on a fifty-year-old tree trimmer who fell twenty feet from a tree and presented with paraplegia at the T-9 level. Plain radiograph showing compression fracture of T-10 with anterior subluxation of T-9 on T-10 and a small fracture at the anterosuperior aspect of the T-10 vertebral body.

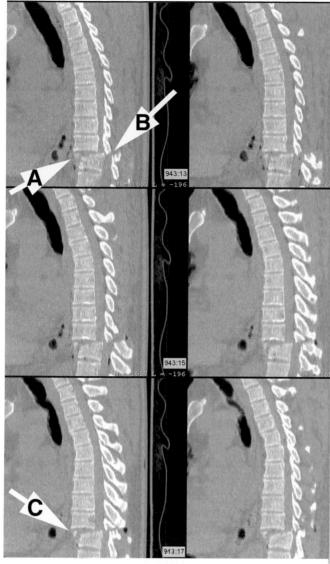

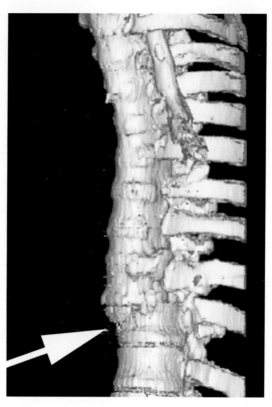

7.18H. 3-D CT scan reconstruction of the previous fracture.

7.18G. Lateral CT scan series reveals posterior displacement and impingement on the spinal cord (arrows A and C), as well as fracture of the posterior elements of T-9 (arrow B).

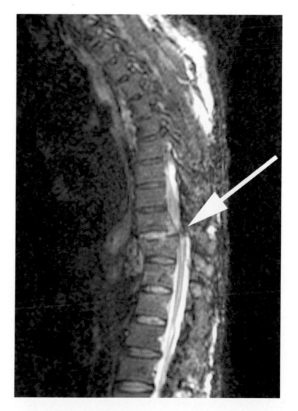

7.18I. T2 weighted MRI of the same patient showing severe compression of the spinal cord at the T-9–T-10 level (arrow).

7.19 Lumbar Compression Burst Fracture

Commentary

Compression fracture of a lumbar vertebra is one of the most common spinal fractures. It occurs in two distinct age groups. The first group is the elderly, in whom anterior vertebral body collapse can occur with relatively minor trauma and often signals underlying bone pathology, such as advanced osteoporosis or metastatic lesions. The second group is made up of younger patients who sustain severe hyperflexion of the lumbar spine, usually during a fall from height. In these patients, associated injuries, such as calcaneal, acetabular, and other lower extremity fractures, mesenteric or renal arterial injury, aortic avulsion, and additional spinal column injuries, are common.

Lumbar compression fracture occurs as a result of acute hyperflexion at the waist, resulting in an anteriorly wedge-shaped vertebral body. The posterior wall of the vertebra is intact, and spinal cord injury is very rare. Collapse of more than 30% of the anterior height may result in progressive collapse of the vertebral body and increasingly severe kyphosis. Consequently, fractures with greater than 30% anterior compression are treated more aggressively. Associated adynamic ileus is commonly associated with these fractures. Radiographically, these fractures appear wedge-shaped with loss of anterior vertebral height on the lateral view. The presence of a burst fracture should be suspected if the AP view shows separation of the pedicles. This finding indicates a burst fracture rather than a wedge compression fracture.

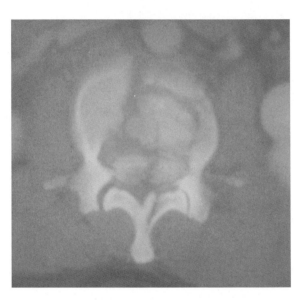

7.19B. CT scan of the same patient: The L-1 vertebral body shows a comminuted fracture (arrow) with intrusion of bony fragments into the spinal canal.

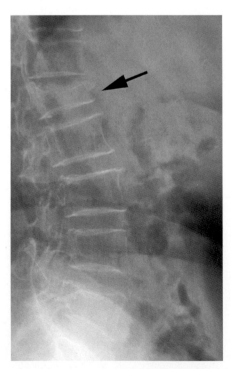

7.19A. Lateral radiograph of the lumbar spine of a suicidal patient who jumped out of a hospital window. It shows an anterior wedge compression fracture of L-1 (arrow).

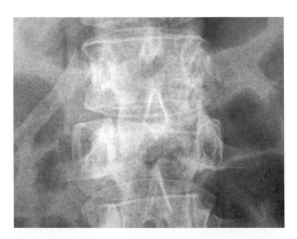

7.19C. Plain radiograph showing close-up view of the L-1 burst fracture with lateral displacement of both pedicles of L-1 compared with T-12.

The extent of fracture comminution may be underestimated on plain radiographs, and a CT scan of the affected vertebra often shows a more extensive fracture. Fractures of the transverse process, lateral mass, or vertebral body in the lumbar spine from L-2 to L-4 may be associated with renal injury. Assessment for the presence of abdominal or retroperitoneal organ injury is indicated by either CT scan or IVP.

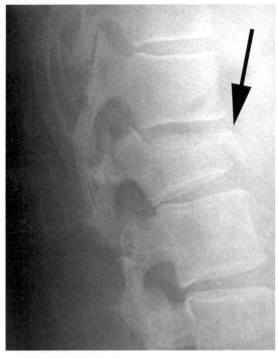

7.19D. Radiograph showing severe compression fracture of L-1 (arrow) with retropulsion of a large fragment into the spinal canal.

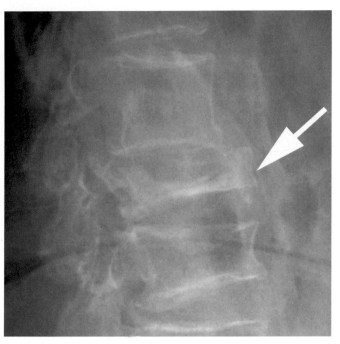

7.19E. Lateral radiograph of the lumbar spine showing severe compression fracture of L-1 (arrow) and less severe fracture of L-2.

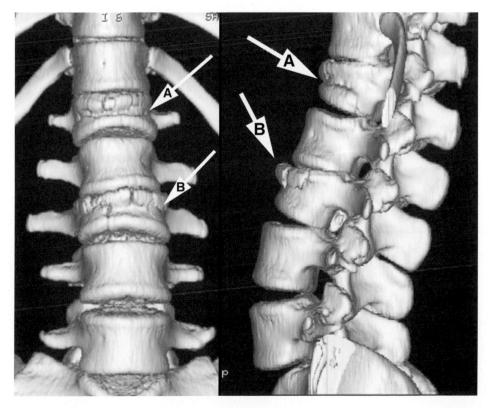

7.19F. 3-D CT scan reconstruction showing anterior wedge compression fractures of L-1 (arrow A) and L-3 (arrow B) on the anterior and lateral views.

7.20 Chance Fracture

Commentary

Chance fracture typically occurs to a rear seat passenger wearing a lap belt, when the car is involved in a front end collision. The patient sustains acute hyperflexion at the waist around the axis of the lap belt. The normal flexion point of the spine is located in the center of the vertebral body. An improperly worn lap belt shifts the flexion point anteriorly and acts as a fulcrum that pries apart the vertebral elements from back to front. There are several variations of Chance fracture, depending on the course of the fracture line. For example, the fracture line may begin in the interspinous ligament and then enter bony elements, only to terminate in a disruption of the disk space. The impact on spinal stability is identical regardless of the exact course of the fracture because both posterior and anterior elements are disrupted. Consequently, this is an unstable fracture.

Because hollow viscera are compressed between the lap belt and the spinal column, Chance fractures are commonly associated with blunt intestinal injury, and patients should be investigated for this possibility.

The presence of a seatbelt sign on the lower abdomen should alert the clinician to the possibility of Chance fracture as well as intestinal injury.

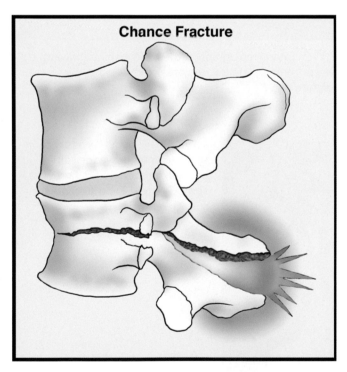

7.20A. Schematic drawing demonstrating classic Chance fracture.

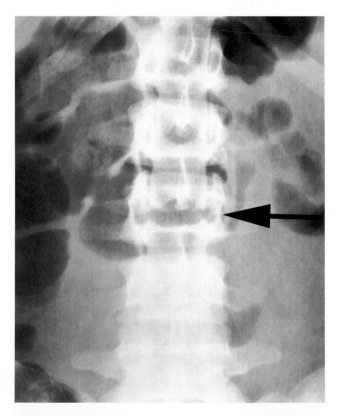

7.20B. Lumbar spine radiograph showing a fracture line coursing through the entire vertebral complex, including the spinous process, laminae, pedicles, and vertebral body. AP radiograph view shown.

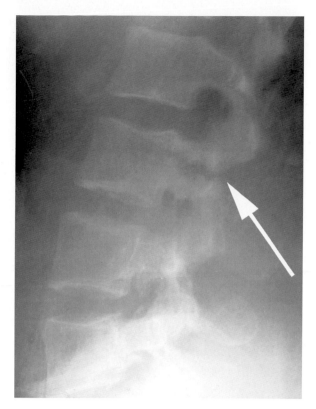

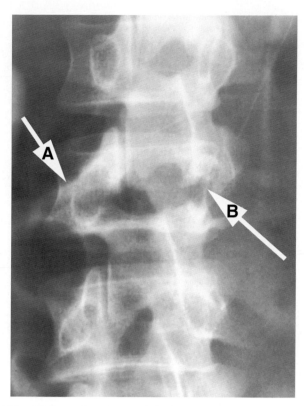

7.20C. Lateral view of Chance fracture (arrow).

7.20D. Oblique showing pedicle fracture (arrow A) and vertebral body fracture (arrow B).

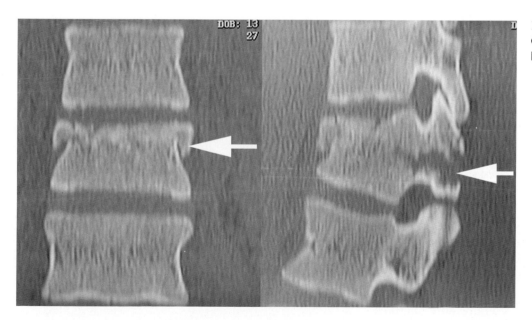

7.20E. CT scan showing Chance fracture on AP and lateral view.

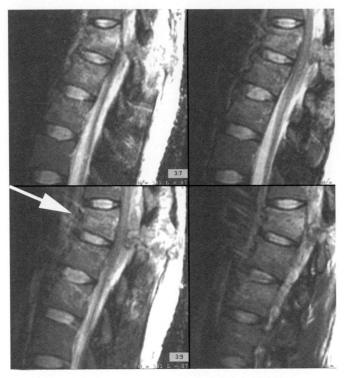

7.20F. T2 weighted MRI lateral view showing Chance fracture with severe disruption of the posterior elements and soft tissues (arrow), as well as complete spinal cord compression and edema.

7.21 Fracture-Dislocation of the Lumbar Spine

Commentary

The spinal cord ends at the level of L-1 or L-2 as the conus medullaris. Nerve fibers supplying the pelvis and lower extremities continue distally as the cauda equina. Injuries to the lower lumbar vertebrae may produce injury to this structure, resulting in the cauda equina syndrome. This syndrome is characterized by the presence of asymmetric weakness and numbness of the lower extremities, often with saddle anesthesia of the perineum, as well as sphincter dysfunction of bowel and bladder. As with compression fractures, injury to the kidneys, ureters, and other retroperitoneal structures must be considered with lumbar fracture-dislocations.

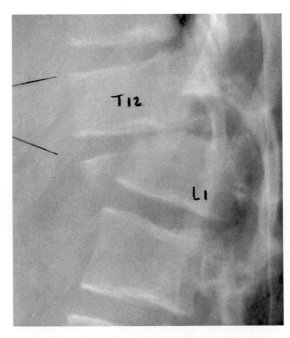

7.21A. Lateral radiograph showing fracture-dislocation of T-12 on L-1.

7.22 Ligamentous Injuries

Commentary

Flexion and extension views of the C-spine are supplementary radiographs that are indicated in patients with increased soft tissue swelling anterior to the vertebral bodies or suspicion of misalignment on the lateral C-spine film. They are contraindicated in patients with apparent neurologic injury or in those whose diagnosis is clear.

The patient must be awake and able to cooperate. He or she should be instructed to actively flex and then extend the neck up to the point of experiencing pain and no further. At the point of maximal voluntary flexion and extension, a lateral radiograph is obtained. The patient's neck should never be passively flexed or extended by the physician during this examination.

Positive findings are increased subluxation of the vertebrae in either flexion (posterior ligaments disrupted) or extension (anterior ligaments disrupted). CT scan is relatively insensitive in detecting ligamentous injuries or misalignment of the spine. MRI may be required to fully delineate the extent of ligamentous injury but is not generally useful in the initial evaluation of the patient.

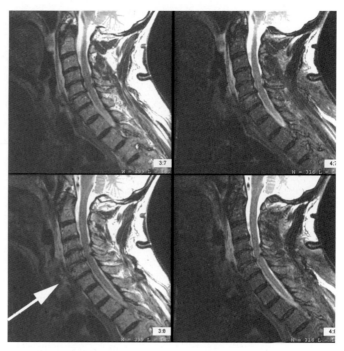

7.22B. T2 weighted MRI showing ligamentous injury and soft tissue edema anterior to the vertebral bodies of C-5 through C-7.

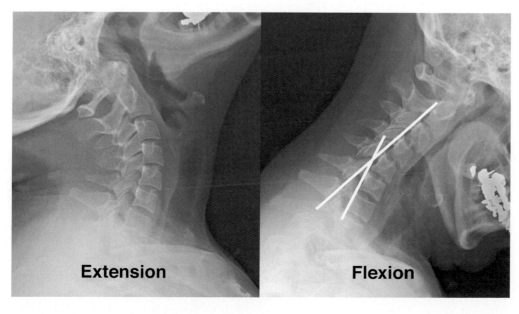

Extension

Flexion

7.22A. Flexion-extension lateral radiographic series. The extension view appears normal, but the flexion view shows significant angulation and anterior subluxation of C-4 on C-5, indicating posterior ligamentous disruption.

7.23 Pediatric Spinal Injury

Commentary

Cervical spine fractures are relatively rare in children because of the inherent flexibility of the pediatric spine. When spinal fractures do occur, the upper cervical vertebrae (C-1 to C-3) are most commonly involved.

The interpretation of spinal radiographs in children is difficult. Soft tissue thickness may vary considerably depending on the phase of respiration. The presence of epiphyses makes the detection of fracture lines difficult. Incompletely calcified vertebrae cause vertebral bodies to appear wedge-shaped, suggesting possible compression fracture. Physiologic anterior subluxation of C-2 on C-3 or C-3 on C-4 occurs in up to 50% of children and persists until midadolescence in 10% of patients. In the presence of apparent subluxation, drawing a line between the posterior spinolaminal line of C-2 through C-3 will demonstrate normal alignment if the spinolaminal line of C-2 lies within 2 mm of this line (Shwischuk's line). Greater distances of C-2 from this line suggest true subluxation.

It is often difficult to obtain adequate open-mouth views of C-1 and C-2 in children because of their small mouths and inability to cooperate. Consequently, it is often necessary to obtain a CT scan of the upper vertebrae in children when the mechanism of injury or physical findings suggest the possibility of spinal injury.

Although it may occur at any age, the syndrome of spinal cord injury without radiographic abnormality (SCIWORA) accounts for approximately one-third of spinal cord injuries in children younger than age eight. Symptoms may be delayed for 24 hours in a significant proportion of these cases. Consequently, obtaining normal radiographs of the spine and a normal neurologic examination at the time of injury does not necessarily exclude delayed spinal cord injury. The presence of any neurologic symptoms such as transient paresthesias at the time of injury requires investigation with either CT scan or MRI. Administration of high-dose steroids for spinal cord injury has not been well studied in children but may be helpful when abnormalities are detected on CT or MRI and when neurologic deficits are present.

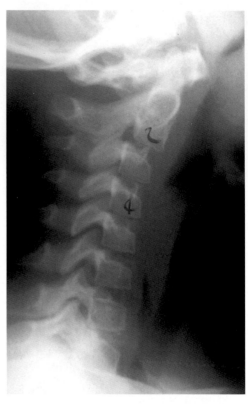

7.23A. Lateral C-spine radiograph showing physiologic subluxation of C-2 on C-3.

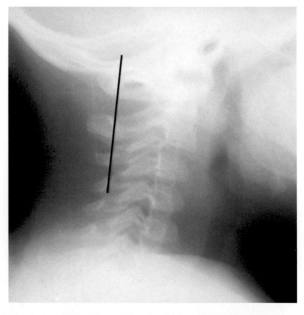

7.23B. Lateral C-spine radiograph showing alignment within Shwischuk's line confirming that the subluxation is physiologic rather than pathologic.

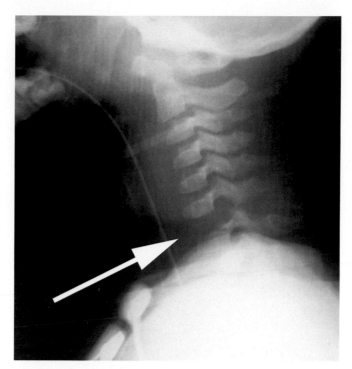

7.23C. Lateral C-spine view of bilateral facet dislocation of C-6 on C-7 and massive anterior soft tissue swelling in a young child.

8 Skin and Soft Tissue Injury

Introduction

The skin, being the largest organ and exposed, is very susceptible to injury, ranging from contusions to deep extensive burns. Furthermore, deeper soft tissue injury can lead to extensive blood loss, tendon injury, neurovascular trauma, and acute compartment syndrome. More than 1.25 million burns are evaluated in emergency departments across the United States annually, and these burns account for about 12,000 deaths each year. Burn injuries to the skin can be cosmetically and functionally devastating, and they account for many years of productive lives lost.

Acute burn evaluation requires special expertise and knowledge, given the unique complications these injuries can have. Careful history is important. Patients involved in closed-space fires with poor ventilation are at especially high risk for inhalational injury and carbon monoxide poisoning. The clinician needs to consider associated blunt trauma injury that may be related to a fall or an attempt to escape the flames. Suicide attempt victims may also have ingested poisons, and thus a coexistent toxicological emergency must be considered.

Clinical Examination

The standard primary survey with ABCDE evaluation is paramount. During this survey, careful attention to facial burns and possible inhalational injury is necessary, as these patients may require immediate airway control. Impaired lung ventilation may be detected by the presence of chest burn eschar or bronchospasm. Signs of shock secondary to third-space fluid loss and/or blood loss from another associated injury may be noted. A brief neurological examination is important to determine the possibility of head or spinal injury, and during the exposure evaluation all clothing should be removed to evaluate the extent of skin and soft tissue injury.

To evaluate burn injury, both the extent and the depth are important to determine. Percentage of body surface area burned can be calculated by using the rule of nines or the Lund-Browder chart. In this calculation, only second- and third-degree burns are included. The presence of skin blisters signifies a second-degree burn, and insensate waxy or charred skin signifies a full-thickness or third-degree burn. Circumferential burn injury can cause inadequate ventilation if it involves the chest or can cause acute compartment syndrome of an extremity. Early detection of this acute limb threat involves careful palpation of the compartments and serial evaluation of neurovascular status.

Deep soft tissue lacerations will need exploration to determine the extent of injury and any possible complications. Foreign bodies need to be excluded and bony injury detected by radiographs. Meticulous tendon and nerve examinations are important to detect subtle injury.

Investigations

History and examination will determine the need for diagnostic tests but common investigations needed in many of these patients are as follows:

1. Arterial blood gas and pulse oximetry. Early detection of hypoxia and/or hypercapnia in patients with inhalational injury is facilitated with these tests.

2. Carbon monoxide (CO) level. Patients in closed-space fires are at high risk for CO poisoning, and thus this level should be included in blood gas analysis.

3. Chest radiography. Though the chest radiograph may be normal in early inhalational injury, it may demonstrate pulmonary abnormalities consistent with pulmonary edema.

4. Doppler stethoscope. In patients with extensive skin burns and extremity edema, peripheral pulses may be difficult to palpate, and a Doppler stethoscope may help detect weak pulses.

5. Compartment pressure measurement. In equivocal cases of suspected compartment syndrome, a bedside compartment pressure can be measured to help clinical management.

6. Flexible bronchoscopy. Bronchoscopy can be done at the bedside to further evaluate the airway in patients with suspected inhalational injury. Visualization of tissue erythema, airway swelling, and carbonaceous material all signify inhalational injury.

General Management

All burn patients should receive supplemental oxygen and be carefully examined for possible inhalational injury. Patients showing any sign of acute inhalational injury should have immediate endotracheal intubation performed to stabilize the airway. Retained clothing and plastics may continue to harbor the burning process, and thus the patient should be completely undressed and all jewelry removed. Dry powders should be brushed off the skin, and other materials such as wet chemicals should be removed with copious water irrigation. Once the skin has been cleansed and fully evaluated, the patient should be promptly dried and covered with warm blankets to prevent hypothermia. Local wound debridement may be done for small burns, but extensive burns should have this process deferred to a burn center. Silver sulfadiazine is commonly used as a topical antimicrobial in burn wound care, and sterile dressings should be used to cover the injury. Tetanus vaccination status should be obtained, and prophylaxis should also be administered when necessary. Careful neurovascular examination of circumferential burn injury is important. Patients demonstrating evidence of acute compartment syndrome should have emergency escharotomy performed before transfer. Adequate analgesia is extremely important in the management of these patients, and thus titrated doses of narcotics and anxiolytics should be liberally used.

Aggressive crystalloid hydration is necessary because of the large amount of third-space fluid shift that occurs with burn injury. In addition to maintenance fluids, patients should receive 2–4 cc/kg/%BSA (body surface area) of lactated Ringer's solution, with half of this amount given in the first eight hours and the remainder in the subsequent sixteen hours. Vital signs, mental status, and central venous pressure measurements should be used to guide and tailor intravenous fluid administration. Urinary output provides a measure of renal blood flow and thus is extremely helpful in guiding intravenous fluids. Adults should maintain a urinary output of 0.5–1.0 cc/kg/hour, and children should maintain a rate of 1.0–1.5 cc/kg/hour. Adequate urinary output is especially important in patients who may have burn-associated rhabdomyolysis.

Extensive burns are optimally referred to a burn center. The following are guidelines for burn center transfer:

- Second- and third-degree burns that are >10% BSA in patients <10 years or >50 years of age
- Second- and third-degree burns that are >20% BSA in any age group
- Second- and third-degree burns that involving the face, eyes, ears, hands, feet, genitalia, or perineum or overlying major joints
- Third-degree burn >5% BSA in any age group
- Significant electrical and chemical burns
- Inhalational injury
- Burn injury in patients with preexisting disorders that could complicate management, prolong recovery, or affect mortality
- Burn injury in patients who will require special social, emotional, or long-term rehabilitative intervention
- Any patient with burns and concomitant trauma (such as fractures) in which the burn injury poses the greatest risk of morbidity and mortality
- Children with burns seen at hospitals without qualified personnel or equipment

Common Mistakes and Pitfalls

1. Missed or delayed diagnosis of inhalational injury. These patients can have progressive airway edema, and delayed airway management may be disastrous.

2. Missed coexistent major blunt trauma. Always consider coexistent blunt trauma, and use liberal imaging modalities to exclude injury if necessary.

3. Mismanagement of circumferential burn injury. Consider acute compartment syndrome in all such injuries. Perform prompt escharotomy or obtain emergent consultation in suspicious cases.

4. Inadequate fluid resuscitation. Burn injury requires aggressive crystalloid administration to maintain hemodynamics and urinary output.

5. Inadequate analgesia and sedation. Large amounts of narcotics and sedative agents are often needed to manage burn patients.

6. Inadequate wound evaluation. All deep soft tissue wounds need proper examination and exploration to exclude tendon, nerve, and vascular injury and the presence of foreign bodies. X-rays should be obtained to evaluate bony structures and to detect radiopaque foreign bodies.

8.1 Burn Zones of Injury

Commentary

Tissue destruction after acute thermal injury is a consequence of heat intensity, duration of exposure, and tissue conductance. This heat injury classically causes three concentric zones of injury in the pathologic model. The central area is where the most intense burn occurs and cells have been coagulated. Thus, this area is termed the zone of coagulation, an area of burn that has definite tissue destruction. The outermost zone is described as the zone of hyperemia and often represents tissue that will survive the injury. This hyperemia will resolve in 7–10 days, but to the inexperienced clinician this may be confused with cellulitis of a burn wound. The intermediate area is the zone of stasis and represents tissue that may or may not survive the burn injury. Progressive tissue loss secondary to dermal ischemia over the following 24–72 hours will determine the extent of injury in this zone. Blood flow may return to this area, but more often progressive thrombosis results in deepening and widening of the necrotic tissue.

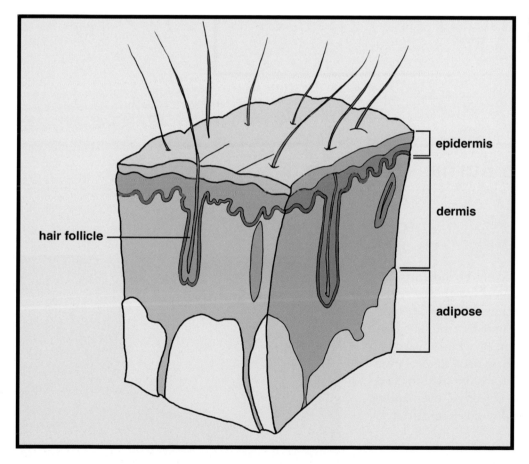

8.1A. Illustration of normal skin layers.

epidermis

dermis

hair follicle

adipose

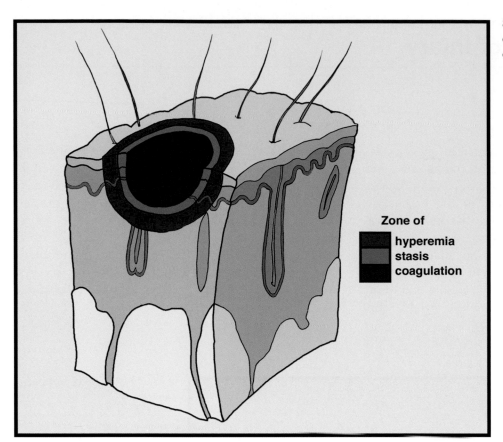

Zone of

hyperemia
stasis
coagulation

8.2 First-Degree Burns

Commentary

Depth of burn injury is classically broken into four types: first degree, the mildest, to fourth degree, the most severe. Bedside examination can help differentiate the depth of burn and thus predict the likelihood of complications, as higher degrees of burn heal much more slowly and are more likely to need surgical intervention. Though common patterns are used in classification, burn depth remains subjective, even among experienced burn surgeons, and serial examinations of the wound are necessary.

First-degree burns are mild injuries to the most superficial layer of epithelium. On examination, there is painful diffuse erythema but without blister formation. A sunburn is a classic example. This type of burn heals well without needing any specific therapy except analgesia. The prognosis is excellent, and good function and cosmesis are the rule.

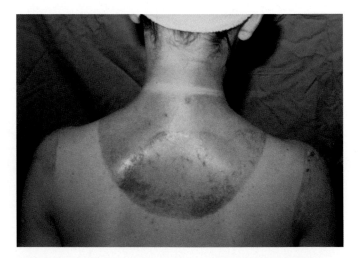

8.2A. This photo depicts a classic first-degree burn with erythema of the skin without blistering. This patient lit a flammable aerosol from a spray can, causing a first-degree flash burn to the exposed areas of skin.

8.3 Second-Degree Burns

Commentary

Second-degree burns involve injury to the dermis layer. Typically, blisters are present, and the wound is extremely painful. These second-degree burns can be classified further into superficial (top one-third dermis) and deep (bottom two-thirds dermis) burns. Superficial burns have pink tissue under the blisters, and deep burns have pink and white mottling of the same areas. The distinction of superficial and deep second-degree burns is important, as deeper sections of the dermis house skin appendages, hair shafts, and sweat and sebaceous glands that initiate reepithelialization of the burned area. Thus, burns affecting these important structures heal more slowly and with poor results. Typically, superficial second-degree burns will heal in less than three weeks, while deep burns heal in three to nine weeks with significant scar formation.

The first step of medical therapy is cleansing the burned tissue of loose debris, blisters, and foreign bodies with saline and sterile gauzes after administration of adequate analgesia. Superficial second-degree burns that are expected to heal within two to three weeks are often treated with topical antibiotic in the form of 1% silver sulfadiazine cream. The wound is then covered with a loose, bulky dressing, with frequent recleansing, reapplication of topical antibiotic, and dressing changes.

Because of slow and poor healing, deep second-degree wounds are considered candidates for early surgical therapy. Tangential excison is performed to remove the necrotic eschar so that the wound is excised down to viable tissue. Ideally, at this point immediate allografting is performed. If a donor site is not available, then fresh or cryopreserved human allograft can provide physiological wound closure until rejection occurs two to four weeks later. Subsequently, the wound can be covered with reharvested allograft.

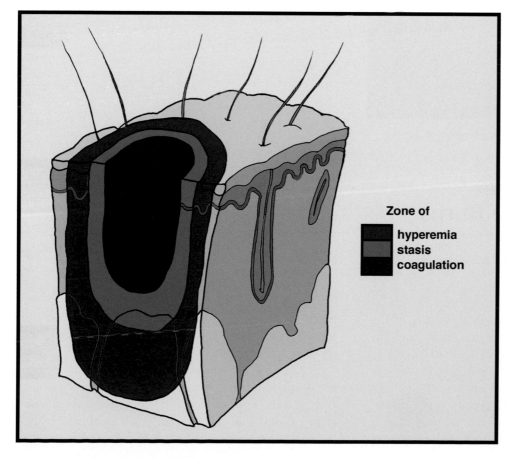

8.3A. Illustration of cross section of a deep second-degree burn of the skin.

Zone of
hyperemia
stasis
coagulation

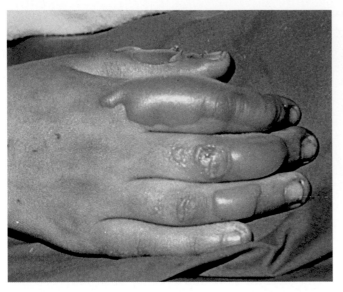

8.3B. Photograph of a hand burn with the classic blistering appearance of a second-degree burn.

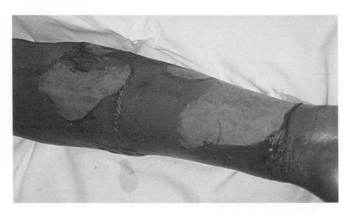

8.3D. Photograph of a superficial second-degree burn to the forearm with debrided blisters.

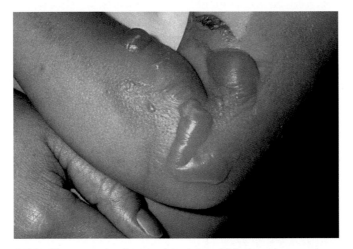

8.3C. Photograph of an accidental scald-induced second-degree burn in a small child.

8.4 Third-Degree Burns

Commentary

Third-degree burns involve the full thickness of the skin, including the epidermis, entire dermis, and the subcutaneous tissue. These wounds are usually easy to recognize by their leathery, firm consistency, absent capillary refill, and absence of sensation to light touch and pinprick. They may also appear waxy white, cherry red, or charred in appearance, and they may be difficult to differentiate from deep second-degree burns. Third-degree or full-thickness burns will also form a classic burn eschar that over days to weeks will separate from the underlying tissue.

Because all the key elements of epithelial growth are destroyed, these wounds can only heal by wound contracture, epithelialization from the wound margins, or skin grafting. Thus, the mainstay of third-degree burn care involves early excision and grafting.

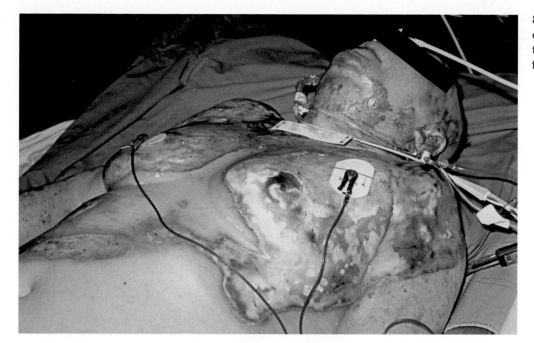

8.4A. Photograph of extensive third-degree burns to the chest in a woman who fell asleep while smoking.

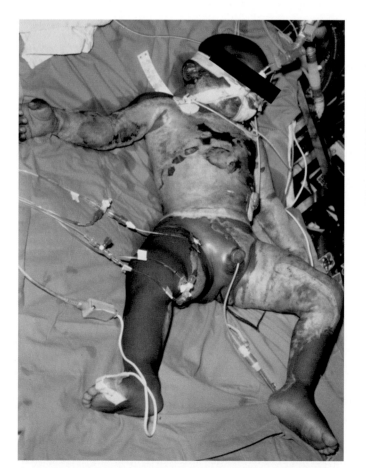

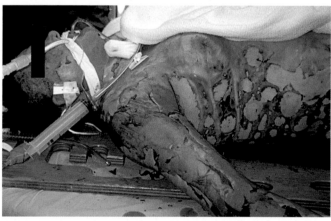

8.4C. Photograph of fatal third-degree burns over the face and chest of a car fire victim.

8.4B. Photograph of large third-degree burns in a child who was standing next to a barbecue that was lit with gasoline.

8.5 Fourth-Degree Burns

Commentary

Fourth-degree burns are extensive burns that are deep to the fascia, muscle, and bone and are often charred in appearance. Complications are common, and extensive surgery, including reconstruction or amputation, is often required.

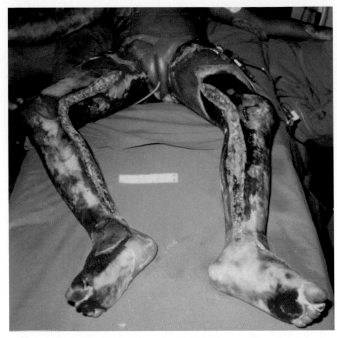

8.5A. Photograph of fourth-degree burns to both legs of a patient involved in a car fire. This patient also had bilateral escharotomies for secondary compartment syndrome of the limbs.

8.6 Extent of Burn Injury

Commentary

Next to depth of injury, the extent of the burn is an important parameter that helps guide burn treatment and predicts mortality. In estimating the burn size, only second-degree or greater burns are included in the calculations. A simple way to roughly determine the body surface area is to use the "rule of nines." In this calculation, each upper extremity and head is 9% while the lower extremities and anterior and posterior trunks are each 18% of the body surface area. The per- ineum accounts for the remaining 1% of body surface area. In children, a modified rule of nines is used. In children, the head is relatively larger and occupies 18%, and the lower extremities account for 14% each. The upper extremities and front and back trunk are the same, respectively, at 9% and 18% body surface area. For estimating small burns, the palm of an adult or child is equal to 1% body surface area and is a useful rule.

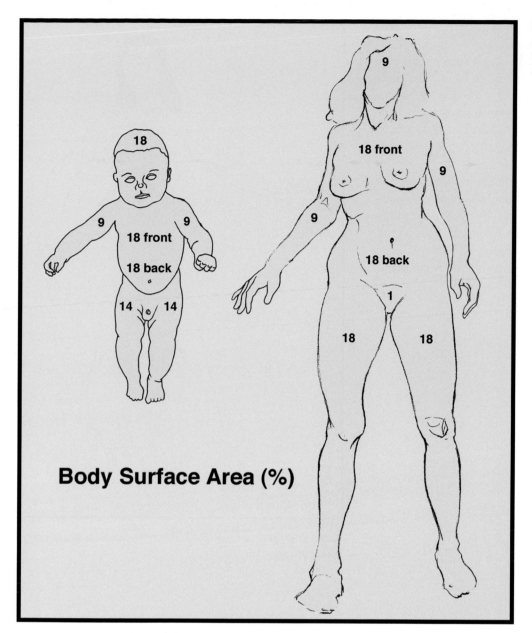

Body Surface Area (%)

8.7 Circumferential Burns

Commentary

Circumferential burns can be complex to manage and are associated with limb-threatening compartment syndrome. If not promptly recognized, edema formation under a tight burn eschar leads to progressive vascular compromise that can produce permanent neuromuscular damage and limb loss. It is important to monitor skin color, capillary refill, Doppler pulses, and sensation on a continual basis in these cases. Compartment pressure monitoring provides objective evidence, and intracompartmental pressures greater than 30 mm Hg mandate escharotomy. Local anesthesia is not needed, as a third-degree burn is insensate, but adjunctive narcotics and anxiolytics are recommended.

The procedure is perfomed using a sterile scalpel or preferably electrocautery to minimize blood loss. Incisions are generally made on the medial or lateral aspects of the limb to avoid injury to nerves and vessels. If unilateral decompression does not lead to adequate tissue perfusion, then escharotomy is performed on the opposite side of the limb.

Circumferential burns of the thorax can lead to diminished chest wall compliance and progressive respiratory distress, often recognized by increasing ventilation pressures and rising CO_2 levels. Chest wall escharotomies are performed along the lateral chest walls and can provide significant decompression that allows improved ventilation.

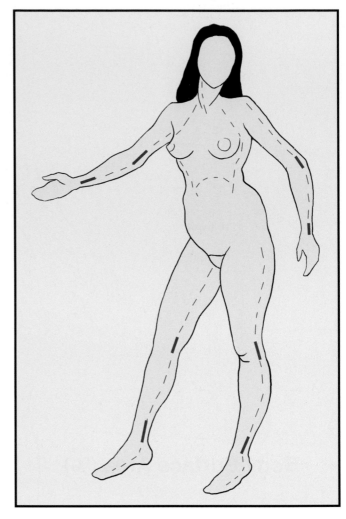

8.7A. Illustration of preferred sites of incision for emergency escharotomy.

8.7B. Photograph of circumferential second- and third-degree burns to the legs in a suicide attempt with gasoline ignition.

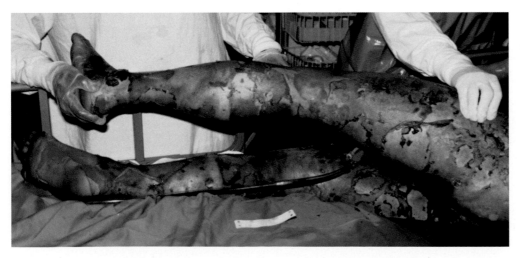

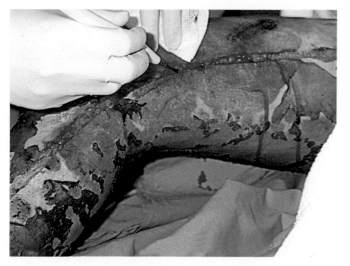

8.7C. Photograph of an escharotomy of the lower extremity in progress with electrocautery.

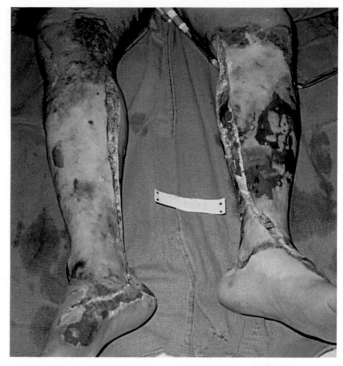

8.7D. Photograph of circumferential burns of the lower extremities requiring extensive escharotomies. This patient was intoxicated while working on his car when a fire erupted.

8.7E. Photograph of extensive truncal and extremity escharotomies from a gasoline fire suicide attempt.

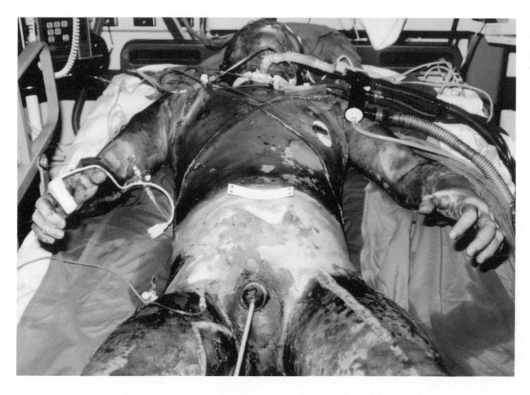

8.8 Scald Burns

Commentary

Scald burns are a very common form of burn injury and are most often from hot water. Water at 60 degrees Celsius can cause a full-thickness burn within three seconds, and regulations to lower hot water tank temperatures have led to a decrease in these types of injuries. Scalds on skin with light clothing tend to be worse than on exposed skin areas, as the clothing tends to retain heat. In a similar fashion, thick soups and sauces also tend to cause deeper dermal injury. Cooking oil and grease may be as hot as 200 degrees Celsius and thus also cause severe injuries. Tar burns are a unique form of scald injury, with similarly high temperatures and adherence to the skin. Removal of tar is facilitated with a petroleum-based ointment. Deliberate scalds are a common form of child abuse, and thus a careful history is important.

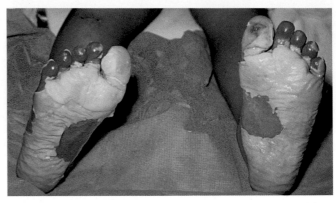

8.8B. Photograph of scald burns to the feet of a young child who accidentally stepped in a hot tub.

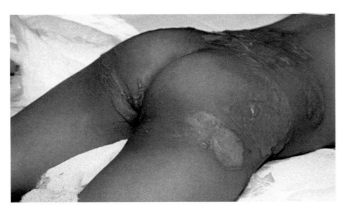

8.8A. Photograph of a scald burn in a child suffering a forced dunking injury. Note the sparing of the buttock area as it is held against the cooler tub floor.

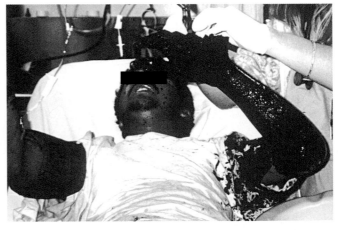

8.8C. Photograph of a tar burn in a construction worker.

8.9 Chemical Burns

Commentary

Chemical burn injury is determined by the agent, concentration, quantity, and duration of skin contact. In contrast to flame burns, chemical burns cause exten- sive biochemical injury rather than thermal injury, and the skin injury may be deceptively minor on ini- tial inspection. The tissue injury continues until the chemical is inactivated with tissue reaction or it is diluted with irrigation. Thus, the most important priority in wet chemical injury is copious tap water or saline irrigation to dilute and remove the offending caustic agent. Eye injuries in particular need extensive saline irrigation to avoid permanent corneal injury. Acid burns tend to be less severe than alkali burns. Acid burn injury forms an impermeable barrier that self-limits its destructive potential, whereas alkalis combine with cutaneous lipids to form a soap that continues to cause tissue damage until neutralized. As a general rule, special neutralizing agents are not needed, although hydrofluoric acid burns are an important exception. In these cases, calcium gluconate should be used topically, subcutaneously, or intra-arterially to help neutralize the fluoride ion.

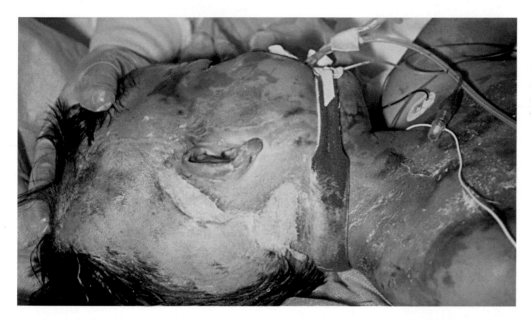

8.9A. Photograph of large second- and third-degree burns from 90% hydrosulfuric acid. This young child accidentally reached for an open container that fell on his face.

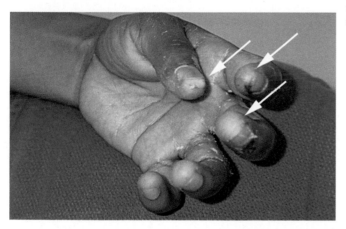

8.9B. Photograph of hydrofluoric acid burn on the hand of a glass etcher.

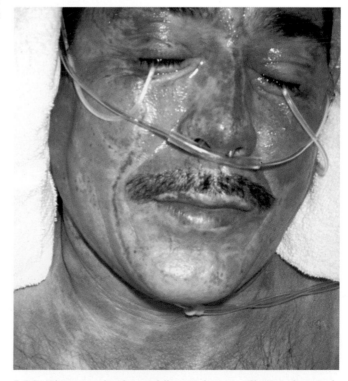

8.9C. Photograph of a middle-aged man suffering chemical burns to his face and eyes from muriatic acid. Morgan lens eye irrigation is being performed.

8.10 Electrical Injury

Commentary

Though electrical injuries are uncommon, they account for disproportionate morbidity and mortality. Conductive high-voltage electrical burns are particularly severe and cause deep tissue injury to muscle, vessels, and nerves that is not visible on direct inspection of the skin. As electrical current meets soft tissue resistance, this energy is converted to thermal energy proportional to the resistance of the tissue and the amperage of the current. Deep thermal injury can also lead to rhabdomyolysis, myoglobinuria, and compartment syndrome, which are common complications in this type of injury. If the current traverses the thorax, ventricular fibrillation or other cardiac arrhythmias may be seen. Patients may also have concurrent thermal injuries secondary to arc burns and ignition of clothing.

Patients suffering acute electrical burns generally require much more fluid replacement than is usually anticipated based on the size of the skin wounds, and urine output needs to be maintained to avoid myoglobinuric renal failure. Early release of compartment syndrome and debridement of deep tissue are important mainstays of treatment, though electrical burns involving deep vessels often require subsequent amputation.

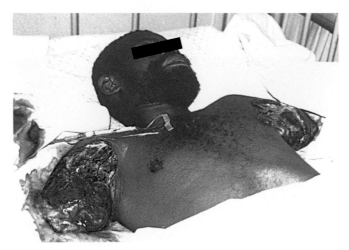

8.10B. Photograph of bilateral arm amputations in a political prisoner tortured by being forced to hold a high-voltage power line.

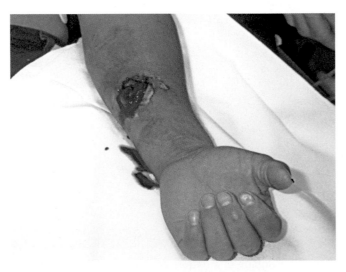

8.10A. Photograph of a high-voltage electrical burn to the forearm of an electrician.

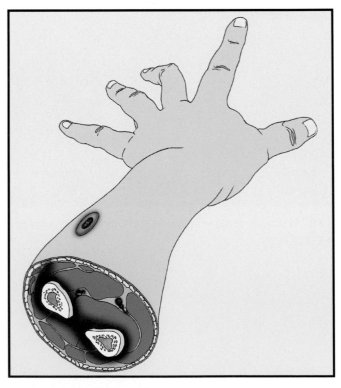

8.10C. Illustration depicting deep neurovascular and tissue injury from a seemingly minor surface electrical burn.

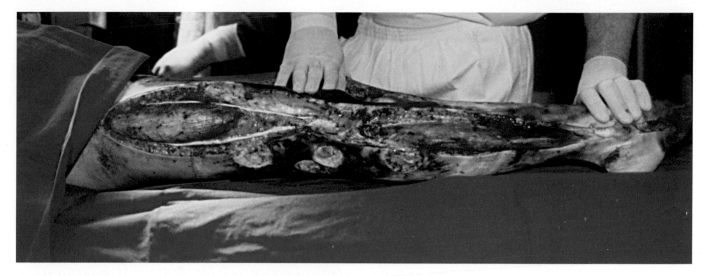

8.10D. Photograph of extensive deep tissue debridement of the leg required in a electrical burn.

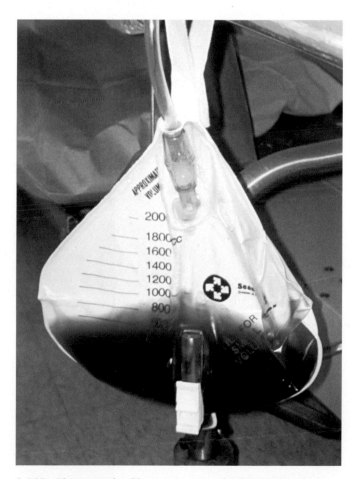

8.10E. Photograph of hyperpigmented urine in electrical burn–induced myoglobinuria.

8.11 Inhalational Injury

Commentary

Smoke inhalational injury should be suspected in all patients in fires that occur within a closed space. Hundreds of toxic substances are present in smoke particles, and inhalation causes direct epithelial damage leading to edema, submucosal hemorrhage, and necrosis, mostly in the lower airways. Microatelectasis and interstitial and alveolar edema subsequently occur and can lead to respiratory failure. One of the most significant early complications is upper airway edema, which, if not treated early with intubation, can lead to airway obstruction.

Patients may present with a combination of cough, shortness of breath, hoarseness, and wheezing. Facial burns and singed facial hairs may be seen, and, if present, carbonaceous sputum is a very specific sign. In questionable cases, fiberoptic bronchoscopy provides direct visualization of the affected airways for definitive diagnosis. Early chest radiographs are often normal, while delayed radiographs show pulmonary edema in advanced cases. Supportive care with humidified oxygen and beta-agonists for wheezing suffice for most minor cases, but intubation and ventilatory support are necessary for serious disease. Of particular note, significant carbon monoxide and cyanide poisoning can lead to lethal inhalations.

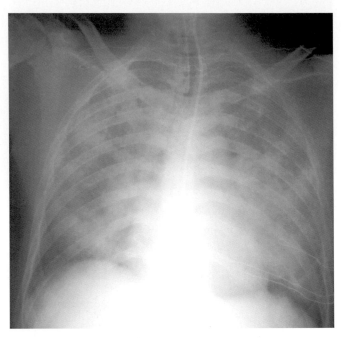

8.11B. Chest radiograph with noncardiogenic pulmonary edema in a patient with severe inhalational injury.

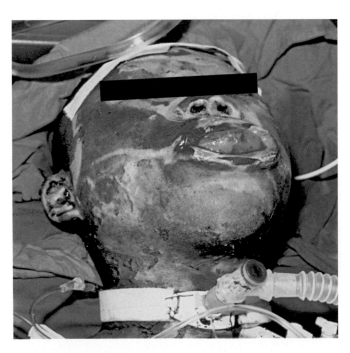

8.11A. Photograph of a facial burn with burned nasal hairs in a young adult with severe inhalational injury.

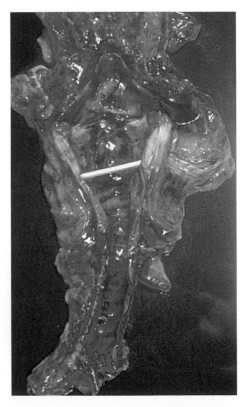

8.11C. Photograph showing the laryngotracheal view of inhalational injury at autopsy. Note the extensive erythema and carbonaceous material throughout the airway.

8.12 Dog Bite Injury

Commentary

About 2 million bite injuries occur yearly in the United States, and 80–90% of these are related to dogs. Most of these bites occur in children and young adults and commonly affect the extremities, although small children are more likely to suffer head and neck bites. Injuries can be severe, and large, aggressive breeds such as pit bulls are commonly implicated in dog bite–related deaths.

Dog bites most often cause avulsions, tears, abrasions, and severe crush injury. Wounds are inoculated with multiple aerobic and anaerobic organisms and thus are at risk for infection, but to a lesser degree than that of cat and human bite wounds. Wound cleansing and high-pressure irrigation are necessary, along with tetanus immunization if indicated. Depending on the locale, rabies vaccination may be indicated, as dogs are common vectors for rabies in many parts of the world. For large wounds, x-rays are important to rule out retained foreign bodies and underlying fracture. Bites from large dogs may produce vascular injury that may be clinically occult at initial evaluation. After appropriate wound care, lacerations can be repaired, especially on the face and neck, where cosmesis is a concern and wound infection less likely.

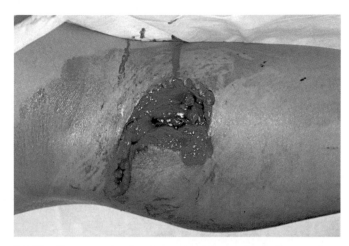

8.12B. Photograph of a chow dog bite to the calf area of the lower extremity.

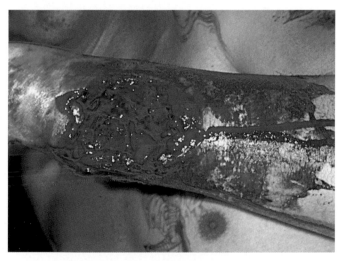

8.12C. Photograph of a German shepherd dog bite to the forearm, with open fracture of the wrist.

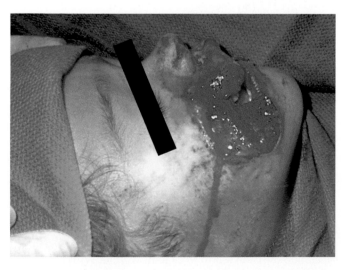

8.12A. Photograph of an extensive facial dog bite involving the lip and cheek of a small child.

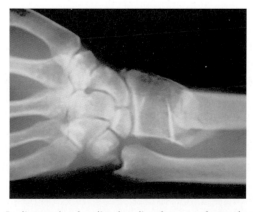

8.12D. Radiograph of a distal radius fracture from dog bite.

8.13 Cat Bite Injury

Commentary

Cat bites account for 5–15% of all bite injuries and most commonly present with a puncture wound on the hand or upper arm. Because these puncture wounds retain inoculated organisms deep in the soft tissues and are difficult to irrigate, cat bites are at high risk for infection. This is compounded by the fact that these wounds usually appear minor initially, and thus patients commonly delay presentation. Because of the high risk of infection, prophylactic antibiotics and close follow-up are necessary to detect complications. Established infections should be treated with antimicrobials effective against *Pasteurella multocida*, the most common infecting organism.

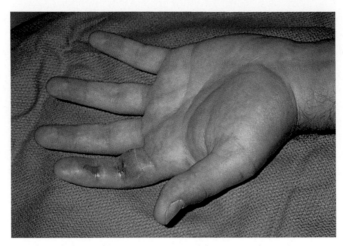

8.13A. Photograph of a flexor tenosynovitis of the index finger complicating a cat bite puncture wound of the hand.

8.14 Human Bite Injury

Commentary

Human bite injuries are serious injuries and most commonly occur on the hand and upper extremities, followed by the head and neck. A crushing and tearing mechanism causes tissue destruction and devitalization, and human saliva, containing up to a hundred different species of organisms per cubic centimeter, is inoculated into the wound. This combination predisposes for the most common complication: wound infection.

Therapy is thus directed to minimize this risk by initially providing adequate wound cleansing and irrigation. In addition, prophylactic antibiotic therapy is necessary in these high-risk wounds. Despite appropriate wound care and prophylactic antibiotics, many human bite injuries to the hand become infected. Any laceration or bite injury over the metacarpals should be considered a human bite. Extensive cellulitis, abscess formation, septic arthritis, and osteomyelitis are common infective complications, and once they are established, parenteral antibiotics and possibly surgical debridement are necessary.

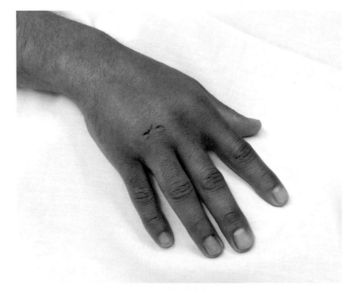

8.14A. Photograph of an early clenched-fist injury with laceration over the fourth MCP joint without signs of infection.

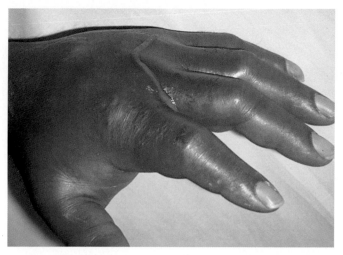

8.14B. Photograph of a clenched-fist injury complicated with acute cellulitis of the hand.

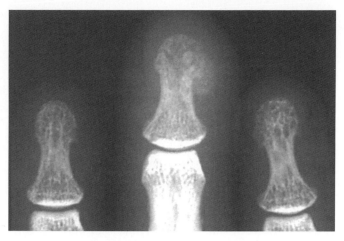

8.14D. Radiograph of distal phalangeal osteomyelitis secondary to a human bite injury.

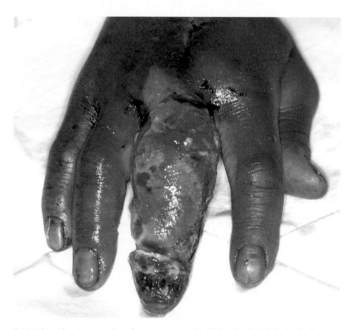

8.14C. Photograph of a severe cellulitis of the third digit from a human bite.

8.15 Retained Foreign Body

Commentary

Retained foreign bodies commonly cause poor wound healing and predispose to subsequent infection. Thus, all lacerations should be carefully examined to rule out the presence of a retained foreign body. If the full wound cannot be clearly visualized, plain radiographs are warranted to rule out a deep foreign body. X-rays reliably detect radiopaque material, but common objects made of wood or plastic will still be missed, and other imaging modalities such as ultrasound or MRI may be necessary in certain cases. Most authors consider glass wounds high risk, given the ability of glass to break into multiple small pieces, and thus liberal use of x-rays to detect retained glass foreign bodies is recommended.

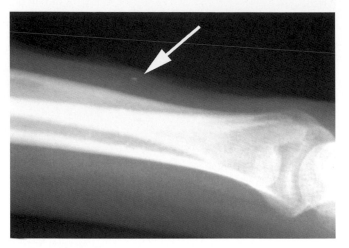

8.15A. Plain x-ray of the forearm with a small retained glass foreign body.

8.16 Major Soft Tissue Injury

Commentary

Major soft tissue injury can pose a serious threat to the trauma patient. These wounds are commonly contaminated and thus need extensive irrigation and debridement. In addition, full exploration of the wound is necessary to ensure that no serious neurovascular injury has occurred and to rule out any retained foreign bodies. Because of the complexity of these wounds, most large soft tissue injuries are best managed in the operating room.

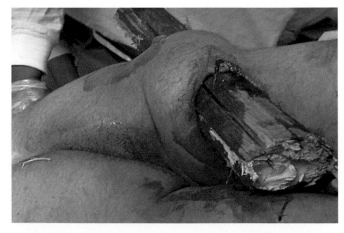

8.16A. Photograph of an impalement of a large pole into the right buttock area of a patient who was ejected from his vehicle.

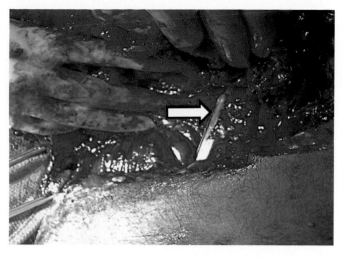

8.16B. Intraoperative photograph of the same patient revealing the proximity of the injury to the sciatic nerve.

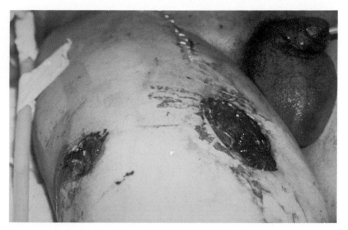

8.16D. Photograph of a high-velocity AK-47 bullet wound injury to the right thigh.

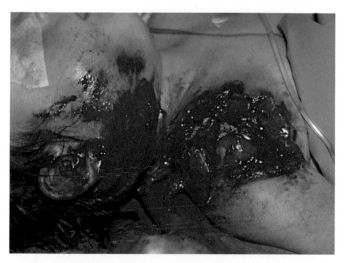

8.16C. Photograph of extensive skin loss and soft tissue injury on the shoulder of a young child suffering a shotgun injury.

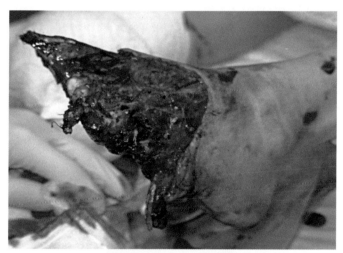

8.16E. Photograph of open fractures and extensive degloving injury to the foot of a patient who was in an auto-versus-pedestrian accident.

8.17 Compartment Syndrome

Commentary

Compartment syndrome is an acute, limb-threatening emergency that occurs when the intracompartmental pressure rises dangerously within a closed osteofascial space. Though this syndrome most often occurs in the calf, it may be seen in any body area. In addition, each major region of the body hosts multiple compartments.

Normal compartment pressure is less than 10 cm of water. As the pressure rises, arterial perfusion diminishes and at a critical point stops completely. The muscle and nerve are at severe risk for permanent injury. Fractures of the mid-shaft tibia are especially at very high risk, though many other etiologies of compartment syndrome exist, such as vascular injuries, burns, excessive exercise, infiltrated infusions, hematomas, tight dressings or casts, and prolonged immobilization or pressure on a limb. In the majority of cases, the rise in compartment pressure is related to tissue edema or intracompartmental bleeding, and the compliance of the fascia and compartment steadily decrease as the intracompartmental pressure rises. At an intracompartmental pressure of 20–30 mm Hg, capillaries are occluded and tissue ischemia results.

Classic teaching includes evaluating for the six Ps associated with compartment syndrome: pain, pallor, paresthesias, poikilothermia, paralysis, and pulselessness. Unfortunately, many of these signs are late, and permanent damage may already have occurred by the time these signs appear. Deep burning pain that is out of proportion to the apparent injury is an important early clue to the condition, along with an increase of the pain on passive stretching of the involved muscle group. Prompt orthopedic consultation is necessary in suspected cases. Compartment pressure measurement is a helpful adjunct in borderline cases and can easily be done by placing a needle pressure transducer within the compartment in question. When compartment syndrome is considered, the pressures of all the compartments in that extremity should be measured. Though compartment pressures help diagnose the syndrome, the patient's clinical symptoms and signs should also be taken into account when making the diagnosis.

Pressures less than 20 mm Hg generally do not cause acute compartment syndrome but may warrant admission and serial examination. Pressures greater than 30 mm Hg are an indication for definitive therapy in the form of fasciotomy. Pressures between 20 and 30 mm Hg are considered to be in a "gray zone" area.

Complications of compartment syndrome include muscle necrosis and infection. Adequate hydration is important, as muscle breakdown can lead to rhabdomyolysis and myoglobinuric renal failure. In the long term, necrotic muscle is slowly converted to an elastic fibrous tissue, which leads to the development of Volkmann's contractures.

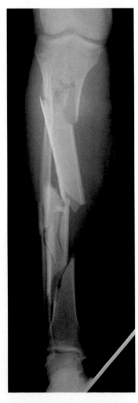

8.17A. Radiograph of a comminuted multisegment tibial shaft fracture at high risk for compartment syndrome.

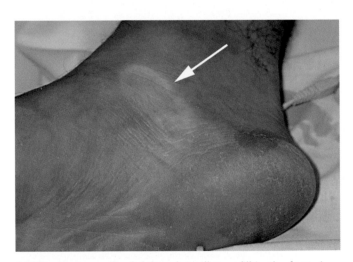

8.17B. Photograph of delayed capillary refill in the foot. A late finding in an acute compartment syndrome.

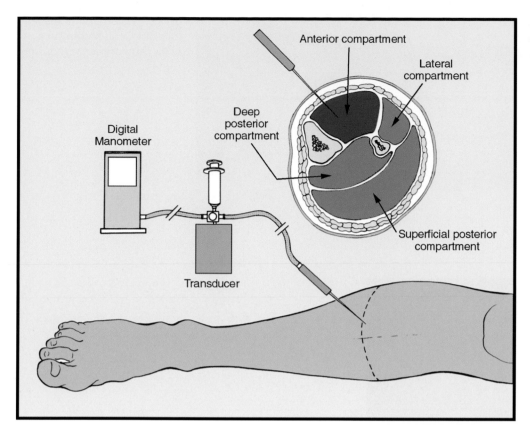

8.17C. Illustration of tibial compartments and pressure monitoring.

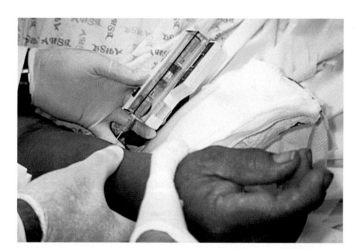

8.17D. Photograph demonstrating compartment pressure monitoring of the forearm.

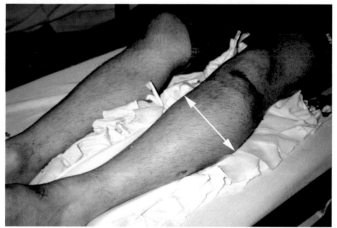

8.17E. Photograph showing a compartment syndrome of the leg from a gunshot wound. Note the asymmetry in calf size.

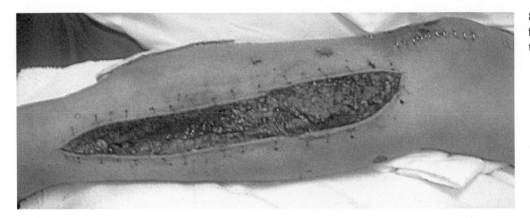

8.17F. Photograph of the leg following a fasciotomy in a tibial compartment syndrome.

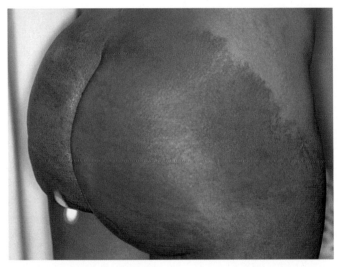

8.17G. Photograph showing an unusual gluteal compartment syndrome of the buttock from a violent beating.

8.18 High-Pressure Injection Injury

Commentary

High-pressure injection injuries to the hand are often occupationally related and have devastating complications. These injuries are commonly the result of paint guns, grease guns, and diesel injectors. Though paint and grease are the most commonly injected chemicals, other substances may be implicated. The injury involves tremendous forces, as the injector guns use pressures of 2,000–10,000 psi, and thus direct hand contact with the paint gun is not necessary.

Physical examination may initially reveal an innocuous-looking wound, though as hours progress, a severe inflammatory process is seen. The affected digit is often swollen and may be pale from associated vascular compromise. Radiographs may reveal discrete opaque areas that can help delineate the extent of deep injury. Emergency therapy includes splinting, tetanus prophylaxis, and broad-spectrum antimicrobial coverage. These injection injuries are extremely serious and have a high rate of amputation and long-term disability. Urgent hand surgery consultation is imperative, as most patients will require emergency operative debridement and decompression.

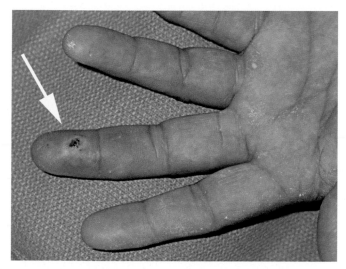

8.18A. Photograph of a high-pressure injection injury of the third digit in a painter.

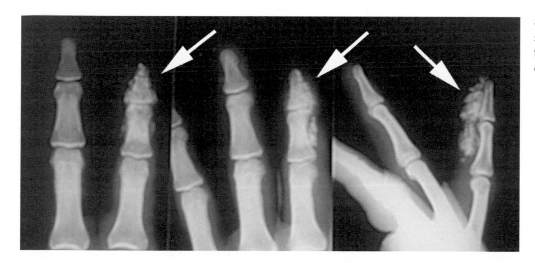

8.18B. Classic radiograph showing paint along the flexor sheath of the fourth digit.

Index